PEDIATRICS, CHILD AND ADOLESCENT HEALTH

CHILD AND ADOLESCENT HEALTH ISSUES

A TRIBUTE TO THE PEDIATRICIAN DONALD E GREYDANUS

PEDIATRICS, CHILD AND ADOLESCENT HEALTH

JOAV MERRICK – SERIES EDITOR –

NATIONAL INSTITUTE OF CHILD HEALTH AND HUMAN DEVELOPMENT,
MINISTRY OF SOCIAL AFFAIRS, JERUSALEM

Positive Youth Development: Theory, Research and Application
Daniel TL Shek, Rachel CF Sun and Joav Merrick (Editors)
2012. ISBN: 978-1-62081-305-8
(Hardcover)

Tropical Pediatrics: A Public Health Concern of International Proportions
Richard R Roach, Donald E Greydanus, Dilip R Patel, Douglas N Homnick and Joav Merrick (Editors)
2012-September.
ISBN: 978-1-61942-831-7
(Hardcover)

Positive Youth Development: A New School Curriculum to Tackle Adolescent Developmental Issues
Hing Keung Ma, Daniel TL Shek and Joav Merrick (Editors)
2012- October. ISBN: 978-1-62081-384-3
(Hardcover)

Understanding Autism Spectrum Disorder: Current Research Aspects
Ditza A Zachor and Joav Merrick (Editors)
2012- November.
ISBN: 978-1-62081-353-9
(Hardcover)

Transition from Pediatric to Adult Medical Care
David Wood, John G. Reiss, Maria E. Ferris, Linda R. Edwards and Joav Merrick (Editors)
2012- November.
ISBN: 978-1-62081-409-3
(Hardcover)

Child and Adolescent Health Yearbook 2012
Joav Merrick (Editor)
2012- November.
ISBN: 978-1-61942-788-4
(Hardcover)

Child Health and Human Development Yearbook 2011
Joav Merrick (Editor)
2012- December.
ISBN: 978-1-61942-969-7
(Hardcover)

Child and Adolescent Health Yearbook 2011
Joav Merrick (Editor)
2013- January. ISBN: 978-1-61942-782-2
(Hardcover)

Child Health and Human Development Yearbook 2012
Joav Merrick (Editor)
2013- March. ISBN: 978-1-61942-978-9
(Hardcover)

Developmental Issues in Chinese Adolescents
Daniel TL Shek, Rachel CF Sun and Joav Merrick (Editors)
2012-September.
ISBN: 978-1-62081-262-4
(Hardcover)

Guidelines for the Healthy Integration of the Ill Child in the Educational System: Experience from Israel
Yosefa Isenberg (Author)
2013 - 3rd Quarter.
ISBN: 978-1-62808-350-7 (Hardcover)

Chinese Adolescent Development: Economic Disadvantages, Parents and Intrapersonal Development
Daniel TL Shek, Rachel CF Sun and Joav Merrick (Editors)
2013 - 3rd Quarter.
ISBN: 978-1-62618-622-4 (Hardcover)

University and College Students: Health and Development Issues for the Leaders of Tomorrow
Daniel TL Shek, Rachel CF Sun and Joav Merrick (Editors)
2013 - 3rd Quarter.
ISBN: 978-1-62618-586-9 (Hardcover)

Adolescence and Behavior Issues in a Chinese Context
Daniel TL Shek, Rachel CF Sun and Joav Merrick (Editors)
2013 - 3rd Quarter.
ISBN: 978-1-62618-614-9 (Hardcover)

Advances in Preterm Infant Research
Jing Sun, Nicholas Buys and Joav Merrick (Authors)
2013 - 3rd Quarter.
ISBN: 978-1-62618-696-5 (Hardcover)

Promotion of Holistic Development of Young People in Hong Kong
Daniel TL Shek, Tak Yan Lee and Joav Merrick (Editors)
2013 - 4rd Quarter.
ISBN: 978-1-62808-019-3 (Hardcover)

Internet Addiction: A Public Health Concern in Adolescence
Artemis Tsitsika, Mari Janikian, Donald E Greydanus, Hatim A Omar and Joav Merrick (Editors)
2013 - 4th Quarter.
ISBN: 978-1-62618-925-6 (Hardcover)

Human Developmental Research: Experience from Research in Hong Kong
Daniel TL Shek, Cecilia Ma, Yu Lu and Joav Merrick (Editors)
2013 - 4th Quarter.
ISBN: 978-1-62808-166-4 (Hardcover)

Chronic Disease and Disability in Childhood
Joav Merrick (Editor)
2013 - 4th Quarter.
ISBN: 978-1-62808-865-6 (Hardcover)

Break the Cycle of Environmental Health Disparities: Maternal and Child Health Aspects
Leslie Rubin and Joav Merrick (Editors)
2013 - 4th Quarter. ISBN: 978-1-62948-107-4 (Hardcover)

Environmental Health Disparities in Children: Asthma, Obesity and Food
Leslie Rubin and Joav Merrick (Editors)
2013 - 4th Quarter.
ISBN: 978-1-62948-122-7 (Hardcover)

Environmental Health: Home, School and Community
Leslie Rubin and Joav Merrick (Editors)
2013 - 4th Quarter. ISBN: 978-1-62948-155-5 (Hardcover)

Child Health and Human Development: Social, Economic and Environmental Factors
Leslie Rubin and Joav Merrick (Editors)
2013 - 4th Quarter.
ISBN: 978-1-62948-166-1 (Hardcover)

Children, Violence and Bullying: International Perspectives
Joav Merrick, Isack Kandel and Hatim A Omar (Editors)
2013 - 4th Quarter.
ISBN: 978-1-62948-342-9 (Hardcover)

Playing with Fire: Children, Adolescents and Firesetting
Hatim A Omar, Carrie Howell Bowling and Joav Merrick (Editors)
2013 - 4th Quarter.
ISBN: 978-1-62948-471-6 (Softcover)

School, Adolescence and Health Issues
Joav Merrick, Ariel Tenenbaum and Hatim A Omar (Editors)
2014 - 1st Quarter.
ISBN: 978-1-62948-702-1 (Hardcover)

Adolescence and Sexuality: International Perspectives
Joav Merrick, Ariel Tenenbaum and Hatim A Omar (Editors)
2014 - 1st Quarter.
ISBN: 978-1-62948-711-3 (Hardcover)

Child and Adolescent Health Yearbook 2013
Joav Merrick (Editor)
2014 - 2nd Quarter.
ISBN: 978-1-63117-658-6 (Hardcover)

Adoption: The Search for a New Parenthood
Gary Diamond and Eva Arbel (Authors)
2014 - 2nd Quarter.
ISBN: 978-1-63117-710-1 (Hardcover)

Adolescence: Places and Spaces
Myra Taylor, Julie Ann Pooley and Joav Merrick (Editors)
2014 - 2nd Quarter.
ISBN: 978-1-63117-847-4 (Hardcover)

Pain Management Yearbook 2013
Joav Merrick (Editor)
2014 - 3rd Quarter.
ISBN: 978-1-63117-944-0 (Hardcover)

Child Health and Human Development Yearbook 2013
Joav Merrick (Editor)
2014 - 3rd Quarter
ISBN: 978-1-63117-939-6 (Hardcover)

Born into this World: Health Issues
Donald E Greydanus, Arthur N Feinberg and Joav Merrick (Editors)
2014 - 3rd Quarter.
ISBN: 978-1-63321-667-9 (Hardcover)

Caring for the Newborn: A Comprehensive Guide for the Clinician
Donald E Greydanus, Arthur N Feinberg and Joav Merrick (Editors)
2014 - 4th Quarter.
ISBN: 978-1-63321-760-7 (Hardcover)

Environment and Hope: Improving Health, Reducing AIDS and Promoting Food Security in the World
I. Leslie Rubin and Joav Merrick (Editors)
2014 - 4th Quarter.
ISBN: 978-1-63321-772-0 (Hardcover)

Pediatric and Adolescent Dermatology: Some Current Issues
Donald E Greydanus, Arthur N Feinberg and Joav Merrick (Editors)
2014 - 4th Quarter.
ISBN: 978-1-63321-853-6
(Hardcover)

Tropical Pediatrics: A Public Health Concern of International Proportions, Second Edition
Richard R Roach, Donald E Greydanus, Dilip R Patel and Joav Merrick (Editors)
2015 - 1st Quarter.
ISBN: 978-1-63463-381-9
(Hardcover)

Child and Adolescent Health Issues (A Tribute to the Pediatrician Donald E Greydanus)
Joav Merrick (Editor)
2015 - 1st Quarter.
ISBN: 978-1-63463-574-5
(Hardcover)

PEDIATRICS, CHILD AND ADOLESCENT HEALTH

CHILD AND ADOLESCENT HEALTH ISSUES

A TRIBUTE TO THE PEDIATRICIAN DONALD E GREYDANUS

JOAV MERRICK
EDITOR

nova publishers
New York

NOTICE TO THE READER

Library of Congress Cataloging-in-Publication Data

ISBN: 978-1-63463-574-5

Library of Congress Control Number: 2014955566

Published by Nova Science Publishers, Inc. † New York

Contents

INTRODUCTION

In: Child and Adolescent Health Issues
Editor: Joav Merrick

ISBN: 978-1-63463-574-5

Chapter 1

A TRIBUTE TO THE PEDIATRICIAN, PROFESSOR DONALD E GREYDANUS

Joav Merrick, MD, MMedSc, DMSc**[*,1,2,3,4,5] **and
***Dilip R Patel, MD, MBA, FAAP, FSAHM, FAACPDM, FACSM, CPHQ, CMQ, CPE**[6,7]*

[1]National Institute of Child Health and Human Development, Jerusalem
[2]Office of the Medical Director, Health Services,
Division for Intellectual and Developmental Disabilities,
Ministry of Social Affairs and Social Services, Jerusalem
[3]Division of Pediatrics, Hadassah Hebrew University Medical Center,
Mt Scopus Campus, Jerusalem, Israel
[4]Kentucky Children's Hospital, University of Kentucky College of Medicine,
Lexington, Kentucky, United States
[5]Center for Healthy Development, School of Public Health,
Georgia State University, Atlanta, United States of America
[6]Department of Pediatric and Adolescent Medicine,
Western Michigan University Homer Stryker MD School of Medicine, Kalamazoo
[7]Department of Pediatrics and Human Development at the Michigan State University
College of Human Medicine, East Lansing, Michigan,
United States of America

INTRODUCTION

In 2015 Donald E Greydanus will round 70 years and, as a pioneer in child and adolescent health, we would like to dedicate this book and this introduction to his many years and contributions in this field.

[*] Correspondence: Professor Joav Merrick, MD, MMedSci, DMSc, Medical Director, Health Services, Division for Intellectual and Developmental Disabilities, Ministry of Social Affairs and Social Services, POBox 1260, IL-91012 Jerusalem, Israel. E-mail: jmerrick@zahav.net.il

Donald E Greydanus was born in Paterson, New Jersey, United States from Dutch and Scotch ancestry. The Greydanus family name can be traced to the early 17th century in Friesland, the Netherlands. The past four centuries have produced a number of Professor Greydanus' and Don is a 20th century example of this ancestral record. Members of this heritage often choose studies in theology (Calvanism), philosophy, or medicine. Under the influence of his nurse mother, Don selected medicine, while an older brother entered the study of theology.

After his medical training in Newark, New Jersey (College of Medicine and Dentistry of New Jersey), Don went to the Mayo Graduate School of Medicine for his post-graduate medical training. Two major events happened in his life during his internship in the early 1970s in Minnesota---he met his future wife and he was inducted into the US Vietnam war (1956-1975). Though he could have postponed his military service, he felt he should answer this call especially since his family had relatives who had served and died in World War II. It was shocking to this young physician Greydanus how American veterans were treated by fellow countrymen, when returning from such an unpopular and controversial war.

When released from the war zone, he returned home, married Kathy Rickheim, and completed residency training in pediatrics at the Mayo Clinic. He finalized his formal studies in pediatrics with a fellowship in adolescent medicine at New York University School of Medicine under the director of the well-known professor Adele Dellenbaugh Hofmann (1926-2001), one of the founders and icons of this field dedicated to youth and a leading force in the development of adolescent medicine in the 20th century.

Academic Work

Admiration for his teachers in medical school and at Mayo sparked an inherent interest in academics that has continued throughout his professional life. He began his scientific writing with members of his teaching faculty at Mayo. For example, his report on generalized cytomegalovirus infection in an infant was published with Professor Gunnar Stickler (1925-2010) in the journal *Infection* (1) and was one of the first in literature to link acute encephalopathy and liver dysfunction in the child to cytomegalovirus infection. Another early publication was with Dr. Gerald Gilchrist and Dr. Omar Burgert that reviewed the hypothalamic syndrome in children with acute lymphocytic leukemia in the Mayo Clinic Proceedings (2). By this time Don realized he had been injected with the condition coined by the Roman writer, Juvenal (60 AD to 127 AD) in Satires: cacoethes scribendi ("Incurable itch to write").

From these early writings professor Greydanus has gone on to become a very well known Professor of Pediatrics at the international level as well as in his own country. He has published an impressive amount of quality scholarship that includes co-editor of 33 medical books, co-editor of 37 medical journal issues, over 300 medical articles (130 articles listed in PubMed), and 200 book chapters. It is not just the numbers, but the extremely high quality of academic work that impresses so many academicians around the world. Professor Greydanus is a very gifted writer who not only looks at the science of a subject but he is able to skillfully utilize words that can challenge and delight the interested reader as well!

INTERNATIONAL WORK

Another reflection of his outstanding international reputation is that professor Greydanus is a highly respected speaker, who has presented at meetings around the world for several decades. I have heard him speak at various global spots including my own country of Israel, specifically in Jerusalem in December 2012. What is awe-inspiring about his lectures is the passion he brings to his talks in addition to the high quality of science that is presented. He is passionate about improving health care for children as well as adolescents and his audience is always cognizant of this well-presented view.

Professor Greydanus has been a member of many committees for national organizations, including the American Academy of Pediatrics (AAP) and the Society for Adolescent Health and Medicine (SAHM). He was Director of Publications for SAHM and Chair of the National Conference and Exhibitions (NCE) for the AAP for a number of years. He was a member of the Planning Committee for the Pediatric Academic Societies for many years and remains an Abstract and Workshop reviewer for them. Professor Greydanus has been a specialty site visitor in Pediatrics for the Accreditation Council for Graduate Medical Education (ACGME) in the past as well as a member of the ACGME Board of Appeals Panel Member for both Pediatrics and Pediatric Adolescent Medicine.

Don has been a keynote speaker and lecturer in many countries. He has been invited by and presented lectures and workshops for a large number of international organizations including the International Congress of Pediatrics, International Pediatric Association, Indian Academy of Pediatrics, Israeli Society for Adolescent Medicine, Portuguese Pediatric Association, Brazilian Pediatric Association, European Pediatric Association, International Academy of Sportology (Tokyo), Israeli Society of Sports Medicine, other societies, and many medical schools around the globe.

Another reflection of the high status his peers have for professor Greydanus is the number of international and national committees he has been part of over the years of his professional life. In the past he has been a consultant in adolescent medicine to UNICEF in Kuwait as well as Taiwan. He has also been a consultant to the World Health Organization in Geneva, Switzerland and currently, is a member of the Scientific Committee for the International Consensus in Pediatrics group. He has been elected an honorary member of various international societies including the Taiwan Society for Adolescent Medicine, the Hong Kong Society for Adolescent Medicine, and the Indian Academy of Pediatrics. Professor Greydanus has been a visiting Professor of Pediatrics for several years at the University of Athens (First Department of Pediatrics, Second Department of Pediatrics, Aghia Sophia Children's Hospital; P & A Kyriakou Children's Hospital).

Other contributions including consultant to the International Pediatric Association (via Professor Swati Bhave MD in India), Excellence in Pediatrics group, and Eu.net.Adb Consortium on Adolescent Internet Addiction (with Artemis Tsitsika MD, PhD in Athens, Greece). He has been a board member for various international journals such as the Asian Journal of Paediatric Practice (Delhi, India), International Journal of Adolescent Medicine & Health (Jerusalem, Israel), International Journal of Child & Adolescent Health (Jerusalem, Israel), Annals of Clinical Pediatrics (Athens, Greece), and others.

Don is or has been a board member for various Journals in the United States including the American Academy of Pediatrics' State of the Art Reviews: Adolescent Medicine (1990 to the present), Seminars in Adolescent Medicine, Adolescent Health Update Journal (American Academy of Pediatrics [AAP]), Journal of Current Adolescent Medicine, and others. As an expert academician, he has reviewed for over 50 scientific journals over the course of his illustrious career in medicine. He was elected to the Alpha Omega Alpha Honor Medical Society (Faculty level) at Michigan State University College of Human Medicine on November 17, 2011.

As an administrator he took over a program that lost its accreditation in pediatrics in 1990, turned it around and had it fully accredited ever since, which has led to countless residents being trained, countless disadvantaged children being cared for, and in July 2014 a medical school established.

Awards

Recognition of his stunning contributions has led to a number of prestigious awards that include:

- American Academy of Pediatrics (1995 Adele Dellenbaugh Hofmann Award for "Distinguished Contributions" in Pediatrics and Adolescent Medicine)
- 2001 Recognition and Appreciation Certificate from the Chair of Pediatrics and Human Development at Michigan State University College of Human Medicine for "tireless efforts in teaching and education of medical students and residents in the discipline of Adolescent Medicine…for his unselfish response to all requests from the Medical School for educational programs across all the campuses and in recognition of praise given to him as a most effective teacher by all those with whom he has come in contact...... and in recognition of his time and effort given in support of the Department as a member of our Department Executive Committee and others….and in recognition of these many efforts in the continuing support of the Department…on behalf of all the faculty and the medical school" (Albert W Sparrow MD, MPH, Chair).
- Michigan State University College of Human Medicine (2003 William B Weil Jr, MD Endowed Distinguished Pediatric Faculty Award ("National and International Recognition, Exemplary Scholarship Activity, Outstanding Professional, and Clinical Service to Pediatrics, Consistent Commitment to Providing Comprehensive and High Quality Healthcare to Children and their Families")
- Charles R. Drew School of Medicine (2004 Stellar Award for Excellence in Pediatric Education for inspiring the King Drew University Pediatric Residents to reach new heights, for his dedication to teaching and countless contributions to furthering the field of Pediatric Resident Education")
- He was recognized by the Mayo Clinic Department of Pediatrics who honored him with their Departmental Honored Alumnus Award on October 5, 2000 for "significant national achievements in Pediatrics."
- 2008 Michigan State University College of Human Medicine Outstanding Community-based Faculty Award ("Strong contributions in the College's educational and community-based research program for bringing distinction and honor to the

College and serving as an outstanding role model for the College of Human Medicine students, residents, and faculty")

- The 2010 Outstanding Achievement in Adolescent Medicine Lifetime Award from the Society for Adolescent Health and Medicine; this is the Society's most prestigious award and is given for a "lifetime of outstanding dedication and service to adolescent health care."
- In 2010 he received the prestigious Doctor Honoris Causa from the University of Athens (Greece) which is an award of the highest distinction at the University of Athens for "Distinguished Academic Achievements in Adolescent Medicine."

Questions about life

When asked about his life, Don notes with joy the recent 40th year wedding anniversary celebration with his wife, Kathy, their four daughters, and 10 grandchildren. When asked about his professional life's contributions, he notes that he has tried to honor his teachers in medical school and graduate medical education. Professor Greydanus has dedicated the last quarter of a century to being a residency program director in pediatrics. When asked, why---he notes that "a residency program director has the wonderful privilege of providing a nurturing milieu for tomorrow's pediatricians who will be caring for children and adolescents well into this century. The US residency program system is funded by the US government and often, as it the case with my program, cares for the indigent population that help these deserving, but disadvantaged children find their own joy and satisfaction in life. Indeed, the highest calling anyone can have, in my view, is to try to help prepare our children to be successful in their adult lives. This is not just a personal religious view, but perhaps, more importantly, a humanitarian view."

Finally, when asked what has sustained his long academic career, he smiles and says: "Doch dyn plicht en lit de lju rabje." This is in honor of his Fresian-Dutch ancestry and essentially means: "Do your duty to your best ability, and let the people criticize you." He notes that "clinicians and academicians can be very critical of one's work. I advise my younger colleagues to do their best work, accept critiques that can improve their contributions, but do not worry about direct criticism that stems from jealousy or negativism."

This book is dedicated to professor Greydanus as he enters the septuagenarian decade of his life! We wish professor Donald E Greydanus a happy birthday and hope for more to come and more work, projects, publications and books together and continuation of our many years of friendship across the ocean and in Kalamazoo. His contributions will be with us for many decades to inspire other pediatricians to "do their best: Doch dyn plicht."

References

[1] Greydanus DE, Smith TF, Stickler GB. Acute encephalopathy with liver dysfunction, chylous ascites and cytomegalovirus infection. Infection 1977;5(4):255-8.

[2] Greydanus DE, Burgert EO, Gilchrist GS. Hypothalamic syndrome in children with acute lymphocytic leukemia. Mayo Clinic Proceed 1978;53(4):217-20.

Section One: Body Shape and Sexual Health

In: Child and Adolescent Health Issues
Editor: Joav Merrick

ISBN: 978-1-63463-574-5

Chapter 2

PERCEPTION OF BODY SHAPE/WEIGHT AND HEALTH: A MEASUREMENT PROBLEM

***Said Shahtahmasebi, PhD*[*,1,2,3] *and Bernadette Cassidy, PhD*[2,4]**

[1]Centre for Health and Social Practice, Wintec, Hamilton, New Zealand
[2]The Good Life Research Centre Trust, Christchurch, New Zealand
[3]Division of Adolescent Medicine, Kentucky Children's Hospital, Lexington, Kentucky, United States of America
[4]Allan Bean Centre, NZ Spinal Trust, Burwood Hospital, Christchurch, New Zealand

Frequently women are targeted by the media through visual images linking body shape with health and healthy behaviour implying a socially ideal body shape/weight. One of the consequences of targeting women in this way is the impact on women's mental health and overall wellbeing. Research in this area often uses subjective variables to observe complex psycho-social and emotional well-being. Subjective variables, due to their temporal dependencies, give rise to additional complexities. This chapter provides a discussion of these complexities, and, uses a secondary data source to illustrate substantive issues related to defining, measuring, and analysing attitudes and perceptions of health and overall wellbeing in relation to body shape.

INTRODUCTION

Culturally, body shape has been associated with health, social status and wealth, and vice versa, promoting a socially idealised body shape/weight for women to aspire to (1). Ideal body shape/weight has varied over the centuries depending on the social norms of the time and the quality of available evidence and information (2, 3). Improvements in our understanding of 'health' has led to a social dealignment where public attitudes shift from previous beliefs and images of healthy body to a new set of images purporting a healthy body

* Correspondence: Said Shahtahmasebi, The Good Life Research Centre Trust, 4 Orkney Street, Strowan, Christchurch 8052, New Zealand. E-mail: radisolevoo@gmail.com

(2, 3). Although, it is common to use a combination of body mass index (BMI) and weight for height as a measure of a healthy body, social norms are driven by social ideals, perceptions and expectations. One of the main feedback effects of linking body image to health is the superimposition of a thin body shape over a variety of healthy body shapes. In other words, there exists an ever widening gap between healthy body shapes and society's idealised body shape (4-6). It is this gap between information and social expectations/perceptions that may, at least in part, be responsible for some modern illnesses such as eating disorders (7-9). The negative and adverse effects of the idealisation of body shape has not had much impact on shifting social norms towards a 'fit' body rather than a thin body. Instead, the negativity is directed at people who do not conform to an ideal body shape.

On the other hand, the media's take on this social issue and the use of media by manufacturers' to promote their products has established in the public mindset a link between an ideal body shape (thinness) and healthiness. A trawl of the literature points to a bias towards women, due to a female-biased media, e.g. the visual portraying of healthiness with the emphasis on appearance (6). It is reasonable to assume that, on average, compared with men women are more adversely affected by the negative feedback from the social idealisation of body shape, resulting in anxiety, eating disorders, and depression (5, 7, 10).

In this chapter we look at the value of subjective psycho-social emotional measurements such as 'happy with body weight' and 'at ease with opposite sex' in informing and providing insight into understanding the link between socially idealised body weight/shape and wellbeing.

HUMAN BEHAVIOR

Human behaviour is a dynamic process. Over and above temporal dependencies and change over time, one of the main features of a process is the feedback effect. For example, the theory of cognitive dissonance may explain some of the variations in attitudes and perceptions over time. Cognitive dissonance explains that individuals align their attitude to their current social state upgrading the satisfaction with both positive and negative attributes of their current state and downgrading those of possible alternatives (11-13). Therefore, it is reasonable to assume that years of exposure to the media's visual emphasis on body shape and healthiness will have had a major influence on shaping individuals' attitudes and perceptions of body shape/weight.

An obvious interventional approach to break the link between body shape and health is to disestablish or at least attenuate the relationship between perceptions of body image and healthiness. For example, Slater et al. (14), describe an experiment that placed warning labels on fashion and women's magazines to inform readers that the images had been digitally enhanced, in order to ameliorate the negative psycho-social effects of idealised media images. Halliwell and Diedrichs (4) reported that a cognitive dissonance intervention in young girls led to fewer girls in their sample reporting body dissatisfaction. Other researchers report similar effects using a simple intervention such as using images of healthy weight models, i.e. the respondent's body ideals were significantly larger than when the same women viewed images of very thin models (5).

Individual characteristics, in part, contribute to temporal dependencies. For example, personality traits such as resilience to peer pressure, through cumulative inertia or cognitive dissonance may produce a different outcome in attitudes to body shape. The reverse may also be true, i.e. temporal dependencies may influence perceptions through individual characteristics. For example, resilience to peer pressure may become internalised so that an idealised body shape may be presumed unobtainable leading to apathy and/or risky behaviour such as smoking, alcohol and drug abuse (15, 16). By the same token, attaining an ideal body shape may be over simplified and over achieved (very thin bodies). Therefore, it is plausible that the increase in the prevalence of obesity or anorexia in the West, e.g. New Zealand, Australia, and the US, is a reaction to these perceptions, i.e. the feedback effect and residual heterogeneity (17).

A major problem in research, policy development, and decision making is the uncritical use of research and information, where the primary source of confusion is in the public mindset. This uncritical behaviour has allowed the media's idealised body shape and healthiness to be used interchangeably. Thus giving rise to terms such as "happy with body shape" or "happy with body weight" as proxy measures for self-assessed body shape and size, self-esteem, confidence, health, or overall wellbeing. Given the dynamics of human behaviour and the notion of cognitive dissonance, the question is whether or not such terminology has anything to do with health. Specifically, do they measure health, an ideal body shape, or much more complex measures of mental wellbeing or overall wellbeing? In other words, being happy with body shape could mean that the respondent's perception of an idealised body shape is similar to that of society/or the media's, or the respondent feels healthy, or, enjoys a high level of wellbeing so that body shape is of little consequence. By the same token, from a practical standpoint, is 'being happy with body shape/weight' sufficient to assume that the respondents' physical shape resembles an ideal weight and shape?

OUR STUDY

Perceptions and attitudes change over time. A longitudinal study is necessary to explore self-reported attitudes and perceptions of the respondent's body in relation to healthy behaviour and health outcomes. A secondary data source was used to relate being happy with body shape and body weight with health related behaviour outcomes, which was the smoking and alcohol drinking habits of adolescents. In 1992, 60 secondary schools in the former Yorkshire Regional Health Authority geographical boundary (UK) agreed to take part in a biennial health related behaviour survey. Years 9 and 11 students (age range 11-16 years) in theschools were surveyed using a health related behaviour questionnaire. The surveys were anonymous and were not linked to previous surveys, i.e. it was not possible to follow change over time in the same individuals. This limitation restricted the analysis to comparative cross-sectional analyses of change in proportion of outcomes of interest (18). The 1994 survey was modified to include a form to be filled in by students who were in their final school year (16+ year olds). The form invited the pupils to indicate their interest in participating in a follow-up survey two years later. Organisational changes within the NHS (National Health Service) during 1994 saw the abolition of the Regional Health Authorities in England and by 1996 the

Yorkshire Regional Health Authority had ceased to exist. However, the survey was conducted as planned and 627 young adults were traced and re-interviewed using the same questionnaire instrument with slight modifications to some questions to suit the 18+ age category, providing two time point data (see (15). The questionnaire covered topics related to the attitudes and behaviour of the pupils with regard to health e.g. physical exercise and out of school activities, nutrition, social contacts, dealing with problems, attitudes to and the use of drugs (including smoking and drinking). The methodology for statistical modelling of the cross-sectional and longitudinal data sets are described elsewhere (15, 16, 18). The outcome variables are binary smoking ('0' non-smoker; '1' smoker) or categorical drinking habits (1- non-drinkers, 2- low drinkers (1-7 units), 3- medium (8-20 units), and 4- heavy drinkers (more than 21 units)). Table 1 shows a list of explanatory variables thought to be related to smoking extracted from the data set and were included in the analysis.

Table 1. Selected variables from the Health Related Behaviour Questionnaire thought to be associated with smoking habits of young people. Bi-variate cross-classification; *p<.05, **p<0.001, ***p<0.00001

Explanatory variables	Smoking
Socio-demographic	**p**
1- Age	***
2- Gender	***
3- Which parents live with	***
4- Where live	***
5- Social class (see §3)	*
Socio-environment	
6- Whether smoker	-
7- Whether drinks	***
8- Whether at least one in family smokes	***
9- Whether relative smokes	***
10- Whether best friend smokes	***
Socio-psychological	
11- Self-esteem	**
12- Whether happy with weight	***
13- Whether happy with body shape	***
14- Whether considers health when choosing food	
14- Whether have a steady partner	***
15- How feels when meeting opposite sex	***
16- How feels when meeting own sex	***
17- Have a drink when have problem	***
How much worry about:	
18- school problems	***
19- money problems	***
20- health problems	***
21- career problems	***
22- problems with friend	***
23- family problem	***
24- the way you look	***

With a binary dependent variable and many independent variables, the common statistical approach is to fit a logistic regression model to the data. The adopted statistical modelling approach allows control for other variables when testing a variable of interest in the model. However, of particular concern is the longitudinal nature of the data set. The logistic regression is essentially a cross-sectional model and fitting such a model to longitudinal data will lead to a well-known specification error and misleading results (19). Furthermore, the model must allow for the possibility that substantial variation between respondents will be due to the omitted variables. The model applied in this paper is the logistic-normal random effects model (15, 16, 18).

FINDINGS

The descriptive analysis shown in table 2suggests that out of the 627 subjects there were 619 valid cases; 62.5% were female and 37.5% were male. The age-effect is fairly straightforward: 22% were smokers in 1994 compared with 33% in 1996; 36% were non-drinkers in 1994 compared with 22% in 1996, which means the proportion of heavy drinkers went up from 6% in 1994 to 17% in 1996.

Table 2. Change in smoking and drinking status over time

a. Smoking status in 1994 by gender (column %s)

1994		**Sex**		**Total**
Freqs (Col %s)		Male	Female	
Smoker	No	188 (81.0%)	296 (76.5%)	484 (78.2%)
	Yes	44 (19.0%)	91 (23.5%)	135 (21.8%)
Total		232 (100%)	387 (100%)	619 (100%)

b. Smoking status in 1996 by gender (column %s)

1996		**Sex**		**Total**
Freqs (Col %s)		Male	Female	
Smoker	No	164 (70.4%)	248 (64.2%)	412 (66.6%)
	Yes	69 (29.6%)	138 (35.8%)	207 (33.4%)
Total		233 (100%)	386 (100%)	619 (100%)

c. Drinking status in 1994 by gender (column %s)

Drinking status		**Sex**		**Total**
		Male	Female	
	Don't drink	83(35.9%)	139(36.0%)	222(36.0%)
	Light drinker	78(33.8%)	160(41.5%)	238(38.6%)
	Moderate drinker	52(22.5%)	70(18.1)	122(19.8%)
	Heavy drinker	18(7.8%)	17(4.4)	35(5.7%)
Total		231(37.5%)	386(62.5%)	617(100%)
Pearson Chi-sq		6.54	(p=0.09)	

d. Drinking status in 1996 by gender (column %s)

Drinks status		Sex		Total
		Male	Female	
	Don't drink	45(19.5%)	88(22.8%)	133(21.6%)
	Light drinker	38(16.5%)	123(31.9%)	161(26.1%)
	Moderate drinker	83(35.9%)	135(35.0%)	218(35.3%)
	Heavy drinker	65(28.1%)	40(10.4%)	105(17.0%)
Total		231(37.5%)	386(62.5%)	617(100%)
Pearson Chi-sq		40	(p=0.0000)	

Only 5% of the sample said they would like to put weight on and 58% said they would like to lose weight, while 37% said they were happy with their weight (see table 3). The distribution of being happy with weight over gender was as expected, e.g. 83% of those who said they would like to lose weight were female, and being happy with their weight was almost equally distributed (51% female, 49% male).

The survey included a number of health related behaviour outcomes such as eating, smoking and drinking habits as well as self-reported fitness levels and physical activities. One of the measures available for eating habits is 'whether consider health when choosing food'. As a guide eating, smoking and drinking habits of the females in the sample for the variable body weight is shown in tables 3-6. Table 3 shows that 58% of females would like to lose weight while 36% said they were happy with their weight. A trend may be observed from the results in table 3; the proportion of those who said they were happy with their weight increases with frequency of health consideration when choosing food (see table 3). Conversely, the proportion of those who said they would like to lose weight increases with frequency of health consideration when choosing food.

Table 3. Female perception of body weight and whether consider health when choosing food

Body Weight	Sometimes	Often	Very often	Total
Would like to put weight on	3 (15%)	8 (4.8%)	9 (4.5%)	20 (5.2%)
Would like to lose weight	7 (35%)	95 (57.2%)	123 (61.2%)	225 (58.1%)
Happy with weight	10 (50%)	63 (38%)	69 (34.3%)	142 (36.7%)
Total	20	166	201	387

A similar pattern can be observed in the results shown in table 4; proportionally more smokers said they would like to lose weight than non-smokers, and, proportionally more non-smoker said they were happy with their weight.

Results in table 5 suggest that the proportion of those who would like to lose weight appears fairly steady over the number of units of alcohol consumed. Conversely, the proportion of those who said they were happy with their weight decreases with the number of units of alcohol consumed.

Table 4. Female perception of body weight and their smoking habits

Body Weight	Non-smoker	Smoker	Total
Would like to put weight on	11 (4%)	9 (6.7%)	20 (5.2%)
Would like to lose weight	139 (55.2%)	86 (63.7%)	225 (58.1%)
Happy with weight	102 (40.5%)	40 (29.6%)	142 (36.7%)
Total	252	135	387

Table 5. Female perception of body weight and their drinking habits

Body Weight	None	1-7 units	8-20 units	>21+	Total
Would like to put weight on	1 (1.1%)	6 (6.4%)	9 (6.6%)	4 (10%)	20 (5.2%)
Would like to lose weight	49 (55.7%)	73 (59.3%)	80 (58.8%)	23 (57.5%)	225 (58.1%)
Happy with weight	38 (43.2%)	44 (35.8%)	47 (34.6%)	13 (32.5%)	142 (36.7%)
Total	88	123	136	40	387

Table 6 shows the distribution of self-image as measured by the variable 'I am glad I am who I am' over body weight. A similar pattern can be observed: the proportion of those who would like to lose weight appears to decrease with levels of agreement with this variable; and, conversely, this proportion decreases increase with agreement.

Table 6. Female perception of body weight and their self-image

	I am glad I'm who I am				
Body Weight	Disagree	Not sure	Agree	Strongly agree	Total
Would like to put weight on	0 (0%)	7 (8%)	11 (6.3%)	2 (1.9%)	20 (5.2%)
Would like to lose weight	17 (94.4%)	60 (68.2%)	88 (50%)	60 (57.1%)	225 (58.1%)
Happy with weight	1 (5.6%)	21 (23.9%)	77 (43.8%)	43 (41%)	142 (36.7%)
Total	18	88	176	105	387

Of course, when taking multicollinearity into account within a statistical modelling framework most of the self-reported and subjective variables such as self-esteem and 'I am glad I am who I am' fail to be significant and do not make it into the model (15, 16, 18).

Clearly there are complex interactions between various subjective variables which make it difficult to assess the meaning of 'being happy body weight' in relation to health, socially idealised weight, or apathy.

The media frequently associates body shape or body weight with health or healthy behaviour and by association the promotion of a practice or a product. There are at least two issues to address: first, has a link been established between body shape/weight and healthy behaviour; and second, do people subscribe to an idealised body shape, or, is the body-shape effect the result of a perceived body shape?

The first issue can be addressed within a statistical modelling framework using health related behaviour outcomes such as smoking and/or drinking as the response variable. The second issue is more complicated because body shape or weight is observed as a measure of how respondents felt about their body shape or weight at the time of the survey. However, if perceived body shape is significant within the same modelling framework, i.e. as a contributing factor to smoking or drinking after controlling for other factors including healthy attitude variables, then it may be interpreted as a direct effect. That is, being happy with one's body weight may indicate a healthy attitude.

For statistical modelling purposes the variable body weight was dichotomised into 'put on/lose weight' and 'happy with body weight'. This variable was included in the list of demographic, social and emotional variables in the longitudinal modelling of teenage smoking and drinking habits (15, 16).

The results (see table 7 and 8) suggest that after controlling for demographic, environmental and socio-psychological factors, and in the presence of the variable 'considers health when choosing food', those who said they were happy with their body weight were less likely to be a smoker than those who wished to lose weight (or put on weight). Conversely, the variable 'happy with body weight' ceased to be significant once age was entered in the model of drinking habits, even before controlling for healthy attitude variables such as 'considers health when choosing food'. It is interesting to note that with this data set females are more likely to be smokers but less likely to be heavy drinkers than males.

It is also interesting to note that those who said they did not have a partner or were not at ease with the opposite sex were less likely to be smokers, but those worrying about problems are more likely to be smokers. These variables are replaced with drug experimentation in the model for drinking patterns.

The fact that psycho-social and emotional variables appear to inversely affect smoking, i.e. not at ease with the opposite sex, or, worrying about problems, suggests the presence of complex interactions between the observed and unobserved variables. Indeed, as shown by the highly significant Scale parameter (ω) there is a lot of variation in data which is left unexplained by observed variables in our models. For example, the variable 'happy with weight' could well be a proxy for 'health' or fitness, on the other hand it could also measure an idealised body weight/shape as perceived by the respondents, or both. By the same token, the variable 'considers health when choosing food' could reflect the perception of a healthy behaviour, but it could also infer a selection bias where those with a perceived idealised body weight respond positively to a healthy behaviour. Both variables could also be referring to the 'feel good' factor perhaps through the respondent's perception of having attained an idealised weight/body, or through feeling fit and healthy.

Therefore, with subjective variables such as 'happy with body weight' it is not always easy to distinguish the body weight aspect from psycho-social and emotional aspects of what these variables measure.

Table 7. Longitudinal teenage smoking patterns: model fitting results; N=619, (>> much greater than, << much less than)

Explanatory Variables	Parameter	Estimate	S. Error	X^2	p
Gender	Male	0.00		1.8	>>0.1
	female	0.43	0.32		
Age				10.5	<0.025
	15 and under	0.00			
	16 years	0.99	0.39		

Explanatory Variables	Parameter	Estimate	S. Error	X^2	p
	17 years	0.74	0.28		
	18 and over	0.86	0.41		
At least one family member smokes				7.4	<0.01
	yes	0.00			
	no	-0.76	0.28		
Drinks				39	<<0.0001
	yes	0.00			
	no	-1.99	0.37		
Best friend smokes				76	<<0.0001
	yes	0.00			
	no	-2.29	0.31		
Consider health when choosing food				6.9	<0.05
	never	0.00			
	sometimes	-0.72	0.41		
	always	-1.28	0.49		
Happy with weight				5.7	<0.025
	put on/lose	0.00			
	happy	-0.63	0.27		
Have a partner				1.3	>>0.1
	yes	0.00			
	no	-0.29	0.26		
At ease with opposite sex				2.1	>>0.1
	yes	0.00			
	no	-0.59	0.41		
Worry about money				5.7	0.05
	never	0.00			
	a little	0.12	0.31		
	a lot	0.72	0.33		
Worry about family problems				2.82	>>0.1
	never	0.00			
	a little	0.42	0.32		
	a lot	0.47	0.31		
Scale (ω)		2.38	0.31		

Table 8. Longitudinal teenage drinking pattern: model fitting results; N=619, (>> much greater than, << much less than)

Explanatory Variables	Parameter estimates	Standard Error	Significance level
Gender			<< .0005
Male	0.00		
Female	0.76	0.14	
Age			.001
14	0.00		
15	-0.29	0.18	
16	-0.66	0.15	
17	-0.74	0.20	
If you drink at home do your parents know?			<< .00005
Do not drink alcohol	0.00		
Parents always/usually know	-2.18	0.22	
Parents sometimes/never know	-1.91	0.27	
Missing	-1.56	0.47	
Is a smoker			<< .0005
No	0.00		
Yes	-0.88	0.16	
Best friend is a smoker			< .0005
No	0.00		
Yes	-0.73	0.14	
Drug experiments: Amphetamines			.05
No	0.00		
Yes	-0.42	0.20	
Drug experiments: cannabis leaf			.001
No	0.00		
Yes	-0.56	0.16	
Drug experiments: ecstasy			.05
No	0.00		
Yes	-0.50	0.21	
Do you consider health when choosing what you eat?			.02
Never	0.00		
Sometimes	0.60	0.22	
Quite often/Always	0.27	0.22	
Scale parameter (ω)	0.72	0.15	

CONCLUSION

The media often associates successful female outcomes, such as self-esteem, confidence and high achieving, with body shape and weight. How important are they and what role do they play? Certainly, cross-sectionally, weight or body shape appears to be related with smoking. For example, young girls who claimed to be happy with their body shape were less likely to be smokers. This variable appears to control for the effects of being happy with body weight. In the absence of objective measures of body shape/weight to compare and contrast - this result could be interpreted in a number of ways. For example the result could indicate that on average, those who responded to this question felt that their body shape fitted the 'ideal' female body shape. It could also indicate a certain level of confidence on the part of the girls. On the other hand, it could also indicate that young girls, on average, were not too worried about whether or not their body shape fitted with the 'ideal' social perception of female body shape.

But these results could be due to omitted variables. In the longitudinal analyses of the same data set, variables body shape and weight were not significant in the model of drinking patterns but worrying and drug experimentation were. Conversely, body weight and worrying about problems were significant in the model of smoking patterns.

The longitudinal modelling indicated that there were substantial variations due to omitted variables that the models could not explain. Overall wellbeing or psycho-social wellbeing omitted from our data set and their effect further confounds the subjective variables such as 'happy with weight', 'at ease with opposite sex', and 'worrying about problems'. The longitudinal modelling showed this phenomena being statistically significant (see scale parameter (ω), table 7 and 8,). Nevertheless, a health link is apparent, but it is not obvious from this dataset whether this may mean that women are more health conscious than men, or, women attach a higher level of importance to an ideal body shape.

It is therefore plausible that the variable "being happy with body shape" may reflect the respondent's state of mind at the time of the interview regardless of actual body shape and weight. This means that, in addition to body shape, the variable "happy with body shape" may well be an indication of this group's insensitivity to social pressures, i.e. social influences that may lead to smoking (20).

As shown in tables 3-6, the alternative to being happy with weight is wishing to lose weight. For a larger proportion the wish to lose weight will be due to pressures to conform to social ideals. One consequence of giving in to pressure is the impact on mental health. It is plausible that one mental health outcome due to emphasis on a socially perceived ideal body shape/weight will be apathy, i.e. to be happy with one's weight in order to counteract the social pressures. Another mental health outcome may be unhealthy behaviour such as the perception that smoking will keep weight down (21,22), and/or eating disorders (7).

IMPLICATIONS FOR POLICY DEVELOPMENT AND FUTURE RESEARCH

Perceptions of a socially idealised body shape or weight is very different to perceived health benefits of acquiring social ideals. As discussed in the background numerous studies suggest that associating body shape or weight with health is a cause of public health concern, particular for women. In terms of developing research to inform policy/behaviour, even in the twenty-first century, women appear to be operating in societies dominated with male-set parameters (23). At least in terms of health and social outcomes trends suggest that women are catching up with men's adverse health and social outcomes, e.g. lung cancer, heart disease, and violence resulting from smoking, alcohol and drug abuse (23). Future research should debate the feminising of health and social parameters, for the reason that although body image appears as a significant factor for health, but longitudinally this effect is no longer significant. This result suggests that, on average, young women acknowledge that social ideals of a body shape are unrealistic and therefore are perceptions only. It is therefore important that future studies of this kind that are related to human behaviour follow a longitudinal design with appropriate longitudinal analytical methodology.

REFERENCES

[1] Cattarin JA, Thompson JK, Thomas C, Williams R. Body image, mood, and televised images of attractiveness: The role of social comparison. J Soc Clin Psychol 2000;19(2):220-39.
[2] Sypeck MF, Gray JJ, Ahrens AH. No longer just a pretty face: Fashion magazines' depictions of ideal female beauty from 1959 to 1999. Int J Eating Disord 2004;36(3):342-7.
[3] Spitzer BL, Henderson KA, Zivian MT. Gender differences in population versus media body sizes: A comparison over four decades. Sex Roles 1999;40(7-8):545-65.
[4] Halliwell E, Diedrichs PC. Testing a dissonance body image intervention among young girls. Health Psychol 2014;33(2):201-4.
[5] Owen R, Spencer R. Body ideals in women after viewing images of typical and healthy weight models. Body Image 2013;10(4):489-94.
[6] Willis LE, Knobloch-Westerwick S. Weighing women down: Messages on weight loss and body shaping in editorial content in popular women's health and fitness magazines. Health Commun 2014;29(4):323-31.
[7] Costa-Font J, Jofre-Bonet M. Anorexia, body image and peer effects: Evidence from a sample of european women. Economica 2013;80(317):44-64.
[8] Hill B, Skouteris H, McCabe M, Fuller-Tyszkiewicz M. Body image and gestational weight gain: A prospective study. J Midwifery Womens Health 2013;58(2):189-94.
[9] Ogden CL, Carroll MD, Kit BK, Flegal KM. Prevalence of obesity and trends in body mass index among us children and adolescents, 1999-2010. JAMA 2012;307(5):483-90.
[10] Heinberg LJ, Thompson JK. Body image and televised images of thinness and attractiveness: A controlled laboratory investigation. J Soc Clin Psychol 1995;14(4):325-38.
[11] McGinnis R. A stochastic model of social mobility. Am Sociol Rev 1968;23:712-22.
[12] Ginsberg RB. Semi-markov processes and mobility. Mathematical Sociol 1971;1:233-62.
[13] Davies R, Flowerdew R. Modelling migration careers using data from a british survey. Geographical Analysis 1992;24:35-57.
[14] Slater A, Tiggemann M, Firth B, Hawkins K. Reality check: An experimental investigation of the addition of warning labels to fashion magazine images on women's mood and body dissatisfaction. J Soc Clin Psychol 2012;31(2):105-22.
[15] Shahtahmasebi S, Berridge D. Teenage smoking: A longitudinal analysis. Int J Adolesc Med Health 2005;17(2):137-55.
[16] Shahtahmasebi S, Berridge D. Teenage drinking patterns: A longitudinal analysis. Int J Adolesc Med Health 2009;21(3):371-85.
[17] Shahtahmasebi S, Berridge D. Conceptualising behaviour in health and social research: A practical guide to data analysis. New York: Nova Science, 2010.

[18] Shahtahmasebi S. Teenage smoking: Some problems with interpreting the evidence. Int J Adolesc Med Health 2003;15(4):307-20.

[19] Davies R, Martin AM, Penn R. Linear modelling with clustered observations an illustratative example of earnings in the engineering industry. Environ Plann A 1988;20:1069-84.

[20] Norton EC, Lindrooth RC, Ennett ST. How measures of perception from survey data lead to inconsistent regression results: Evidence from adolescent and peer substance use. Health Econ 2003;12(2):139-48.

[21] Bresnahan MJ, Zhuang J, Sun S. Influence of smoking norms and gainâ€"loss antismoking messages on young chinese adults. Nicotine Tob Res 2013;15(9):1564-71.

[22] Loken B. Heavy smokers', light smokers', and nonsmokers' beliefs about cigarette smoking. J Appl Psychol 1982;67(5):616.

[23] Shahtahmasebi S, Shahtahmasebi R, Cassidy B. Trends in women's smoking and health outcomes: Lessons that should have been learned from trends in men's smoking. In: Tolson KP, Veksler EB, eds. Smoking and women's health research. New York: Nova Science, 2008:277-302.

In: Child and Adolescent Health Issues
Editor: Joav Merrick

ISBN: 978-1-63463-574-5

Chapter 3

MEDIA EXPOSURE AND WEIGHT CONCERN?

***Olusegun T Afolabi, MBChB, MPH, FMCPH*[*,1]*,
Bamidele Bello, BSc,MPH*[2]*,
Macellina Y Ijadunola, MBChB, MPH, FWACP*[1]*,
Christopher O Alabi, MBChB*[1]*,
Chinedu E Akabueze, MBChB*[1]
and Oluwaseun A Alabi, MBChB[1]**

[1]Department of Community Health
[2]Population and Reproductive Health Programm,
Obafemi Awolowo University, Ile-Ife, Nigeria

The changing face of media has increased the length of time children spend before the television screen. There has been increasing evidence of the positive relationship between the length of time spent watching television and increased BMI in children. Studies have implicated childhood obesity as a predictor of premature death from endogenous causes and a positive association with death from all causes. Studies conducted among children in Nigeria have shown a prevalence of between 9-14% and 4-5% for overweight and obesity respectively in both sexes. This study explores association between screen/media exposure and body weight. This was a cross-sectional study conducted among 600 primary school pupils in south west Nigeria using interviewer administered questionnaire and anthropometric measurements of the pupils. Data were analysed using SPSS version 16 soft ware. Data were summarised with univariate, bivariate and multivariate analysis using frequency tables, chi-square and multinomial logistic regression respectively. P was significant at <0.05. Ownership of television in the household was 94%, only 29% of the pupils had a mobile phone while only 12% could use the internet. Two-thirds of the pupils were underweight while 6.6% and 2.4% were overweight and obese respectively. The association between nutritional status and gender, were statistically significant (p=0.003 and 0.001 respectively), while that between nutritional status and internet exposure was not statistically significant (p=0.98). Media exposure and snacking between

* Correspondence: Olusegun T Afolabi, MBChB, MPH, FMCPH, Department of Community Health, Obafemi Awolowo University, Ile-Ife, Osun State, Nigeria. E-mail: temitopesegun@yahoo.com

meals were predictors of nutritional status. Though a preponderant part of our sample were under weight, obesity and overweight are becoming common.

INTRODUCTION

The changing face of media has increased the length of time children spend before the screen. Research suggests that children may be spending more time watching television than they spend in school (1). Despite the advantages of media/television viewing which include improved knowledge, imagination (2), reduced risk of low overall social-emotional competence (3), amongst others, increased screen time has been linked to poor mental health (2, 4, 5), poor academic performance and cognitive outcomes (2,6,7), poor body image (8,9), sleep problems (10) and poor dietary intake (11) including overweight and obesity (12-14). Overweight and obesity are growing threats to public health (15) and are increasingly becoming as prevalent as infectious diseases even in developing countries (16-19). Over the past few years, childhood overweight and obesity issues have attracted great concerns due to its adverse health implication even in adulthood (20,21). Studies have implicated childhood obesity as a predictor of premature death from endogenous causes (20) and a positive association with death from all causes (21). Studies conducted among children in Nigeria have shown a prevalence of between 9-14% and 4-5% for overweight and obesity respectively in both sexes (22-26).

There has been increasing evidence of the positive relationship between the length of time spent watching television and increased BMI in children (12-14) and adolescents (12, 27). This has been explained through various mechanisms including high intake of energy dense food and low consumption of vegetables (28-30), reduction in time spent on more physical activities (31,32), reduced sleep time (33, 34) and exposure to food (35,36). Several studies have considered the effect of video games and or internet/computer use on a number of health related outcomes including attention problems (37), disturbed sleep pattern (11), but very few (38) had looked into their influence on the BMI where he observed no relationship between video game/computer use and BMI even though they observed a positive relationship with increased television viewing. This association has been widely studied across the globe, however, one study that examined the association between television viewing and BMI among Nigerian children and adolescents was a global study that made use of secondary data and Nigeria was one of the countries studied (12). In addition, currently, there is paucity of data from Nigeria on the association between BMI and the media beyond the television. Therefore, this study explores association between screen/media (TV, DSTV, internet, Computer, electronic games, mobile phones) exposure and body weight.

OUR STUDY

The study was conducted in Ife Central Local Government Area (LGA) of Ile-Ife, a semi-urban settlement in Osun State, southwest Nigeria. In this descriptive cross-sectional study, 600 primary school students were selected using sample size formula for cluster sampling with a design effect of 1.5; prevalence of obesity set at 50%; level of confidence 95% and precision of 0.05 from ten schools through a multi-stage sampling technique. At the first stage, the schools were stratified into public and private schools. There were 91 registered primary schools in the LGA (42 public and 49 private schools), five private and public primary schools each were selected by simple random sampling technique. At the second stage a total of 300 respondents each from private and public schools were selected by a systematic sampling technique by calculating the kth interval until 600 students were recruited from primary two to primary six representing 60 from each class level. Parents of the recruited children were also selected to participate in the study. Consent was obtained for parents' participation in the study while child assent and parental consent were obtained for the child respondent. The survey response rate was 89% and 72% for private schools and public school children respectively. Only children whose parent gave consent and completed the study instrument were included in the sample.

Data were collected using pre-tested, semi-structured, interviewer-administered questionnaire for children and self-administered questionnaire for their parents. The child instruments obtained information on socio-demographics, media/screen viewing time as well as nutrition and nutritional status of the child respondent. The parent survey instrument asked questions specifically about the target child's feeding practices, physical activity, television viewing habits and weight perception as well as parents' socio-demographic information. As part of the parents' survey instrument, the amount of time a child spends on media devices (television, DVD/video, computer/video game, mobile phone, DSTV/HiTV and the internet) was evaluated with questions separately for weekdays and weekend days. Total time per week and average daily time were computed and respondents were categorised into three groups: <60min per day, 61 -120 min per day or >120 min per day. Also included were questions to evaluate the Childs' eating pattern which included consumption of fizzy drinks, fruits and vegetables, frequency of snacking and a 24hr dietary recall. Child's physical activity was measured by asking parents structured questions on the kind of recreation activity the child engaged in at home and the average number of hours spent on the activity.

As concern has been raised about the validity and reliability of parent/caretaker's report of their children's screen time (39), a procedure that is being used by several studies (4, 32, 40), this study in addition to parents' report utilised children's recognition of TV characters and internet logos and provision of their exact names as a proxy measure for media exposure. This measure was first used in 1970 (41) to assess the effects of Sesame Street on children and has subsequently been used by other studies among pre-school in several countries (39, 42, 43). Children were presented with a card containing sixteen pictures (six cartoon characters, five sport/movie stars and five computer related logos). Media exposure scores were based on the number of characters and logos the child recognised and named correctly. We compared this measure of exposure—recognition of characters and logos—with traditional parental report of children's exposure.TV exposure was a composite score with pupils who were able to recognise 6 or more of the 11 TV characters scored as having excess TV exposure while recognition of 3 or more of the 5 internet characters was scored as excess internet exposure.

Body Mass Index, BMI, (kg/m2) of the child respondents were calculated using measurement obtained by weighing the child on a bathroom scale while wearing light clothing at the time of the survey. Their heights were also measured from the top of their head to the sole of the feet, bare footed, with the child standing against a stadiometer. Age- and sex-specific growth charts and relative cut-off points were used to define nutritional status of the children (44).

Ethics approval was obtained from the Institute of Public Health Institutional Review Board. Letters were sent to the study schools to obtain permission for the conduct of the study. Information letters as well as consent forms were sent to parents/caregivers through their children/wards availing them of details of the study. Children with returned consent forms and who gave assent to participate were recruited into the study and given the parents' instruments to be completed by their parents/caregivers in their various homes. Children who returned the parents instrument by agreed dates were interviewed on the children instrument and their anthropometric measurements obtained.

Data were analysed using SPSS version 16 with univariate, bivariate and multivariate analysis using frequency tables, chi-square and multinomial logistic regression respectively. P was significant at <0.05.

OUR FINDINGS

Table 1 shows that a little over two-fifth (42.0%) of pupils were aged 9-10 years and slightly over a quarter (26.1%) between 7 and 8 years. Over half of the pupils were female and ownership of television set was almost universal (94%) while only 29% of the pupils had mobile phones with only 12% being able to use the internet.

Table 1. Sociodemographic characteristics of pupils

Variable	Frequency (N=482)	Percentage
Age group		
5-6	21	4.4
7-8	126	26.1
9-10	203	42.1
11-12	97	20.1
>=13	35	7.3
Sex		
Male	232	48.1
Female	250	51.9
Have television at home	453	94.0
Have mobile phone	140	29.0
Know how to use internet	60	12.4

Over two-thirds (68.5%) of interviewed pupils were underweight while 6.6% and 2.5% were overweight and obese respectively (see table 2).

Table 2. Nutritional status of pupils

Nutritional status	Frequency (N=482)	Percentage
Underweight	330	68.5
Normal	108	22.4
Overweight	32	6.6
Obese	12	2.5

There was a statistically significant relationship between gender and nutritional status (p=0.003) with 74% of males being underweight compared to 63% of females and more females were obese (4.4%) compared to just 0.4% of male pupils (see table 3).

Table 3. Nutritional status of pupils by gender

Gender	**Nutritional Status**				Total	Statistics
	Normal (N=108)	Overweight (N=32)	Obese (N=12)	Underweight (N=330)	(N=482)	
Male	48 (20.6%)	11 (4.7%)	1 (0.4%)	172 (73.8%)	232 (100%)	χ^2=14.19 P=0.003
Female	60 (24%)	21 (8.4%)	11 (4.4%)	158 (63.2%)	250 (100%)	

There was a statistically significant association between media exposure and nutritional status (p=0.001) with 10% and 4% of those with excess media exposure being overweight and obese compared to 4% and 1% of those with standard exposure to media while internet exposure was not statistically associated with nutritional status (p=0.96) (see table 4).

Table 4. Nutritional status of pupils by media and internet exposure

Internet Exposure	**Nutritional Status**				Total (N=482)	Statistics
	Normal (N=108)	Overweight (N=32)	Obese (N=12)	Underweight (N=330)		
Standard	97 (22.1%)	29 (6.6%)	11 (2.5%)	302 (68.8%)	439 (100%)	χ^2=0.30 P=0.96
Excess	11 (25.6%)	3 (7.0%)	1 (2.3%)	28 (65.1%)	43 (100%)	
Media Exposure						
Standard	56 (20.3%)	11 (4.0%)	3 (1.1%)	206 (74.6%)	276 (100%)	χ^2=16.84 P=0.001
Excess	52 (25.2%)	21 (10.2%)	9 (4.4%)	124 (58.3%)	206 (100%)	

Snacking between meals was statistically significantly associated with nutritional status (P<0.001) with lesser proportion of pupils who snacked between meals (63%) being underweight compared to 80% of those who do not snack between meals (see table 5).

Table 5. Nutritional status of pupils by consumption of snacks between meals

Snack between meals	**Nutritional Status**				Total	Statistics
	Normal (N=108)	Overweight (N=32)	Obese (N=12)	Underweight (N=330)	(N=482)	
Yes	88 (27.7%)	23 (7.2%)	7 (2.2%)	200 (62.9%)	318 (100%)	χ^2=16.61 P<0.001
No	20 (12.2%)	9 (5.5%)	5 (3.0%)	130 (79.3%)	164 (100%)	

The multinomial logistic regression showed that snacking between meals and media exposure were predictors of nutritional status with pupils with excess media exposure and not snacking between meals being two and a half times more likely to be overweight than pupils with normal body weight while for the underweight pupils more media exposure reduced the likelihood two folds compared to normal weight pupils and pupils who do not snack in between meals were thrice more likely to be underweight (see table 6).

Table 6. Correlates of nutritional status of pupils

Overweight	B coefficient	Odds ratio	95% Conf Interval
Intercept	-2.94	-	-
Snack between meals (ref Yes)	0.87	2.38	1.02-5.58
Internet exposure (ref poor)	-0.45	0.64	0.18-2.25
Media exposure (ref poor)	0.93	2.54	1.14-5.63
Underweight			
Intercept	0.43	-	-
Snack between meals (ref Yes)	1.17	3.23	1.80-5.80
Internet exposure (ref standard)	0.07	1.07	0.47-2.43
Media exposure (ref standard)	-0.59	0.56	0.34-0.91

*Ref: Normal body weight pupils.

DISCUSSION

In this study, there was a significant association between excess TV exposure and BMI/nutritional status, but not with internet exposure. The significant association between TV viewing and BMI was in line with several previous studies (12, 45, 46). As with other cross-sectional studies, we were unable to ascertain if this association is causal or whether TV viewing may be a marker of other dietary lifestyle that may influence BMI as may be suggestive in this study as more of the children with normal BMI were in the class of excess TV viewing (25.6%) compared to those with standard TV view (20.6%) and also a higher percentage of children with standard TV viewing (74.3%) were underweight compared to 59.6% among those with excess TV viewing. This is not suggestive of better nutritional practice among children with excess TV viewing but could be indicative of their more sedentary lifestyle and/or high consumption of energy dense food and snacks associated with TV viewing (29, 30, 47). This argument can be supported by higher prevalence of obesity among pupils who snacked in-between-meals as observed in this study.

As the percentage of pupils with normal BMI in the class of excess TV viewing was higher compared to their counterpart with standard TV viewing one could infer that the habit of excessive TV viewing and or its associated dietary practice had helped them in attaining a normal BMI particularly since the percentage of pupils who were underweight and had standard TV view were almost twice as high as those with excess TV viewing.

The prevalence of obesity was highest among female students with excess TV viewing. The relationship between excess TV viewing and BMI when disaggregated by sex only remained significant for females. This reaffirms the findings of stronger association between TV viewing and obesity among females in previous studies (14, 45). Hancox and Poulton

(14) in their study found stronger and consistently statistically significant association in girls while in boys, the associations were consistently positive, but were generally weaker and often not statistically significant, particularly at the older ages.

One unanticipated, but important outcome of the study was the high prevalence of underweight (68.6%) co-existing with overweight (6.6%) and obesity (2.4%) among the study population. This supports the result of several studies that has found the problem of over-nutrition occurring simultaneously with under-nutrition in many developing countries including Nigeria (19, 24, 48).

There are a number of important limitations to this study. First is the cross-sectional design which shows association and not causality or temporality. The association between excess TV viewing cannot be said to be the cause of obesity among the study population. Also, recall bias may not be excluded, as the pupils had to recall their snacking pattern and frequency. Thirdly, social desirability bias may not be excluded, as pupils may under or over-estimate their frequency of snacking and physical activity respectively.

The major strength of this study is that till date, it is the only study conducted in Nigeria primarily on the effects of prolonged TV viewing on BMI. The only other study was a global study which utilised secondary data (12). Additional strengths of this study are its measure of TV viewing of character recognition as opposed the traditional parental report and the study participants from both public and private school hence affording us the opportunity of a generalizable result.

CONCLUSION

This study showed a positive association between excess TV viewing and BMI among primary school pupils in a Nigerian sample. Our result is in accordance with previous global evidence however, providing concrete data for Nigeria. Our findings suggest that although excess TV viewing contributed to the attainment of a normal BMI among primary school children, the habit of excessive TV viewing has its associated risk of obesity.

ACKNOWLEDGMENTS

We are grateful to the children and parents who participated in this study and to the school authorities for allowing us to undertake the study in their school. We also appreciate the effort of the head teachers of the schools for granting access to the schools in the data collection process and Ms. Omowumi Dairo, who searched for relevant articles.

REFERENCES

[1] Strasburger VC. Children, adolescents and television. Pediatr Rev 1992; 13:144–51.

[2] Thakkar RR, Garrison MM, Christakis DA. A systematic review for the effect of television viewing by infants and pre-schoolers. Pediatrics 2006;118:2025-31.

[3] Intusoma U, Mo-suwan L, Ruangdaraganon N, Panyayong B, Chongsuvivatwong V. Effect of television viewing on social-emotional competence of young Thai children. Infant Behav Dev 2013;36:679-85.

[4] Parkes A, Sweeting H, Wight D, Henderson M. Do television and electronic games predict children's psychosocial adjustment? Longitudinal research using the UK millennium cohort study. Arch Dis Child 2013;98:341-348.

[5] Tin SP, Ho DS, Mak KH, Wan KL, Lam TH. Association between television viewing and self-esteem in children. J Dev Behav Pediatr 2012;33(6):479-85.

[6] Sharif I, Wills TA, Sargent JD. Effect of visual media use on school performance: A prospective study. J Adolesc Hlth 2010;46(1):52.

[7] Zimmerman F J, Christakis DA. Children's television viewing and cognitive outcomes: A longitudinal analysis of national data. Arch Pediatr Adolesc Med 2005;159:619-25.

[8] Mulgrew K E, Volcevski-Kostas D, Rendell PG. The effect of music video clips on adolescent boys' body image, mood and schema activation. J Youth Adolescence. doi 10.1007/s10964-013-9932-6

[9] American Academy of Pediatrics, Committee on Public Education. Children, adolescents, and television. Pediatrics 2001;107:423-6.

[10] Thompson DA, Christakis DA. The association between television viewing and irregular sleep schedules among children less than 3 years of age. Pediatrics 2005;116;851.

[11] Van den Buck J, Eggermont S. Media use as a reason for meal skipping and fast eating in secondary school children. J Hum Nutr Dietet 2006; 19:91-100.

[12] Braithwaite I, Stewart AW, Hancox RJ, Beasley R, Murphy R, Mitchell EA, et al. The worldwide association between television viewing and obesity in children and adolescents: Cross sectional study. PLoS ONE 2013;8(9):e74263. doi:10.1371/journal.pone.0074263

[13] Jackson DM, Djafarian K, Stewart J, Speakman JR. Increased television viewing is associated with elevated body fatness but not with lower total energy expenditure in children. Am J Clin Nutr 2009;89:1031–6.

[14] Hancox RJ and Poulton R. Watching television is associated with childhood obesity: but is it clinically important? Int J Obesity 2006:30:171-5.

[15] Popkin BM, Gordon-Larsen P. The nutrition transition: worldwide obesity dynamics and their determinants. Int J Obes Relat Metab Disord 2004;28:(3):S2–9.

[16] Wang Y, Lobstein T. Worldwide trends in childhood overweight and obesity. Int J Pediatr Obes 2006;1:11-25.

[17] Hossain P, Kawar B, El Nahas M. Obesity and diabetes in the developing world – a growing challenge. N Engl J Med 2007;356:213-5.

[18] Chhatwal J, Verma M, Riar SK. Obesity among pre- adolescent and adolescents of developing country (India). Asian Pacif J Clin Nutr 2004;13(3):231-5.

[19] De Onis M, Blössner M. Prevalence and trends of overweight among pre-schoolchildren in developing countries. Am J Clin Nutr 2000;72: 1032-9.

[20] Franks PW, Hanson RL, Knowler WC, Moffett C, Enos G, Infante AM, et al. Childhood predictors of young- onset type 2 diabetes. Diabetes 2007;56:2964-72.

[21] Gunnell DJ, Frankel SJ, Nanchahal K, Peters TJ, Davey Smith G. Childhood obesity and adult cardiovascular mortality: a 57y follow-up study based on the Boyd Orr cohort. Am J Clin Nutr 1998;67:1111-8

[22] Izuora AN, Animasahun BA, Nwodo U, Ibeabuchi NM, Njokanma OF, Renner JK. Assessment of overweight and obesity among Nigerian children and adolescents using triceps skin-fold thickness and body mass index. Clin Obes 2013;3:103-11.

[23] Sabageh AO, Ojofeitimi EO. Prevalence of obesity among adolescents in IleIfe, Osun state, Nigeria using body mass index and waist hip ratio: A comparative study. Niger Med J 2013;54:153-6.

[24] Chinedu SN, Eboji OK, Emiloju OC. Trends in weight abnormality of school children and adolescents in Nigeria. J Med Sci 2012;12:239-43.

[25] Senbanjo IO, Adejuyigbe EA. Prevalence of overweight and obesity in Nigerian preschool children. Nutr Health 2007;18(4):391-9.

[26] Ansa VO, Odigwe CO, Anah MU. Profile of body mass index and obesity in Nigerian children and adolescents. Niger J Med 2001;10:78-80.

[27] Steffen LM., Dai S, Fulton JE., Labarthe DR. Overweight in children and adolescents associated with TV viewing and parental weight. Am J Prev Med 2009;37(1S):S50-5.

[28] Ramos E, Costa A, Araujo J, Severo M, Lopes C. Effect of television viewing on food and nutrient intake among adolescents. Nutrition 2013;29:1362-7.

[29] Salmon J, Campbell KJ, Crawford DA. Television viewing habits associated with obesity risk factors: a survey of Melbourne school children. Med J Aust 2006;184:64-7

[30] Vereecken CA, Todd J, Robert C, Mulvihill C, Maes L. Television viewing behaviours and associations with food habits in different countries. Public Health Nutr 2006;9:244-50.

[31] Hamer M, Stamatakis E, Mishra G. Psychological distress, television viewing, and physical activity in children aged 4 to 12 Years. Pediatrics 2009;123;1263-8.

[32] Robinson TN. Reducing children's television viewing to prevent obesity: a randomised controlled trial. JAMA 1999;282:1561-7.

[33] Haines J, McDonald J, O'Brien A, Sherry B, Bottino CJ, Schmidt ME, et al. Health habits, happy home: Randomised trial to improve household routines for obesity prevention among preschool aged children. JAMA Pediatr 2013 Nov;167(11):1072-9.

[34] Garmy P, Nyberg P, Jacobsson U, Sleep and television and computer habits of Swedish school-age children. J Sch Nurs. 2012;28(6):469-76.

[35] Halford J CG, Boyland E J, Hughes G M, Stacey L, McKean S, Dovey TM. Beyond-brand effect of television food advertisements on food choice in children: the effects of weight status. Public Health Nutr 2007;11(9):897–904.

[36] Halford JCG. Gillespie J, Brown V, Pontin EE, Dovey TM. Effect of television advertisements for foods on food consumption in children. Appetite 2004;42:221-5.

[37] Swing EL, Gentile DA, Anderson DA, Walsh D. Television and video game exposure and the development of attention problems. Pediatrics 2010;126:214-21.

[38] Wake M, Hesketh K, Waters E. Television, computer use and body mass index in Australian primary school children. J Paediatr Child Health 2003;39:130-4.

[39] Rimal RN, Figueroa ME, Storey JD. Character recognition as an alternate measure of television exposure among children: Findings from the Alam Simsim Program in Egypt. J Health Commun 2013;18(5):594-609.

[40] Manios Y, Kourlaba G, Kondaki K, Grammatikaki E, Anastasiadou A, Roma-Giannikou E. Obesity and television watching in preschoolers in Greece: The GENESIS Study. Obesity 2009;17(11):2047-53.

[41] Ball S, Bogatz GA. The first year of Sesame street: An evaluation. Princeton, NJ: Educational Testing Service, 1970.

[42] Borzekowski DLG, Henry H. The impact of Jalan Sesama on the educational and healthy development of Indonesian preschool children: An experimental study. Int J Behav Dev 2011;35(2):169-79.

[43] Borzekowski DLG, Macha J. The role of Kilimani Sesame in the healthy development of Tanzania preschool children. J Appl Dev Psych 2010; 31(4):298-305.

[44] Cole TJ, Bellizzi MC, Flegal KM, Dietz WH. Establishing a standard definition for child overweight and obesity worldwide: international survey. BMJ 2000;320(7244):1240-3.

[45] Ray-Lopez JP, Vicente-Rodriguez G, Biosca M, Moreno LA. Sedentary behaviour and obesity development in children and adolescents. Nutr Metab Cardiovasc Dis 2008;18:242-51.

[46] Gortmaker SL, Must A, Sobol AM, Peterson K, Colditz GA, Dietz WH. Television viewing as a cause of increasing obesity among children in the United States, 1986–1990. Arch Pediatr Adolesc Med 1996;150: 356-62.

[47] Phillips SM, Bandini LG, Naumova EN, Cyr H, Colclough S, Dietz WH, Must A. Energy-dense snack food intake in adolescence: londitudinal relationship to weight and fatness. Obes Res 2004;12:461-72.

[48] Caballaro B. A nutrition paradox: Underweight and obesity in developing countries. N Engl J Med 2005;325:1514-6.

In: Child and Adolescent Health Issues
Editor: Joav Merrick
ISBN: 978-1-63463-574-5

Chapter 4

HUMAN PAPILLOMAVIRUS (HPV) VACCINE AND PARENTS

***Nemica Thavarajah, BSc**[*,1,2]**, Edward Chow, MBBS**[1]*
***and Jose Arocha, PhD**[2]*
[1]Odette Cancer Centre, Sunnybrook Health Sciences Centre,
University of Toronto, Toronto, Ontario, Canada
[2]Faculty of Applied Health Sciences, University of Waterloo,
Waterloo, Ontario, Canada

The primary objective of this chapter was to explore the literature to determine common factors that influence parental decision making regarding uptake of the HPV vaccine for their sons and daughters. A systematic literature review was conducted using MEDLINE, EMBASE, and PsychINFO databases to identify studies published between January 2011 and October 2013 reporting factors influencing parental decision making regarding uptake of the HPV vaccine for their children. A total of 19 studies regarding parental decision making for the HPV vaccine for daughters and/or sons and fit the eligibility criteria were retrieved. The sample size of the studies retrieved ranged from 20 to 8652 parents. The most prevalent factors (found in five or more studies) in order of most to least prevalent included knowledge on prophylaxis; concerns with safety and/or side effects; trust in health provider, and/or government, and/or school; sexual health; positive parental attitudes; insufficient information; influence of family and/or friends; and parent-child communication. Many factors influence parental decisions in regards to providing consent for their children to receive the HPV vaccine. Future efforts should focus on addressing these factors to improve uptake of the HPV vaccine by implementing focused strategies and decision aids to help parents make informed decisions.

---

* Correspondence: Nemica Thavarajah, BSc, Department of Radiation Oncology, Odette Cancer Centre, Sunnybrook Health Sciences Centre, 2075 Bayview Avenue, Toronto, ON M4N 3M5, Canada. E-mail: nemica.thavarajah@gmail.com

INTRODUCTION

The human papillomavirus (HPV) is the most common sexually transmitted infection (STI) worldwide, with about 75% of Canadians developing at least one HPV infection in their lifetime (1, 2). A greater risk of exposure are attributed towards individuals who are sexually active at an earlier age, with the highest prevalence of HPV being among people between the ages of 15 and 24 (2, 3).

HPV infections are often asymptomatic, but the most obvious symptom is the development of genital warts (2, 4). However, HPV has also been known to be linked to various cancers, accounting for 5.2% of cancers worldwide (4). More specifically, HPV accounts for the cause of almost all cervical cancers, 88% of anal cancers, and 50% of penile cancers (4). HPV has also been known to cause some vaginal cancers, vulvar cancers, and head and neck cancers (2). Pap screening in women are helpful in detecting abnormal cervical cells before said cells become cancerous. The HPV test is another procedure that can help detect infections and precancerous lesions. The HPV test can detect HPV-types that are of high oncogenic risk through detection of the epithelial and cervical cells (5). Although the HPV test is more sensitive than the pap test, the HPV test is currently not standard, routine, or available for men. However, even though the pap test is a standard routine, 15% of Canadian women claim to have never received a pap test and 30% of Canadians have not been screened within the past three years (4).

Unfortunately there is currently no cure for HPV; however, the HPV vaccine can help protect again certain types of HPV infections (6). For instance, Gardasil and Cervarix are licensed vaccines that help protect against specific HPV-types. Cervarix protects against types 16 and 18, while Gardasil protects against types 6, 11, 16, and 18 (4). The government of Canada allocated $300 million in 2006 towards the implementation of provincial universal HPV vaccination programs for girls between the ages of nine and 16 (7). The grade eight vaccination program was introduced in Ontario in 2007 which offers an optional HPV vaccine to girls with the consent of their parents. The vaccine (Gardasil) is administered in a three-dose treatment schedule with the first dose being baseline, followed by a second dose two months after baseline, and a third dose six months after baseline (2). Although the public vaccination program has been implemented throughout Canada, the HPV vaccine uptake rate varies across the country from as low as 50% in Alberta, to as high as 86% in Quebec (8).

The HPV infection also remains an important issue in men as both men and women can be infected with HPV. Men can transmit HPV to sexual partners; however, there are currently no routine tests to screen men. Furthermore, there is currently no publicly funded HPV vaccination program for boys in Ontario (2). There has been much debate about implementing a publicly funded HPV vaccination program for boys (4). Whether the issue is increasing uptake of the HPV vaccine in boys or girls, the key common underlying factor is the obtainment of parental consent. Considering HPV is an STI, the most effective point of administration of the HPV vaccine is before becoming sexually active. Thus, parents play a critical role in ensuring optimal uptake of the HPV vaccine in children by providing consent (4). However, several studies have shown that there are many factors that influence parental decision making when it comes to providing consent for their children to uptake the HPV vaccine (1, 3, 6). There are a variety of factors that are often rooted in parental knowledge, beliefs, and attitudes (4). As such, it is important to identify and address these factors to improve vaccination rates across Canada, and worldwide. The primary objective of this study was to explore the literature to determine common factors that influence parental decision making regarding uptake of the HPV vaccine for their sons and daughters. A secondary objective was to further examine common sources of information available to parents regarding the HPV vaccine and the effectiveness of its use.

OUR STUDY

A systematic literature review was conducted using MEDLINE (1948 to October 2013), EMBASE (1980 to week 42 of 2013), and PsychINFO (2002 to October 2013) databases to identify studies reporting factors influencing parental decision making regarding uptake of the HPV vaccine for their children. Search terms 'HPV' or 'human papillomavirus' were coupled with 'parental decisions' or 'parent decision' or 'decision making' or 'decision aids' and 'vaccine' or 'vaccination' to extract relevant literature.

A total of 465 studies were retrieved, 135 of which were from MEDLINE, 261 from EMBASE, and 39 from PsychINFO. All abstracts and titles of the identified articles were screened in accordance to the eligibility criteria. Articles included in the review were peer-reviewed, published between January 2011 and October 2013, and empirical studies that focused on factors influencing parents' decisions regarding HPV vaccines. The start date of January 2011 was selected because prior literature reviews included studies up to 2011 (1, 3, 6). Articles that were editorials, literature reviews, did not include parents in the study sample, or were not published in English, were excluded. A total of 446 studies retrieved did not fit the eligibility criteria or were excluded due to duplicates.

OUR FINDINGS

A total of 19 studies, published between 2011 and 2013, regarding parental decision making for the HPV vaccine and fit the eligibility criteria were retrieved, as summarized in table 1 (9-27). The sample size of the studies retrieved ranged from 20 to 8652 parents. Most study samples were primarily composed of mothers, ranging from 63% of participants to 100%. The types of study designs utilized in these studies included focus groups, structured interviews, semi-structured interviews, and surveys. Twelve studies focused solely on parental decision making for the uptake of the HPV vaccine in their daughters (10-12, 14, 16-20, 23, 24, 27), three studies focused solely on sons (9, 21, 25), and four studies involved both sons and daughters (13, 15, 22, 26). There was a wide geographical range of study locations, including Canada, USA, Peru, Vietnam, South Africa, England, Netherlands, Australia, and China. A detailed list of identified factors that influenced parental decision making in these studies are listed in Table 1. Figure 1 also shows the common factors found among studies. The most prevalent factors (found in five or more studies) in order of most to least prevalent included knowledge on prophylaxis; concerns with safety and/or side effects; trust in health provider, and/or government, and/or school; sexual health; positive parental attitudes; insufficient information; influence of family and/or friends; and parent-child communication.

Table 1. Studies identifying factors that influence parental decision making with regards to the uptake of the HPV vaccine for their children

Study (year)	Location	Study design	Study about daughters or sons	Number of parents (% of parents that are mothers)	Factors	Ref.
Alexander et al. (2012)	Indiana, USA	Semi-structured interviews	Sons	21 (81%)	- recalling information provided by health provider - concerns about safety - realization that son may soon become sexually active - protection of son - concerns about side effects - misconceptions about protection against STIs	[9]
Allen et al. (2012)	Boston, USA	Focus groups	Daughters	64 (72%)	- insufficient information - varied preferences for involvement in decision making - concerns about safety of HPV vaccine - mistrust of pharmaceutical companies and medical providers - preferred sources of information	[10]
Bartolini et al. (2012)	Peru	Structured interviews	Daughters	48 (100%)	- community sensitization meetings with parents - understanding HPV vaccine is an accepted form of prevention - recognizing HPV vaccine can prevent cervical cancer - trusted teachers, schools, and health personnel - free HPV vaccine - positive media reports on HPV vaccine - support from other parents and health personnel - joint parent decision-making - educational materials - influence of daughter's opinion - concerns about side effects - consent process as a barrier - insufficient information (in media) - leaving decision to be made solely by father - belief that HPV vaccine might encourage promiscuity - unclear information	[11]
Cover et al. (2012)	Vietnam	Focus groups and structured interviews	Daughters	133 (67%)	- perception of health benefits and risks - trust in a government program - economic benefits - concerns about safety	[12]

Study (year)	Location	Study design	Study about daughters or sons	Number of parents (% of parents that are mothers)	Factors	Ref.
					- concerns about side effects - misconceptions and suspicions about HPV vaccination - age-related concerns of daughter - seeking guidance from family, friends, leaders, and media	
Dorell et al. (2013)	USA	National immunization survey	Both daughters and sons	8652 (unspecified)	- news coverage - school requirement - family - friends - books, magazines, or information from a library - Internet - television shows or talk shows - drug company advertisements	[13]
Francis and Katz (2013)	Johannesburg, South Africa and Ohio, USA	Focus groups	Daughters	43 (95%)	- knowledge about HPV and cervical cancer - who makes health decisions in family - parent-child communication about sexual health - concern about children's health - cost of HPV vaccine - sexual abuse - lack of enough HPV vaccination information via educational programs/ materials	[14]
Francis et al. (2011)	South Africa	Focus groups	Both daughters and sons	24 (100%)	- mother-daughter communication about sexuality - gender roles in healthcare decision making - knowledge about HPV and cervical cancer - overall acceptance of HPV vaccine	[15]
Griffioen et al. (2012)	USA	Semi-structured interviews	Daughters	32 (100%)	- mother's health beliefs and experiences - interactions with family, friends, and clinicians - exposure to media and marketing	[16]
Henderson et al. (2011)	England, UK	Semi-structured interviews	Daughters	26 (100%)	- perceived protection of HPV vaccine against cervical cancer (complete or partial) - misconception that HPV vaccine will replace need for future cervical cancer screening - lack of awareness of information about HPV vaccine	[17]
Hertweck et al. (2013)	USA	Surveys	Daughters	68 (100%)	- mother's attitude - mother's subjective norms - mother's perceived behavioural control	[18]

Table 1. (Continued)

Study (year)	Location	Study design	Study about daughters or sons	Number of parents (% of parents that are mothers)	Factors	Ref.
Hofman et al. (2013)	Netherlands	Focus groups	Daughters	36 (94%)	- perceiving cervical cancer as a severe disease - perceived susceptibility of child to HPV - having experienced significant others with cancer - perceived HPV vaccination effectiveness/relevance - possibility of serious side effects	[19]
Hughes et al. (2011)	Philadelphia, USA	Semi-structured interviews	Daughters	20 (100%)	- perception that children are currently not at risk - concerns about safety and efficacy of HPV vaccine	[20]
Katz et al. (2012)	Ohio, USA	Self-administered surveys	Sons	111 (88%)	- confidence in ability to talk to son about HPV vaccine - belief in effectiveness of HPV vaccine - unaware of son's sexual activity - unaware of HPV related disease that can affect males	[21]
Lechuga et al. (2012)	Wisconsin, USA	Surveys [note: also asked about format preferences for info]	Both daughters and sons	150 (100%)	- concerns about safety and effectiveness of HPV vaccine - anticipated relief of protective effects of HPV vaccine - concerns about HPV vaccine leading to engaging in sexual activity at an earlier age	[22]
Morales-Campos et al. (2013)	Texas, USA	Focus groups	Daughters	24 (100%)	- gaps in knowledge - fears/concerns about safety of HPV vaccine - socio-cultural communication practices (parents not communicating with daughters about sexual health) - prevention of cervical cancer - physician's recommendation	[23]
Okoronkwo et al. (2012)	Thunder Bay, Canada	Surveys	Daughters	188 (92%)	- distrust in use/effects of HPV vaccination - positive attitudes towards HPV vaccination - religious beliefs - knowledge about HPV vaccination	[24]
Perkins et al. (2013)	Boston, USA	Semi-structured interviews	Sons	120 (80%)	- positive attitude towards HPV vaccine - perceived barriers to HPV vaccine - attitudes towards male sexuality - attitudes towards vaccination during early adolescence - opinions on school-entry requirements for HPV vaccine	[25]

Study (year)	Location	Study design	Study about daughters or sons	Number of parents (% of parents that are mothers)	Factors	Ref.
Savas et al. (2012)	Texas, USA	Surveys	Daughters	99 (92%)	- awareness and knowledge about HPV vaccine - perceived HPV vaccine efficacy - perceived susceptibility - HPV vaccine may cause future health problems - health provider communication - health provider recommendation	[27]
Zhang et al. (2013)	China	National survey	Both daughters and sons	2895 (63%)	- concerns about safety - concerns about effectiveness of HPV vaccine - cost - perceptions of daughters being too young for cervical cancer - prior knowledge about HPV, cervical cancer, and genital warts - age of child - should be decided by children themselves - prior consultation regarding HPV vaccines - fear of cervical cancer	[26]

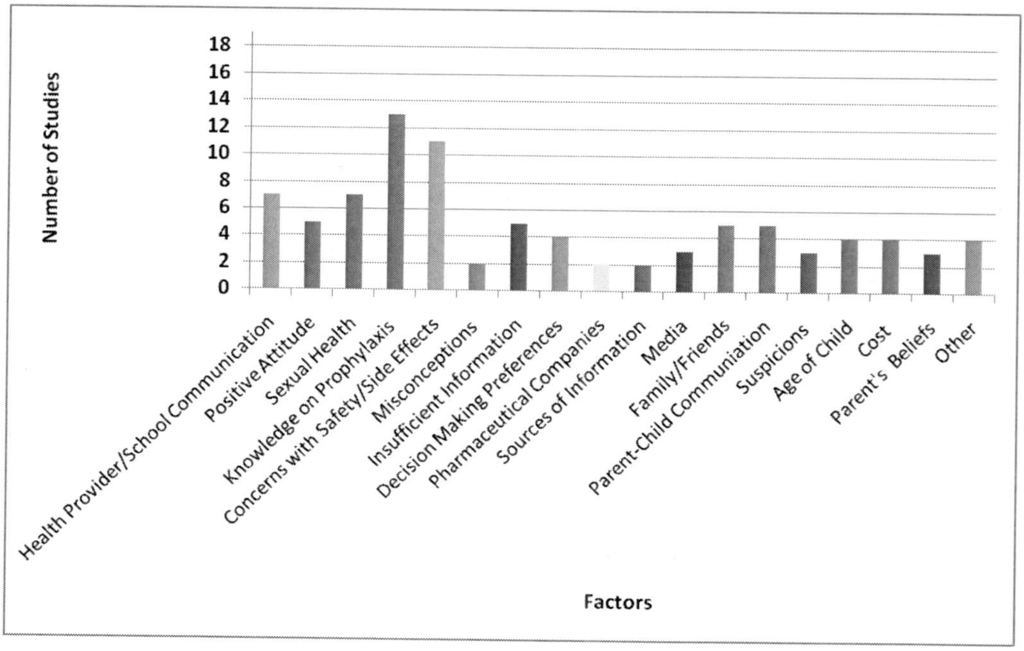

Figure 1. Common factors influencing parental decisions regarding uptake of the HPV vaccine for their children.

Knowledge on prophylaxis

A total of 13 studies identified knowledge on the prophylactic effects of the HPV vaccine as being a critical factor influencing parental decision making in regards to the uptake of the HPV vaccine for their children (9, 11, 12, 14, 15, 17, 19, 21-24, 26, 27). For instance, understanding that the HPV vaccine can help prevent serious complications like cervical cancer played an important factor in the decision making process (11). Furthermore, parents having sufficient knowledge regarding HPV in general, genital warts, and/or cervical cancer tended to increase the acceptability of the HPV vaccine (26). There was also increased acceptance among parents when they understood and realized their child may soon become sexually active and thus become vulnerable to HPV infections (19).

Concerns with safety/side effects

Eleven studies identified concerns with safety and/or side effects as a major factor influencing parental decision making for the HPV vaccine (9, 11, 12, 19, 20, 22, 23, 25-28). Concerns with safety and/or side effects of the HPV vaccine were typically factors that discouraged parents from the vaccination. For instance, some parents feared that the HPV vaccine would cause infertility in their children (11). Other parents were more concerned about the long-term side effects due to the newness of the vaccine (19).

Trust in health provider/government/school

A total of seven studies identified trust in a health provider, and/or government, and/or school was a critical factor in parental decision making for the HPV vaccine (9, 11, 12, 16, 23, 26, 27). For instance, many parents accepted the HPV vaccine if the information was relayed by credible and trusted teachers and health providers (11). Furthermore, parents often find trust and comfort in the advice of their family physicians and thus were more likely to accept the HPV vaccine if their physician recommended it (23). Some parents, in countries such as Vietnam, were also influenced by the fact that the HPV vaccination program was a publicly funded government program with the impression that if the government implemented the vaccine, then the vaccine must be effective and necessary (12).

Sexual health

Seven studies identified sexual health as a key factor in parental decision making (9, 11, 14, 21-23, 25). For instance, some parents were discouraged from uptake of the HPV vaccine in their children due to the belief that the HPV vaccine would condone their children becoming sexually active (23). Furthermore, some parents were unaware of their child's sexual activity and would not consider it an issue, whereas others realized their child may soon become sexually active (9, 21).

Positive attitude towards HPV vaccine

Five studies in total identified positive attitudes towards the HPV vaccine as a key factor in parental decision making (9, 15, 24, 25, 27). The general belief that vaccines are important and that children should stay up to date with recommended vaccines contributed towards acceptance of uptake of the HPV vaccine. Furthermore, positive attitudes towards the effectiveness of the HPV vaccine were also often correlated with acceptance of the HPV vaccine by parents (24).

Insufficient information

A total of five studies identified parents having insufficient information on the HPV vaccine as a major factor influencing their decision making (10, 11, 14, 21, 23). Some parents believed they did not have sufficient information about the HPV vaccine to make an informed decision about consenting to vaccinate their children (10). Furthermore, many parents did not understand what HPV is and were unsure of the types of questions to ask their health providers to find out more information (14).

Influence of family and friends

Five studies identified the influence of family and friends as a key factor that influenced parental decision making regarding the HPV vaccine (11-13, 16, 19). Many parents typically sought advice from family members and friends to help reinforce their decision on whether or not to consent to vaccinate their child (12). Some parents' decisions were also influenced by family members with a history of cervical cancer in the sense that they wanted to prevent their child from developing cervical cancer (16).

Parent-child communication

Five studies also identified parent-child communication as a major factor that influenced parental decision making for the HPV vaccine (11, 14, 15, 21, 26). For instance, the strength of parent-child communication regarding sexual health played an important role in some parental decisions, with stronger communication leading to an increased likelihood of accepting the HPV vaccine (15). Some parents in China; however, felt that the decision about the HPV vaccine should be made by children themselves (26).

Other factors influencing parental decision making

Apart from the factors discussed, there were several other factors that were prevalent in four or less studies and influenced parental decision making regarding the HPV vaccine as seen in Figure 1. For instance, some parents had misconceptions about the HPV vaccine such as the misconception that the HPV vaccine protects against all STIs (9, 17). Decision making preferences in terms of who makes the decisions in the family (i.e. mother versus father) also played a role in decision making (10, 11, 14, 15). Some parents had suspicions about the HPV vaccine, such as the suspicion of the HPV vaccine being a part of a clinical experiment (12, 24, 26). Age of the child also played a role in parental decision making in the sense that some parents believed their child was too young to become sexually active or be at risk of contracting an HPV infection (12, 20, 25, 26). Whether the HPV vaccine was publicly funded or not also influenced parental decision making because having to pay for the HPV vaccine resulted in parents feeling less inclined to accept the vaccine compared to if the cost of the vaccine was covered by the government (11, 12, 14, 26). The beliefs of parents, such as religious beliefs, also influenced some parents' decisions (16, 18, 24). Information about the HPV vaccine that was portrayed in the media influenced decision making for some parents as well (11, 13, 16). Another factor that influenced parental decision making was the sources where parents were obtaining information from, such as the format or type of source (10, 11). Some parents were also concerned about the pharmaceutical companies that were linked to the HPV vaccines (10, 13). Remaining factors included fears, concerns with the consent process, and other minor factors that were not identified in more than one study (11, 25-27).

Discussion

The field of research pertaining to parental decision making regarding uptake of the HPV vaccine for their children has become increasingly important, especially when considering the risks associated with HPV infections and suboptimal vaccination rates (4). Identifying and addressing influential factors in parental decision making for the HPV vaccine in current and future studies may play an influential role in improving vaccination rates and overall prevention of HPV infections, genital warts, cervical cancers, and other associated cancers. It is interesting to note that despite the wide range of geographical locations of studies, similar factors were found to influence parental decision making for the HPV vaccine.

In general, the same types of factors were found to influence parents' decision in vaccinating their daughters in comparison to sons. However, slightly more concerns about sexual health were brought up in studies focusing on sons (9, 21, 25). It is recommended that increased awareness about HPV in males should be brought to attention (21). A recent article published in the Toronto Star has discussed the need for publicly funded HPV vaccination programs for boys in Ontario. A growing number of doctors, parents, and health officials have been asking for gender-neutral HPV vaccination programs. Australia has become the first country this year to initiate a publicly funded HPV vaccination program for boys, and Prince Edward Island has recently announced that they will also soon be implementing a gender-neutral vaccination program (29). Publicly funded gender-neutral HPV vaccination programs would be beneficial for parents as it would remove the cost factor in the decision making process. Furthermore, it would help encourage the importance of vaccinating both males and females to protect against the transmission and infection of HPV and other serious complications.

Although generally not discussed in the literature, there are several decision making models that may play a role in the types of decisions made by parents. For instance, in regards to heuristics and biases, the framing effect may influence decision making. The way information regarding the HPV vaccine are framed could influence parental decisions (30). Cognitive decision making is another model that could play a role. For instance, knowledge-based decision making are commonly used by parents when obtaining information from a variety of sources to formulate an opinion on the HPV vaccine. Furthermore, the cognitive framework for medical decision making includes three types of knowledge: factual, conceptual, and procedural. Parents may gain facts without in-depth understanding (factual knowledge) from sources they find on their own such as websites or information from family and friends. Integration of new knowledge with prior knowledge to create a deeper understanding (conceptual knowledge) often occurs when parents receive reputable information from reputable sources such as their family physician (31). Evidence-based decision making can also apply to parents when using reputable sources such as information from government sources, for example. Finally, clinical decision support, such as the use of decision support aids, can be largely influential in helping parents make informed decisions (32).

Although the studies included in this literature review did not discuss the decision aids in detail that helped parents make decisions, it is important to recognize that decision making aids may play a large factor in a parent's decision to vaccinate their child against HPV. For instance, a study conducted by Pias-Peleteiro et al. (33) examined the standard web-based Google search by conducting cross-sectional studies of results of 14 web searches. The authors revealed that although 72% of websites offered information favorable towards the HPV vaccine, the most common types of websites retrieved were blogs or forums. Such websites are often incomplete, poorly structured, and lack adequate citations and credible criteria. The authors concluded that such information available on the Internet are not necessarily specialized in providing valid scientific information and could lead parents to poorly grounded statements or opinions (33).

A study conducted by Madden et al. also looked at websites as decision aids for parents regarding the HPV vaccine. Results of their study revealed that the top website searches were academic or non-profit sources (35%) and government agencies (27%). The authors recommended that health professionals designing websites regarding the HPV vaccine should include more information about the low risk of side effects as a barrier that can be overcome, benefits of the HPV vaccine, and susceptibility of HPV, to name a few (34). Improving the validity and reliability of information regarding the HPV vaccine online could ultimately help improve parental decision making factors such as misconceptions and having insufficient information about the HPV vaccine.

Fiks et al. (35) explored the use of clinician and family focused interventions to help parents make decisions regarding the HPV vaccine. The clinician-focused intervention involved three parts including education, electronic health record-based alerts, and audit or feedback. The family-focused intervention involved educational telephone calls to parents. Both interventions focused on improving overall uptake of the HPV vaccine. The authors found that the clinician-focused intervention was the most effective for having parents initiate the HPV vaccine for their children. However, the family-focused intervention helped to promote completion of the vaccine (35). This coincides with results found in the literature as trust in healthcare providers was a key factor that promoted increased acceptance of the HPV vaccine among parents (9, 11, 12, 16, 23, 26, 27).

Pamphlets are also a very common decision making aid for parents to gain more information on the HPV vaccine. A study conducted by Rosen et al. explored the uses of different informational pamphlets for women deciding about the HPV vaccine. Participants were randomized to receive either a long or short informational pamphlet about HPV. The authors found that providing more information (longer pamphlet) resulted in increased uncertainty which was often followed by increased anxiety (36). The Society of Obstetricians and Gynecologists of Canada (SOGC) has released a quick guide to facts on sexuality and HPV that are distributed at clinics. The pamphlets include information regarding STIs, facts and myths about HPV, and information regarding other applications, videos, games, and social media available online for further information (2). Pamphlets are an effective way of addressing parental decision making factors such as clearing up misconceptions regarding the HPV vaccine, and improving awareness with valid information on the prophylactic effects of the vaccine.

The strengths of the studies included within this literature review are that the studies generally included relatively large sample sizes, there was a variety of studies involving decision making for daughters and/or sons, and there was a wide geographical range of locations for studies included. The limitation was that studies did not focus on whether or not parents followed through with consenting their child to receive the HPV vaccine, and rather only focused on whether they hypothetically agreed with the HPV vaccine or not.

Overall, this literature review has revealed significant factors that have commonly appeared in the literature, which can be applied to future interventions aimed at improving parental consent rates of the HPV vaccine for their children. For instance, more clinician and/or school based communication about the prophylactic effects and minimal side effects of the HPV vaccine should be implemented. A more focused intervention to communicate about the HPV vaccine, and particularly about sexual health, would also be helpful to help clear up misconceptions among parents and prevent having parents gain misguided information from non-reputable sources. For example, school-based seminars led by healthcare providers and school staff could be implemented for parents and children. Such seminars could be organized to provide information to both children and parents through different types of media (i.e. pamphlets, videos, etc). These seminars would address the major factors influencing parental decision making such as providing information by trusted school staff and healthcare providers on prophylaxis, safety, side effects, and sexual health. Furthermore, these seminars would encourage parent-child communication and reduce misconceptions from recommendations of family and friends as they would also be present at the seminar receiving the same information. Other recommendations could include using simple language to communicate information to parents through a variety of different user-friendly sources like social media. Furthermore, eventual public funding of the HPV vaccine is recommended for males to eliminate the cost factor of parental decision making and to increase awareness of the importance in uptake of the HPV vaccine in males.

CONCLUSION

The HPV vaccine is important in both males and females in preventing HPV infections, genital warts, and specific cancers, such as cervical cancer. Many factors influence parental decisions in regards to providing consent for their children to receive the HPV vaccine. Major factors found in the literature include knowledge on the prophylactic effects of the HPV vaccine; concerns with safety and/or side effects; trust in the health provider, government, or school; sexual health, parents having a positive attitude towards the vaccine; having insufficient information; influence of family or friends; and parent-child communication. Future efforts should focus on addressing these factors to improve uptake of the HPV vaccine by implementing focused strategies and decision aids to help parents make informed decisions.

REFERENCES

[1] Trim K, Nagji N, Elit L, Roy K. Parental knowledge, attitudes, and behaviours towards human papillomavirus vaccination for their children: A systematic review from 2001 to 2011. Obstet Gynecol Int 2012;2012:921236.

[2] The Society of Obstetricians and Gynaecologists of Canada. Your Quick Guide to Facts on Sexuality and HPV. Ottawa, ON: Society Obstetricians Gynaecologists Canada, 2012.

[3] Walhart T. Parents, adolescents, children and the human papillomavirus vaccine: a review. Int Nurs Rev 2012;59(3):305-11.

[4] Rosberger Z, Perez S, King L, Franco EL. Public perception: A significant challenge in the battle against HPV. Oncol Exchange 2013;12(2):16-20.

[5] Mayrand MH, Duarte-Franco E, Rodrigues I, Walter SD, Hanley J, Ferenczy A, et al. Human papillomavirus DNA versus Papanicolaou screening tests for cervical cancer. N Engl J Med 2007;357(16):1579-88.

[6] Bartlett JA, Peterson JA. The uptake of Human Papillomavirus (HPV) vaccine among adolescent females in the United States: a review of the literature. J Sch Nurs 2011;27(6):434-46.

[7] Steben M. Do you approve of spending $300 million on HPV vaccination? yes. Can Fam Physician 2008;54(2):174.

[8] Eggertson L. Provinces weighing HPV vaccination of boys. CMAJ 2012;184(5):E250-1.

[9] Alexander AB, Stupiansky NW, Ott MA, Herbenick D, Reece M, Zimet GD. Parent-son decision-making about human papillomavirus vaccination: a qualitative analysis. BMC Pediatrics 2012;12:192.
[10] Allen JD, De Jesus M, Mars D, Tom L, Cloutier L, Shelton RC. Decision-making about the HPV vaccine among ethnically diverse parents: Implications for health communications. J Oncol 2012;2012:401979.
[11] Bartolini RM, Winkler JL, Penny ME, LaMontagne DS. Parental acceptance of HPV vaccine in Peru: A decision framework. PLoS One 2012;7(10):e48017.
[12] Cover JK, Nghi NQ, LaMontagne DS, Huyen DT, Hien NT, Nga le T. Acceptance patterns and decision-making for human papillomavirus vaccination among parents in Vietnam: an in-depth qualitative study post-vaccination. BMC Public Health 2012;12:629.
[13] Dorell C, Yankey D, Kennedy A, Stokley S. Factors that influence parental vaccination decisions for adolescents, 13 to 17 years old: National Immunization Survey-Teen, 2010. Clin Pediatr 2013;52(2):162-70.
[14] Francis SA, Katz ML. The HPV vaccine: A comparison of focus groups conducted in South Africa and Ohio Appalachia. Matern Child Health J 2013;17(7):1222-9.
[15] Francis SA, Battle-Fisher M, Liverpool J, Hipple L, Mosavel M, Soogun S, et al. A qualitative analysis of South African women's knowledge, attitudes, and beliefs about HPV and cervical cancer prevention, vaccine awareness and acceptance, and maternal-child communication about sexual health. Vaccine 2011;29(47):8760-5.
[16] Griffioen AM, Glynn S, Mullins TK, Zimet GD, Rosenthal SL, Fortenberry JD, et al. Perspectives on decision making about human papillomavirus vaccination among 11- to 12-year-old girls and their mothers. Clin Pediatr 2012;51(6):560-8.
[17] Henderson L, Clements A, Damery S, Wilkinson C, Austoker J, Wilson S, et al. 'A false sense of security'? Understanding the role of the HPV vaccine on future cervical screening behaviour: a qualitative study of UK parents and girls of vaccination age. J Med Screen 2011;18(1):41-5.
[18] Hertweck SP, LaJoie AS, Pinto MD, Flamini L, Lynch T, Logsdon MC. Health care decision making by mothers for their adolescent daughters regarding the quadrivalent HPV vaccine. J Pediatr Adolesc Gynecol 2013;26(2):96-101.
[19] Hofman R, van Empelen P, Vogel I, Raat H, van Ballegooijen M, Korfage IJ. Parental decisional strategies regarding HPV vaccination before media debates: a focus group study. J Health Commun 2013;18(7):866-80.
[20] Hughes CC, Jones AL, Feemster KA, Fiks AG. HPV vaccine decision making in pediatric primary care: a semi-structured interview study. BMC Pediatrics 2011;11:74.
[21] Katz ML, Kam JA, Krieger JL, Roberto AJ. Predicting human papillomavirus vaccine intentions of college-aged males: an examination of parents' and son's perceptions. J Am Coll Health 2012;60(6):449-59.
[22] Lechuga J, Swain G, Weinhardt LS. Perceived need of a parental decision aid for the HPV vaccine: content and format preferences. Health Promot Pract 2012;13(2):214-21.
[23] Morales-Campos DY, Markham CM, Peskin MF, Fernandez ME. Hispanic mothers' and high school girls' perceptions of cervical cancer, human papilloma virus, and the human papilloma virus vaccine. J Adolesc Health 2013;52(5Suppl):S69-75).
[24] Okoronkwo C, Sieswerda LE, Cooper R, Binette D, Todd M. Parental consent to HPV vaccination for their daughters: The effects of knowledge and attitudes. Can J Hum Sex 2012 2012;21(3-4):117-26.
[25] Perkins RB, Tipton H, Shu E, Marquez C, Belizaire M, Porter C, et al. Attitudes toward HPV vaccination among low-income and minority parents of sons: a qualitative analysis. Clin Pediatr 2013;52(3):231-40.
[26] Zhang S-, Pan X-, Wang S-, Yang C-, Gao X-, Wang Z-, et al. Perceptions and acceptability of HPV vaccination among parents of young adolescents: A multicenter national survey in China. Vaccine 2013 2013;31(32):3244-9.
[27] Savas LS, Fernandez ME, Jobe D, Carmack CC. Human papillomavirus vaccine: 2-1-1 helplines and minority parent decision-making. Am J Prev Med 2012;43(6 Suppl 5):S490-6.
[28] Allen JD, Othus MK, Shelton RC, Li Y, Norman N, Tom L, et al. Parental decision making about the HPV vaccine. Cancer Epidemiol Biomark Prev 2010;19(9):2187-98.

[29] Teotonio I. Ontario asked to publicly fund HPV vaccine for boys. Toronto Star 2013 Oct 4.

[30] Bornstein BH, Emler AC. Rationality in medical decision making: a review of the literature on doctors' decision-making biases. J Eval Clin Pract 2001;7(2):97-107.

[31] Patel VL, Arocha JF, Kaufman DR. A primer on aspects of cognition for medical informatics. J Am Med Inform Assoc 2001;8(4):324-43.

[32] Clayton PD, Hripcsak G. Decision support in healthcare. Int J Biomed Comput 1995;39(1):59-66.

[33] Pias-Peleteiro L, Cortes-Bordoy J, Martinon-Torres F. Dr Google: What about the human papillomavirus vaccine? Human Vaccines Immunotherapeutics 2013;9(8):1712-9.

[34] Madden K, Nan X, Briones R, Waks L. Sorting through search results: a content analysis of HPV vaccine information online. Vaccine 2012;30(25):3741-6.

[35] Fiks AG, Grundmeier RW, Mayne S, Song L, Feemster K, Karavite D, et al. Effectiveness of decision support for families, clinicians, or both on HPV vaccine receipt. Pediatrics 2013;131(6):1114-24.

[36] Rosen NO, Knauper B, Di Dio P, Morrison E, Tabing R, Feldstain A, et al. The impact of intolerance of uncertainty on anxiety after receiving an informational intervention about HPV: a randomised controlled study. Psychol Health 2010;25(6):651-68.

In: Child and Adolescent Health Issues
Editor: Joav Merrick

ISBN: 978-1-63463-574-5

Chapter 5

LACTATION EDUCATION AND BREASTFEEDING DURATION

Kelly Eichmann, PhD, Timothy Baghurst, PhD* and Chris Jayne, MEd
Health Science, State Center Community College District, California and Health and Human Performance, Oklahoma State University, Stillwater, Oklahoma, United States of America

Although the benefits of breastfeeding for both mother and infant are numerous, a large number of women choose not to breastfeed. The purpose of this chapter was to determine whether regular postpartum follow-up by a certified lactation Consultant (CLC) or Certified lactation Educator (CLE) increased the duration mothers breastfed their infants. Ninety-four (Control = 54; Experimental = 40) breastfeeding mothers completed a 24-week study in which participants in the experimental condition received 9 follow-up support telephone calls by either a CLC or CLE. These calls were used to elicit possible breastfeeding problems, offer solutions, identify factors that may have influenced the mother's decision to initiate and continue breastfeeding, and to identify why mothers would decide to discontinue breastfeeding. Follow-up by a CLC or CLE did not yield significantly longer durations in breastfeeding. However, gender of the breastfeeding infant, hospital discharge with supplemental formula, and the use of pacifiers were found to influence breastfeeding duration. In addition, both groups breastfed longer than the national average indicating that specific hospital protocols can positively influence breastfeeding duration. Findings are discussed and practical implications for health practitioners are provided.

INTRODUCTION

The promotion of breastfeeding is due to the nutritional and immunologic benefits of human milk for the infant as well as the physiological and social benefits of lactation for the mother.

* Correspondence: Timothy Baghurst, PhD, 189 Colvin, Oklahoma State University, Stillwater, OK 74078, USA. E-mail: tbaghurst@live.com

Breastfeeding has been recognized as the preferred form of infant nutrition (1, 2). The American Academy of Pediatrics (AAP) recommends exclusive breastfeeding is the ideal nutrition and sufficient to support optimal growth and development for the first four to six months after birth. Further, mothers should continue breastfeeding after age appropriate solid foods have been introduced until mutually exclusive for both mother and infant (3).

Since its establishment in 1948, the AAP has been a strong supporter of breastfeeding as the most beneficial method of infant feeding (3). The continuing challenge for promoters of breastfeeding is to communicate the importance of exclusive breastfeeding for a minimum of six months. Introductions of age appropriate solid foods and juices in tandem with breastfeeding should follow for the first year of life (4, 5).

Despite the well-known benefits of breastfeeding, rates have continued to decline. Beginning in the 1880s, breastfeeding practices began to rapidly decline in the United States due largely to two seemingly unrelated factors. First, mothers as a whole became fearful of the "germ-theory", published in the 1880s, along with lay magazines publishing common breastfeeding problems. Second, pediatricians searching for a solution to re-establish themselves in the medical community took on a promotional stance for the use of infant formula.

These two groups unintentionally popularized infant supplementation use in the United States and the number of women breastfeeding has not recovered from the onset of this trend that started over 130 years ago (6).

The highest rates of breastfeeding continue to occur among the higher socio-economic groups, middle class, white, affluent, and college educated. Non-participants are generally those registered with Women, Infant, and Children (WIC) programs, stay-at-home-mothers, and women who delivered full-term infants of normal birth weight greater than 2,500 grams. Several barriers may inhibit women from breastfeeding and include maternal expectation, returning to work, infant behavior, social acceptance, and cultural beliefs. Frequently women are disenchanted with the experience of breastfeeding. This, coupled with the increased demands on women, results in breastfeeding often being discontinued regardless of the benefits.

Additional barriers include lack of consistent and accurate information about breastfeeding, hospital discharge of breastfeeding mothers with formula, public assistance programs such as WIC providing free formula, and diminishing social acceptance of breastfeeding (7-12).

Barriers to breastfeeding

Societally, over the past few decades breastfeeding has been portrayed as taboo. Cultural attitudes towards modesty and the sexual association of breasts have limited women in their ability to breastfeed in public. The notion that breastfeeding somehow limits the bonding experience for fathers has also made a significant impact on women choosing to breastfeed (8, 13), and the use of pacifiers has also been shown to decrease the duration mothers breastfeed (14).

Benefits of breastfeeding

The benefits of breastfeeding are well known and numerous. Breastfed infants have shown a decreased incidence of several health-related problems when compared to bottle-fed infants which include a significant decrease in the number of hospital admissions, incidence and severity of diarrheal illness, respiratory tract infections, atopic skin disorders, and urinary tract infections (1, 4). Additional studies have shown that breastfed infants have a reduced risk for chronic diseases that may be limited by long-term breastfeeding include obesity, allergies, and heart disease (4, 13). Further, infants exclusively breastfed for 4 months have shown a fifty-percent decrease in the number of ear infections, gastrointestinal disorders, and the onset of insulin dependent diabetes mellitus. Finally, a plethora of empirical evidence shows that breastfeeding enhances intellectual, visual, and oral development (4, 7, 13, 15).

Breastfeeding also provides benefits for mothers. The immediate postpartum benefits include increased levels of oxytocin, resulting in less bleeding and more rapid uterine contraction (13, 15). In addition, less menstrual blood loss over the months after delivery, earlier return to pre-pregnancy weight, delayed return of ovulation leading to a natural increased spacing between siblings, decreased bone loss, reduced risk of ovarian and breast cancer, and improved diabetic control have been observed (1, 7, 13-15). Mothers also benefit from breastfeeding financially, as purchasing high cost formula is not required. In addition, a decreased absenteeism from work due to fewer infant illnesses is another economic benefit (7, 12).

Health care interventions

There is amble research to support that accurate and appropriate encouragement from health care professionals can improve rates of breastfeeding initiation and duration. Past research shows that physicians have discouraged breastfeeding by providing formula at discharge and imposing rigid feeding schedules, yet reports have also shown that physician intervention can improve the initiation and duration of breastfeeding (1, 7, 10).

Most women make the decision to breastfeed prior to conception or delivery and early education through prenatal infant feeding classes is one step toward breastfeeding success. Promoting breastfeeding through the community and professionals is the key to changing the attitudes towards breastfeeding and correcting misinformation (2, 5, 7, 9, 15).

The most popular misconception the public has regarding breastfeeding is that infant formula feeding is just as good as breastfeeding. It has been suggested that formula manufacturers have promoted this notion and, combined with the lack of breastfeeding role models to combat such allegations, the myth has perpetuated (2, 15). Thus, in order to rebut this allegation, health care providers need to promote the benefits of breastfeeding for the infant as well as the mother.

Early postpartum support is crucial to the success of breastfeeding for several reasons. First, the suckling reflex is strongest during the first thirty minutes of life and a delay of the first feeding may result in the infant having difficulty latching on to the mother's breast. This is most likely to happen if the infant was given a bottle prior to nursing. Second, the infants sucking stimulates the mother's milk supply. Therefore, feeding on demand and regular feedings at night when levels of prolactin are highest are most effective to establish and increase milk supply, which in turn prevents engorgement (8).

Breastfeeding is not instinctive and must be taught and learned. Due to the long-time decline of breastfeeding, family role models are not available for new breastfeeding mothers. Knowledge and support is needed from health care providers who support breastfeeding to increase the duration women breastfeed their infants (9). Therefore, prior to hospital discharge it is recommended that a qualified staff member supervise a breastfeeding interaction to ensure that the baby is latching on properly and to show the mother various breastfeeding positions and techniques. Outpatient follow-up is also necessary for encouragement and support of breastfeeding. Early detection and correction of breastfeeding problems is crucial breastfeeding success (15).

Study purpose

Researchers have identified support as an important factor in the duration mother's breastfeed their infants. However, although family support, society, a physician, and nurses may be helpful, routine specialist support through the crucial early weeks postpartum and follow-up throughout the first six months of life may positively impact the continuation of breastfeeding following discharge. Therefore, the purpose of this study was to determine whether postpartum follow up by a certified lactation consultant (CLC) or certified lactation educator (CLE) would increase the duration of breastfeeding during the first six months.

OUR STUDY

Participants were obstetrical patients between the ages of twenty and thirty-five who gave birth at a hospital located in the Western United States and planned to breastfeed their infants. In addition, participants had delivered a normal, single infant, at least 37 weeks gestation with a birth weight above 2,500 grams, and had no severe medical conditions or complications. Women participating in WIC and mothers who planned to exclusively bottle-feed were excluded from the study. Ethnic background, race, and religious preference were not specified; however, all participants had to be able to read and speak English in order to read the consent form and receive lactation follow-up calls via telephone.

Instruments

Data for the study was collected by the CLC/CLE using a pre-determined list of questions designed to gather information about the participants' breastfeeding behaviors. The questions included both closed and opened ended questions with ordered and unordered responses. The primary researcher and the lactation staff developed the questions used in the study. A small random sample of breastfeeding mothers from the hospital where the study took place were selected to field test the questions. Appropriate changes were made to the questionnaire based on feedback obtained during the field test. A research committee reviewed the questions for reliability, for which it was deemed appropriate to be used for data collection. The final survey was 34 questions but the number of questions answered varied depending on if and when the participant had stopped breastfeeding. The survey included items such as “Did you use the formula you received?”, “How often is your baby nursing in a 24 hour period?”, and “Are you pumping?”

Procedure

Following IRB approval, potential participants were approached during their post-partum follow-up appointments at the Maternal Infant Lactation Clinic (MILC). Each potential participant was interviewed to determine if they planned to breastfeed or bottle-feed. Those mothers that intended to breastfeed and agreed to participate in the study were randomly assigned to either a control or experimental group. To insure confidentiality, participants were identified by their hospital medical record number (MRN).

As part of the routine hospital breastfeeding support protocol, participants in the control group were contacted by a CLC or CLE 48 to 72 hours following discharge, and during routine postpartum MILC follow up appointments. At the post-partum appointment, breastfeeding support classes were made available to the control group as well as telephone numbers for both the CLEs and CLCs on staff. The staff initiated no additional contact until the twenty-fourth week postpartum. At this time the lactation educator called the study participants in the control group to determine if they were still breastfeeding, the length of time that they breastfed their infant, and completed the follow-up questionnaire.

Participants in the experimental group were followed for 24 weeks and provided the same routine hospital MILC protocol. This protocol included a post-partum follow, and breastfeeding support classes, conducted by a CLC or CLE. The experimental group received additional regular follow-up contact via telephone by one of the five lactation educators from the hospital’s lactation clinic. Contact by a CLE was initiated one week after the routine MILC Clinic appointment. Additional follow-up calls were made at weeks 2, 4, 8, 12, 16, 20, and 24 postpartum, making up the experimental intervention. Special needs or problems with regards to breastfeeding were referred to the CLC for follow-up. At each follow-up interval, one of the CLEs called each participant in the experimental group to determine the length of time each had breastfed her infant. The follow-up questionnaire was also completed via telephone at the end of the 24 week period.

RESULTS

Participant demographics by group are presented in table 1. Chi-square analyses of these variables yielded no significant differences ($p < .05$). All participants were between 20 and 40 years of age, with a mean age of 28.87 years. All the subjects delivered normal, single infants, between 37 and 42 weeks gestation, with a mean gestational age of 39.55 weeks. The birth weights of the infants ranged from 5.8 to 10.02 pounds, with a mean weight of 7.48 pounds. None of the participants experienced any severe medical conditions or complications.

Table 1. Subject demographic characteristics

Characteristics	Control Group (n = 54)	Experimental Group (n = 40)
Mean Maternal Age (years)	28.87 +/- 6.02	27.95 +/- 5.68
Mean Gestation Age (weeks)	39.68 +/- 1.30	39.35 +/- 1.02
Mean Birth Weight (pounds)	7.61 +/- .936	7.28 +/- 1.11
Type of Delivery		
Cesarean	4 (7.4 %)	7 (17.5 %)
Vaginal	50 (92.6 %)	33 (82.5 %)
Marital Status		
Married	47 (87.0 %)	37 (92.5 %)
Unmarried	7 (13.0 %)	3 (7.5 %)
Ethnicity		
White	25 (46.3 %)	28 (70.0 %)
Black	3 (5.6 %)	2 (5.0 %)
Hispanic	20 (37.0 %)	6 (15.0 %)
Other	6 (11.1 %)	4 (10.0 %)
Annual Gross Income		
< $30,000	13 (24.1 %)	9 (22.5 %)
$30,000-$50,000	18 (33.3 %)	18 (45.0 %)
> $50,000	23 (42.6 %)	13 (32.5 %)
Education Level		
High School	15 (27.8 %)	8 (20.0 %)
Associates Degree	17 (31.5 %)	15 (37.5 %)
Bachelors Degree	19 (35.2 %)	14 (35.0 %)
Graduate Degree	3 (5.6 %)	3 (7.5%)
Breastfeeding Experience		
Yes	36 (66.7 %)	23 (57.5 %)
None	18 (33.3 %)	17 (42.5 %)
Infant Sex		
Female	34 (63.0 %)	17 (42.5 %)
Male	20 (37.0 %)	23 (57.5 %)

Breastfeeding duration

The mean age of the breastfeeding mothers were 28.96 years of age in the control group and 27.75 years of age in the experimental group. The mean length of gestation was 39.70 weeks in the control and 39.35 in the experimental groups. The mean birth weight of participants' infants was 7.61 pounds in the control and 7.29 pounds in the experimental group. An analysis of covariance was used to determine the mean length of time each group breastfed. The unadjusted duration of breastfeeding for the control group was 20.40 weeks compared to 21.42 weeks for the experimental group. After adjusting for significant dependent variables (i.e., covariates or group differences) which included sex of the breastfeeding infant and supplemental formula given at discharge, the duration of breastfeeding for the control group was 20.22 weeks versus 22.26 weeks for experimental group participants. Though an increase in duration among the experimental group, this finding was non-significant ($p = 0.45$) and after covariant adjustments still remained non-significant ($p = 0.26$).

Additional analyses

Of the total 94 subjects who initiated breastfeeding their infants at birth, 64 (68.1%) of the participants were still breastfeeding at 6 months. More participants (75%) were still breastfeeding at six months in the experimental group, but it was not a significant difference to the 63% within the control group.

Of the 54 infants of mothers in the control group, 34 (63.0%) were female and 20 (37.0%) were male compared with 17 (42.5%) female and 23 (57.5%) male infants in the experimental group. Pearson's Chi-Square Analysis compared birth gender differences yielding significant differences (p = .04).

Throughout the study, participants were asked if their infants were using a pacifier. Pearson's Chi Squares were used to analyze differences between the control and experimental groups with regards to the use of pacifiers and whether supplemental formula was sent home with the participants at discharge.

There were significant differences (p = .04) between pacifier use by group where the experimental group were more likely to use pacifiers (85.0%) than the control group (66.7%). Participants were asked at the conclusion of the breastfeeding study whether or not the hospital had sent supplemental infant formula home with them when they were discharged. A significantly (p = .003) greater number of participants from the experimental group (90%) were discharged with formula in comparison to the control group (63.0%).

DISCUSSION

The purpose of this study was to determine whether follow-up procedures by a lactate specialist could positively impact breastfeeding duration of mothers. Findings indicated that while the duration of breastfeeding is slightly increased by the additional follow up by a CLC or CLA, it did not significantly impact breastfeeding duration. However, both control (63%) and experimental (75%) groups using the MILC clinic and hospital protocols exceeded the national goal set by Healthy People 2020 of 50% duration of breastfeeding after 6 months (16). These findings suggest that pre-birth and in-hospital education can significantly impact breastfeeding intentions and success.

Part of the hospital's routine breastfeeding support protocol includes contact by a CLC or CLE 48 to 72 hours following discharge and during routine postpartum MILC follow up appointments. At the post-partum appointment, breastfeeding support group classes are made available to the breastfeeding mothers, and contact information is given to provide support upon request by the nursing mothers.

The American Academy of Pediatrics recommends breastfeeding from birth to 4 to 6 months of age (17). In addition, Healthy People 2020 set a goal of 74% initiation of breastfeeding and 43.5% to 6 months (16). The participants in this study met and exceeded these standards and goals. Additionally, this study surpassed the breastfeeding trends reported in the ongoing periodic mail survey conducted by Ross laboratories. In 2000, Ross Mothers Survey (RMS) concluded that 68.4% of the women surveyed initiated breastfeeding; 70.1% in 2002 initiated breastfeeding; and 64.7% in 2004 initiated breastfeeding (18). In addition, 31.4% of the mother's surveyed continued breastfeeding to 6 months in 2000 (18) versus

47.2% in 2009 (19). Participants in this study exceeded the breastfeeding trends nationwide, suggesting the post-partum support is an essential component to the initiation and continuation of breastfeeding duration. This assertion can be further supported by an extensive systematic review which demonstrated that breastfeeding education and support significantly increased breastfeeding initiation rates. Moreover, the assessment revealed an increase in the established breastfeeding rates, with continued post-partum individual and group follow-up (20).

Additional variables

There were additional variables that may have impacted our findings such as the gender of the breastfeeding infant, hospital discharge with supplemental formula, and the use of pacifiers. There were also marginally significant differences in infant gender between the two groups. Literature suggests that female infants tend to breastfeed longer (21); thus, since there were significantly more female infant participants in the control group this could have affected the outcome of this study. Currently, there are very few studies specifically focused on the duration of breastfeeding and gender of the breastfed infant. However, at least three research studies observed that male infants are weaned earlier than female infants (21, 22). Conversely, 18.3% more participants within the experimental group used pacifiers with their infants. Research literature strongly suggests that infants who do not regularly use pacifiers breastfeed longer (10-14, 23, 24).

The most interesting finding occurred when comparing the two groups regarding whether supplemental formula was sent home with the participants. A number of studies suggest that mothers who are given supplemental infant formula when leaving the hospital are much more likely to use formula and, ultimately, breastfeed less. They are also more likely to discontinue breastfeeding earlier than those who are not given supplemental infant formula upon discharge from the hospital (23-26). Although a significantly greater number of participants (27%) in the experimental group were provided with formula, they still breastfed for a longer duration suggesting that the use of lactation educators should not be discounted.

Limitations for future study

When designing, implementing, and evaluating a research study, controlling for limitations may increase the validity and robustness of the study's outcomes. Generally, researchers strive to decrease the number of limitations in their studies in an effort to increase validity and worthiness. Nonetheless, all research studies are prone to some error. Limitations of this study include: a) self-reported data collected by the CLC/CLA; b) no long-term measures were set to assess sustained long-term breastfeeding durations; c) sample selection was based on participants willingness to sign consent forms; d) sample size was relatively small; and e) the testing instrument was designed specifically for this study. The use of self-reporting data are historically unreliable and unpredictable and long-term studies are more likely to provide a more realistic outcome result of the intervention. Sampling was limited due to the requirement of informed consent and a larger sample size may have yielded a more true outcome of the intervention.

CONCLUSION

In sum, this study highlights the importance of breastfeeding education prior to and during a mother's hospital stay. It is encouraging that participants receiving long-term consultation breastfed for a longer duration, but future research studies are needed to determine whether lactation support affects the duration of male infant breastfeeding specifically. Other studies utilizing the same proportion of mothers who use pacifiers and who are given supplemental formula at discharge should be conducted to determine the true effects of lactation intervention on the duration of breastfeeding.

REFERENCES

[1] Freed GL, Clark SJ, Sorenson J, Lohr JA, Cefalo R, Curtis P. National Assessment of Physicians' Breast-feeding knowledge, attitudes, training, and experience. JAMA 1995;273:472-6.

[2] Nutrition Committee of the Canadian Pediatric Society and the American Academy of Pediatrics Committee on Nutrition and Breastfeeding. Pediatrics 1978;62:591-601.

[3] American Academy of Pediatrics, American College of Obstetricians and Gynecologists. Guidelines for Perinatal Care, 3rd ed. Elk Grove Village, IL: American Academy of Pediatrics, 1992.

[4] Freed GL. Breast-feeding: Time to teach what we preach. JAMA 1993;269:243-5.

[5] Saarinen UM. Prolonged breast-feeding as prophylaxis for recurrent otitis media. Acta Paediatr Scand 1982;71:567-71.

[6] Wolf J. Low breastfeeding rates and public health in the United States. Am J Public Health 2003;93:2000-10.

[7] Murtaugh MA. Optimal breast-feeding duration. J Am Diet Assoc 1997;97:1252-4.

[8] Ryan AS. The resurgence of breastfeeding in the United States. Pediatrics. 1997;99(4):e-12.

[9] Ross Laboratories Mothers' Survey, 1993.

[10] Frank DA, Wirtz SJ, Sorenson JR, and Heeren T. Commercial discharge packs and breast-feeding counseling: effects on infant feeding practices in a randomized trial. Pediatrics 1987;80:845-54.

[11] Jones EG, Matheny RJ. Relationship between infant feeding and exclusion rate from child care because of illness. J Am Diet Assoc 1993;93(7):809-11.

[12] Ryan AS, Lewandowski G, Krieger FW. The recent decline in breast-feeding in the United States, 1984 through 1989. Pediatrics 1991;88:719-27.

[13] Black RF. Transmission of HIV-1 in the breast-feeding process. J Am Diet Assoc 1996;96:267-74.

[14] Ryan AS, Martinez GA. Breast-feeding and the working mother: a profile. Pediatrics 1989;83:524-31.

[15] Position of The American Dietetic Association: promotion of breast-feeding. J Am Diet Assoc 1997;97:662-8.

[16] Healthy People 2020. National Health Promotion and Disease Prevention Objectives. Washington, DC: US Department of Health and Human Services, Public Health Services, DHHS publication PHS91-50212, 1991.

[17] American Academy of Pediatrics Work Group on Breastfeeding. Breastfeeding and the use of human milk. Pediatrics 1997;100:1035-9.

[18] Ross Production Division. Mothers survey. Columbus, OH: Abbott Laboratories, 2007.

[19] Centers for Disease Control and Prevention: Report Card, 2012. Retrieved from http://www.cdc.gov/breastfeeding/pdf/2012breastfeedingreportcard.pdf

[20] Haroon S, Das K, Salam R, Imdad A, Bhutta Z. Breastfeeding promotion interventions and breastfeeding practices: a systematic review. BMC Public Health 2013;13:S20.

[21] Pande H, Unwin C, Haheim L. Factors associated with the duration of breastfeeding: Analysis of the primary and secondary responders to a self-completed questionnaire. Acta Paediatr 1997;86:173-7.

[22] Perez-Escamilla R, Lutter C, Segall m, Rivera A, Trevino-Siller S, Sanghvi T. Exclusive breastfeeding duration is associated with attitudinal, socioeconomic and bicultural determinants in three Latin American countries. J Nutr 1995;125:2972-84.

[23] Dungy CI, Christensen-Szalanski J, Losch M, Russell D. Effect of discharge samples on duration of breastfeeding. Pediatrics 1992;90:233-7.

[24] WHO/UNICEF meeting on infant and young child feeding. WHO Chron 1979;33:435-43.

[25] Evans CJ, Lyons NB, Killien MG. The effect of infant formula samples on breast-feeding practice. J Obstet Gynecol Neonatal Nurs 1986;15:401-5.

[26] Ross Products Division. Updated breast-feeding trends: 1987-1995. Available from: Ross Laboratories. 625 Cleveland Ave. Columbus, OH 43216.

SECTION TWO: WORK, STUDY AND HEALTH ISSUES

In: Child and Adolescent Health Issues
Editor: Joav Merrick

ISBN: 978-1-63463-574-5

Chapter 6

CONCEPTS OF WORK, STUDYING, AND LEISURE TIME IN ADOLESCENTS

Lea Ferrari*[*], *PhD, Laura Nota, PhD, Salvatore Soresi, PhD and Maria Cristina Ginevra, PhD

Department of Philosophy, Sociology, Education and Applied Psychology,
University of Padua, Padua, Italy

Participation in work, school and leisure activities provides young people with important opportunities to develop their vocational identities and career pathways; it also plays a crucial role in their school-to-work transition processes. Three studies to devise the Working, Studying, and Leisure Time Questionnaire, which assesses adolescents' concepts of work, studying, and leisure time were conducted. The first study served to formulate the instrument's items and to verify its factorial structure; the second used confirmatory factor analysis to test the instrument's multidimensional structure; and the third evaluated its discriminant validity and factorial structure invariance across gender. Results showed that the questionnaire is an effective and multidimensional measure for collecting data on adolescents' concepts of work, study, and leisure time. It can also serve school and vocational guidance purposes and in screening adolescents whose ideas of work, studying, and leisure time poorly reflect current labor market demands. Finally, suggestions for intervention are provided.

INTRODUCTION

There is a general consensus that work, at least in Western society, is today extremely fluid and job stability now pertains to the past. In fact noumerous forms of employment such as time-limited contracts exist and cross-company worker mobility are frequent (1). Vocational guidance psychology has responded to these changes by proposing theories and models that account for the dynamism, non-linearity, diversity, and contextual-individual specificity of work life. Specifically the social constructionist approach and the life designing perspective

[*] Correspondence: Lea Ferrari, Department of Philosophy, Sociology, Education and Applied Psychology, University of Padua, via Belzoni 84, 35121 Padua, Italy. E-mail: lea.ferrari@unipd.it.

underscore people's active role in constructing their lives and consequently suggest we need to more closely examine their ideas about work, study, and leisure time, and the meaning(s) they attribute to these aspects of human existence (2).

Work is generally considered an activity carried out to produce goods or services; its meaning is determined by a given society's values and beliefs; and it fosters the development of a professional identity (3). A more recent definition of work underscores it is a multidimensional social and cultural construct, which plays a key role in people's lives. It is also a means for survival and power, for social connection, and for self-determination, and it has a crucial impact on people's psychological health and well-being (4).

Recently qualitative studies have shown that peoples' ideas about work vary in function of contextual and cultural factors (3). People with lower incomes and educational levels, and who belong to the manual labor class less frequently consider work an intrinsically interesting activity and tend to place greater emphasis on the economic benefits (5).

A qualitative study examined answers to the question "What is your definition of work?" for 467 Italian adolescents (6) in the process of selecting their university faculty. Work resulted characterized by outcomes associated with economic benefits (70.7%), psychological advantages (33.4%), and the satisfaction of social values (14.8%). Consistent with the multiple sets of meaning observed by Chaves et al. (5), work was also defined in terms of positive ("pleasant/enjoyable", "interesting") (9.4%) and negative characteristics ("tiring, requires sacrifices", etc.) (9.6%). Gender differences also emerged, with boys valuing earnings and viewing work mostly as a means to obtain economic advantages, and girls seeing work as a means to obtain psychological advantages, such as fulfilling their own interests and personal achievement.

With respect to the concepts of school and education, actual world of work requires competencies that differ considerably from the knowledge and skills demanded in the previous century. Better reading, writing, and math abilities as well as good interpersonal skills and at least two years of post high school-diploma training are required to have job success (7). To be ready to compete for jobs in the 21st century, students must be able to develop strategies for achieving success, starting from the formal languages schools should be teaching them.

Hence, education and training are crucial, and the greater awareness young people have of the link between education and work, the more they will invest in their own school life (8). Hull-Blanks et al. (9) observed that boys focused more on work benefits, such as money or prestige than girls did, who conversely saw job goals and the specific roles they would be allowed to fill as having higher priority. Nota et al. (10) asked adolescents "What is your definition of work?", "What is your definition of study?", "Do you think that school/education is related to your future as an adult?". Work and education resulted highly similar in terms of psychological benefits, personal and professional development advantages, as well as positive and negative aspects. Thirty percent youth linked their education to their future job opportunities and to skills and abilities they could use to the benefit of their future careers. Twenty-five percent described the relation in terms of the acquisition of knowledge and skills they could use to obtain a more general cultural education. Another 30% stated that only some of the disciplines they were studying at school would influence their future lives; lastly, 5% saw no relation between the two.

As concern leisure time, it is generally viewed in terms of unpaid activities that originate from free choice, are intrinsically satisfying, determine optimal physiological activation, and which generally imply a degree of personal commitment. Snir and Harpaz (11) reviewed several longitudinal studies and found that people today tend to attribute more importance than previously to the value of leisure time in their lives, with a parallel decline in the number of hours dedicated to work. Leisure activities frequently involve the same psychological, social and behavioral skills required on the job, and when people find themselves employed in jobs that are below their original expectations, leisure time can compensate these work shortcomings (12). The link between leisure time and work is also currently influenced by the growing dual awareness that some jobs are no longer exclusively places of production, but offer creative opportunities for fulfillment, and that some leisure time activities are no longer dedicated exclusively to relaxation and to self-expression, but can quite easily take on a productive nature (13). Given their positive influence on mental health, on satisfaction levels, and on psychological growth, these occasions can foster a greater sense of self-efficacy and can positively influence people's quality of life (14, 15). Armstrong and Rounds (16) found a link between students' extracurricular activity participation and the RIASEC model of interests, especially with respect to computer activities and arts and crafts, which perfectly fit the model (more so than other activities, such as collecting and team sports). Nota et al. (17) surveyed a group of 120 high school adolescents, who responded to the question, "Do you think that what you do now in your leisure time may be related to your adult life in the future?". They answered that what they did would help them: develop useful and satisfying social relationships (3.4%), maintain a sense of well-being (10.1%), allow them to cultivate interests to use in their future work lives (18.5%), and foster their overall individual development (4.3%). Approximately 45% responded that there was no relation. Hence, young people view participation in school- and extracurricular activities as presenting important opportunities for them to develop their vocational identities and career pathways, and as playing a crucial role in the school-to-work transition (18).

In summarizing, research on the topic suggests that adolescents' ideas about work, study, and leisure time can actually impact their life designing, including their short and long term educational and career decisions. The importance of focusing on many of people's life spheres, and not only on their concepts of work and their employment role is an emerging theme in Guidance Psychology (i.e. 2, 4, 19). This view highlights the need to take on a more holistic perspective of career development, in the attempt to meet people's current needs and to help them develop and maintain psychologically healthy lives. A better understanding of the ways in which adolescents construct their concepts of work, education, and leisure time can help career counselors assist them in their transition to the labor market, and can more generally support their transition to adulthood thereby (6).

We therefore developed the Work, Study, and Leisure Time Questionnaire (WSLT) for adolescents, with the aim of designing an instrument that could parsimoniously pinpoint – more so than with previously used qualitative procedures (5, 6, 17) – work, study, and leisure time concepts to better understand the different meanings young people attribute to them. Three studies were conducted with three independent samples of adolescents: the first study formulated the instrument's items and tested its psychometric characteristics, such as reliability and construct validity; the second examined the WSLT structure's stability; the third verified the invariance of the factorial structure between boys and girls and the instrument's discriminant and convergent validity.

STUDY 1

The first study's goals were (a) to generate a range of items to adequately represent adolescents' concepts of work, study, and leisure time, in the first phase, and (b) to examine the questionnaire's factorial structure and reliability in the second.

Phase 1. In the process of generating the items we referred to several qualitative studies we had developed over recent years (6, 10, 17), which had asked participants to describe their definitions of work, study, and leisure time. We then conducted qualitative analyses to establish categories that would validly and reliably describe the participants' concept of work, study, and leisure. The results from this phase yielded the following categories: Work could be classified by referring to outcomes associated with (a) Economic Advantages, (b) Psychological Advantages, (c) Social Needs Satisfaction, and (d) an Enhancement of Skills and Knowledge. Study could be classified by referring to (a) the Pursuit of Future Career-Work Goals, and (b) Preparation for the World of Work. Both work and study could be represented by (e) Positive and (f) Negative aspects. Leisure time could be classified as time that allowed one (a) to Rest and Relax, (b) to Have Fun and Enjoy participating in pleasant activities, (c) Satisfying one's Own Interests and Helping one Achieving Self-fulfillment, and (d) an Extra-Work activity. A group of items were generated for each category. Two independent expert raters, with experience in qualitative analysis and questionnaire construction, evaluated the items in terms of clarity of wording, category representativeness, and the extent to which item differences were clear. Thus, 37 items deemed by both raters as being representative were included in the instrument. A five-point Likert scale, with values ranging from 1 ("Completely disagree") through 5 ("Completely agree"), was selected as the response format, as it is a frequently used procedure with adolescents.

Phase 2. We expected to observe a factorial structure in line with the categories to which we had referred in developing the instrument, and to achieve internal consistency indices of at least. 60 (20).

Participants

The total sample was composed of 940 North-Italian students, aged 15 to 19 years (M = 16.9, SD = .55), for a total of 386 boys and 554 girls. In this sample, 277 students were in their third year of high school, and 663 in their fourth year.

Instruments

In this first study, we used the preliminary version of the 37-item instrument developed as described above, to analyze the participants' concepts of work, study, and leisure time.

Procedure

Participants were asked to participate in school-based vocational guidance activities and fill in a battery of measures in group testing sessions conducted in a small group format by specialized psychologists, in classrooms and in training contexts. Students were informed that they would be given a personalized report on their individual results once the data had been processed.

RESULTS (STUDY 1)

Preliminary analyses. A preliminary asymmetry and kurtosis verification showed all items to have satisfactory values (e.g., Skewness values of 2 or less and Kurtosis values of 4 or less; 21).

Construct validity. A principal axis factoring (PAF) analysis in SPSS was conducted on the 37 WLST items to estimate the number of factors. The factorability was supported by Bartlett's test of sphericity, χ^2 (666, N = 940) = 9538.5, p < .0001, and the Kaiser-Meyer-Olkin measure of sampling adequacy of .87 (22). Parallel analysis (23) and scree analysis of the eigenvalues were used to determine the number of factors to extract from the data. These analysis suggested an initial six-factor solution that was carefully examined with both orthogonal and oblique rotations on the items. Following the suggestions by Pett et al. (24), ten items should not be considered, as they loaded on more than one factor simultaneously. The final run of PAF on the six-factor oblique solution with 27 items accounted for 51.89% of the total variance (see table 1).

The first factor referred to Leisure Time as an Occasion for Personal and Social Needs Satisfaction (LTOPSNS, α = .79). The second factor pertained to the idea of Work as a Stimulating and Gratifying Activity (WSGA, α = .73). The third factor concerned Working and Studying as Activities that Entail Effort and Fatigue (WSAEEF, α = .68). The fourth factor referred to the idea of Work as an Activity that Makes it Possible to Obtain Economic Benefits (WAMPOEB, α = .75). The fifth factor referred to the concept of Studying as Preparation for Work (SPW, α = .66). The sixth factor referred to Work as a Way to Contribute to the Good of Society (WWCGS, α = .61).

Descriptive statistics and Intercorrelations among factors. Table 2 illustrates that the 6 factors representing the dimensions had different means and that the standard deviations indicated appropriate within-dimension variance. The intercorrelations, ranging from .07 to .39, indicated some overlapping but distinct factors nonetheless.

CONCLUSION (STUDY 1)

The preliminary analysis showed satisfactory discriminant validity for all items. Our construct validity expectations were also confirmed and the exploratory factor analysis identified six factors with factor loadings of >.40. The factors were moderately interrelated (.07-.39) and showed acceptable levels of internal consistency (.61-.79) (20).

Table 1. Items, component loading, and communality estimates (z) from PAF; loading and intercept values for each indicator from the strong invariance model

							Equated Estimates	
	1	2	3	4	5	6	Loading (SE)	Intercept (SE)
28. Leisure involves above all pleasant and amusing activities	**.772**	-.013	-.033	-.018	-.002	.091	1.00	3.94 (.05)
23. Leisure is above all a time in which you can do what you like	**.692**	.045	.004	-.013	-.014	.000	.97 (.07)	3.88 (.05)
27. Leisure must above all guarantee the satisfaction of your own interests	**.692**	-.035	-.023	-.070	-.007	-.020	.71 (.07)	3.74 (.05)
36. Leisure is above all a time to spend with your friends	**.688**	.022	-.015	-.074	.115	.118	1.11 (.08)	3.69 (.06)
34. Leisure is above all a time without rules and commitments	**.606**	.077	.252	.178	-.019	-.026	.91 (.08)	3.61 (.05)
31. Leisure is above all a time free from work and study duties	**.592**	-.152	-.088	-.110	-.004	-.008	.91 (.07)	3.97 (.05)
20. Leisure must above all be a time you devote to yourself	**.570**	.051	.019	.050	-.158	-.074	.74 (.09)	3.20 (.06)
37. Work is above all a training ground for your personal growth	-.066	**-.726**	.099	-.005	.016	.073	1.00	3.11 (.05)
25. Work is above all stimulating	-.040	**-.718**	.033	.121	-.005	.084	1.34 (.11)	3.47 (.05)
30. Work is above all a gratifying activity	.045	**-.681**	-.006	.105	-.039	.111	1.18 (.12)	3.62 (.05)
32. Work must above all allow you to satisfy your own aspirations	.248	**-.550**	-.149	-.053	-.122	-.030	.94 (.11)	3.80 (.05)
16. Work is above all a 'training ground' to develop competencies and skills	-.061	**-.527**	-.025	-.190	-.131	.037	.94 (.11)	3.48 (.05)
9. Study is above all a demanding and fatiguing activity	.054	-.169	**.687**	-.081	.090	-.073	1.00	3.12 (.06)
13. Work is above all a duty you can't escape	-.065	.106	**.672**	-.037	-.173	.081	.71 (.09)	3.57 (.05)
12. Work is above all commitment and fatigue	.012	-.173	**.651**	-.083	-.052	.062	.81 (.09)	3.41 (.05)
26. Study is above all a boring and uninteresting activity	.078	.072	**.607**	-.106	.145	-.070	.46 (.08)	2.83 (.05)
15. Work is above all the repetition of boring things	-.003	.248	**.537**	.109	-.170	.111	.54 (.08)	2.37 (.05)
3. Work must above all allow you to get what is needed for yourself and your family.	-.059	.107	.005	**-.843**	-.041	.124	1.00	3.87 (.05)
4. Work must above all allow you to earn wages that can secure a decent life	.048	.064	.118	**-.807**	.040	-.002	1.19 (.11)	4.04 (.05)

	1	2	3	4	5	6	Equated Estimates	
							Loading (SE)	Intercept (SE)
21. Work must above all guarantee your financial security	.103	-.058	.106	**-.665**	-.137	-.065	1.16 (.11)	3.86 (.05)
22. Study allows you above all to be trained for your future job	.035	-.040	-.078	-.068	**-.768**	.011	1.00	3.52 (.05)
17. Work is above all the natural continuation of the school you have attended	-.104	.064	.030	.099	**-.704**	.174	.57 (.08)	2.79 (.05)
35. Study must above all allow you to learn what you need to enter the world of work	.146	-.059	-.054	-.155	**-.581**	-.002	.76 (.08)	3.48 (.05)
18. Study must guarantee above all the achievement of desired qualifications	.085	-.192	.154	-.090	**-.561**	-.152	.84 (.08)	3.62 (.05)
8. Work must above all allow you to so something useful for others too	.060	.046	-.146	-.025	-.037	**.730**	1.00	3.48 (.05)
29. Work must above all contribute to the development of society	.082	-.152	.084	-.004	-.089	**.683**	1.18 (.12)	3.36 (.06)
10. Work is a tangible way to participate in the life of your nation	-.029	-.159	.131	-.055	.061	**.662**	1.07 (.11)	3.35 (.05)

Table 2. Fit indices for the nested sequence in the multiple factor analysis

Model	χ^2	*df*	*P*	$\Delta\chi^2$	Δ *df*	*p*	RMSEA	RMSEA 90% CI	CFI	NNFI	Mean Girls	Mean Boys
Configural invariance[1]	1209.42	618	<.001	-	-	-	.060	.055-.065	.91	.90		
Weak invariance[1]	1235.27	639	<.001	-	-	-	.060	.055-.065	.91	.90		
Strong invariance[1]	1309.76	660	<.001	-	-	-	.061	.056-.066	.91	.90		
Homogeneity of Variance/covariance[2]	1332.09	681	<.001	22.33	21	.38	.060	.055-.065	.91	.90		
Latent mean invariance[2]	1352.76	666	<.001	42.99	6	< .001	.064	.059-.069	.89	.89		
LTOPSNS mean invariance	1329.76	661	<.001	19.99	1	<.001	.063	.058-.068	.89	.89	4.21	3.95
WSGA mean invariance	1320.12	661	<.001	10.35	1	<.05	.063	.058-.068	.90	.89	3.28	3.11
WSAEEF mean invariance	1319.51	661	<.001	9.74	1	<.05	.062	.057-.067	.90	.89	2.92	3.10
WAMPOEB mean invariance	1311.53	661	<.001	1.77	1	.18	.062	.057-.067	.90	.89	3.94	3.86
SPW mean invariance	1310.15	661	<.001	.039	1	.53	.062	.057-.067	.90	.89	3.56	3.54
WWCGS mean invariance	1309.83	661	<.001	.06	1	1.00	.062	.057-.067	.90	.89	3.49	3.47

Note. Each nested model contains its constraints, plus the constraints of all previous, tenable models.

[1]Evaluated with the RMSEA model test.

[2]Evaluated with χ^2 difference test.

Legend: LTOPSNS = Leisure Time as an Occasion for Personal and Social Needs Satisfaction; WSGA = Work as a Stimulating and Gratifying Activity; WSAEEF = Working and Studying as Activities that Entail Effort and Fatigue; WAMPOEB = Work as an Activity that Makes it Possible to Obtain Economic Benefits; SPW = Studying as Preparation for Work; WWCGS = Work as a Way to Contribute to the Good of Society.

Table 3. Means and SD, and intercorrelations among the six factor of the WSLT and my life as a student and self-determination scale

	Mean	SD	2	3	4	5	6	a	b	c	d	e	f	g	h	i	L	m
1. LTOPSNS	3.82	.63	.17**	.20**	.30**	.30**	.08**	.05	.23**	.09	.02	.02	-.01	.20**	-.01	.04	.14**	.15**
2. WSGA	3.61	.61	-	-.07*	.20**	.34**	.40**	.29**	.15**	.16**	.09	.08	.21**	.17**	.17**	.12*	.15**	.15**
3. WSAEEF	2.92	.66		-	.30**	.20**	.11**	-.18**	.01	.01	-.05	.01	-.26**	-.12*	-.17**	-.19**	-.09	-.13*
4. WAMPOEB	3.95	.71			-	.31**	.14**	.02	.21**	.04	.04	-.05	-.09	.15**	-.03	.05	.14**	.09
5. SPW	3.35	.68				-	.31**	.31**	.08	.11*	.06	.08	.12	.16	-.01	.09	.02	-.04
6. WWCGS	3.41	.75					-	.29**	.04	.09	.06	.17**	.22**	.13*	-14**	.06	-.02	.06

Note: ** $p \leq .01$ * $p = .05$.

Legend: a. Satisfaction with the School Experience; b. Satisfaction with Opportunities to Make Decisions Autonomously; c. Satisfaction with Relationships with Class Mates; d. Satisfaction with Current Life Conditions; e. Satisfaction with Relationships with Family Members; f. Satisfaction with Praise Received when Due; g. Satisfaction with Help Availability; h. Self-Determination about Expressing and Making Use of Abilities and Decisions; i. Self-Determination about Future Decisions; l. Self-Determination about Leisure Time; m. Self-Determination about Expressing Ideas and Feelings. LTOPSNS = Leisure Time as an Occasion for Personal and Social Needs Satisfaction; WSGA = Work as a Stimulating and Gratifying Activity; WSAEEF = Working and Studying as Activities that Entail Effort and Fatigue; WAMPOEB = Work as an Activity that Makes it Possible to Obtain Economic Benefits; SPW = Studying as Preparation for Work; WWCGS = Work as a Way to Contribute to the Good of Society.

STUDY 2

The goal of study 2 was to test the multidimensional structure of the WSLT using confirmatory factor analysis, with a maximum likelihood estimation method (25).

Participants

The total sample was composed of 413 North-Italian students, aged 15 to 19 years (M = 16.9, SD = .56), for a total of 182 boys and 231 girls; 131 students were in their third year, and 282 in their fourth year of high school.

Instrument and procedure

Instrument and procedures replicated those in Study 1.

RESULTS (STUDY 2)

Confirmatory factor analysis of the WSLT. Following the suggestions by Schermelleh-Engel et al. (26), we examined multiple indices to assess the fit of our model to the data: the Comparative Fit Index (CFI), the Nonnormed Fit Index (NNFI), the Root Mean Square Error of Approximation (RMSEA), and the Standardized Root Mean Squared Residual (SRMR; 25). The hypothesized six-factor model showed acceptable fit: $\chi^2(309, n = 413) = 683.72$; $p < .001$; CFI = .92; NNFI = .92; RMSEA =.056 (CI_{90} =.050–.061); SRMR = .068. As shown in Figure 1, all of the factor loadings ranged from .40 to .76 and were significant ($p < .001$), suggesting that the six factors were well represented by the items thereby.

CONCLUSION (STUDY 2)

Study 2 was conducted to examine the stability of the factor structure of the WSLT's 27-item factorial structure. The confirmatory factor analysis results indicated that the six-factor structure from Study 1 was stable in a large North-Italian sample.

STUDY 3

A third study was conducted: (a) to analyze the WSTL's measurement invariance across gender, and (b) to evaluate the instrument's discriminant validity. Regarding our first aim, we followed a hierarchical set of steps from a less restrictive model to a more restrictive one, to test measurement invariance, and therefore, by starting from determination of a baseline model, then by adding equivalence constraints in the models across groups. This procedure yielded nested models ranging invariance measurement level (27): (a) Configural Invariance;

(b) Weak Invariance; (c) Strong Invariance. After ascertaining factorial invariance, we examined the homogeneity of the variances and covariances to verify if the entire covariance structure is invariant across groups and has the same parametric structure. We also tested the equivalence of the latent construct means to verify if means of factors are significantly different across groups. With respect to latent means differences, based on the above mentioned studies reporting gender differences, we expected that girls would be more focused on the psychological and intrinsic aspects of the constructs than boys would, and that boys would report more extrinsic aspects than girls would.

Our second goal was to examine WSLT construct validity, as it relates to quality of life and self-determination. We predicted positive and higher correlations between positive aspects of work and study with quality of life, especially in terms of school experience, tendency to assume responsibility toward one's professional choices (locus of control), and self-determination about future decisions.

Participants

The total sample was composed of 500 North-Italian students, aged 15 to 19 years (M = 16.94, SD = .57), for a total of 250 boys and 250 girls.

Instruments

In addition to the WSLT, the measures of My Life as a Student and the Self-Determination Scale were used.

My Life as a Student (28) was administered to measure quality of life as experienced by students aged 15 to 19 years. This instrument consists of 26 items (e.g. "I am really happy with the school I am attending", "I am a free individual who can actually plan his/her own life in an autonomous way) requiring respondents to use a five-point Likert scale (1 = "Not at all" and 5 = "Very much") to indicate the extent to which each item's statement describes the student's usual way of thinking and behaving. The scale domains comprise: Satisfaction with the School Experience; Satisfaction with Opportunities to Make Decisions Autonomously; Satisfaction with Relationships with Classmates; Satisfaction with Current Life Conditions; Satisfaction with Relationships with Family Members; Satisfaction with Praise Received when Due; and Satisfaction with Help Availability. Cronbach's alphas for the standardization sample ranged from .65 to .86.

The Self-Determination Scale (29) is a self-report instrument measuring four domains allowing for the expression of self-determination. The instrument consists of 20 items (e.g. "About my abilities: I am sure I will exploit them in full vs. I am sure I will not exploit them in full", "About emotions: I always express them freely vs. I never express them freely") requiring respondents to use a seven-point Likert scale (ranging from 1 = high levels of self-determination, to 7 = low levels) to best describe themselves in terms of each item. The domains yielding subscale scores were: Self-Determination about Expressing and Making Use of Abilities and Decisions; Self-Determination about Future Decisions; Self-Determination about Leisure Time; and Self-Determination about Expressing Ideas and Feelings. Cronbach's alphas for the standardization sample ranged from .73 to .80.

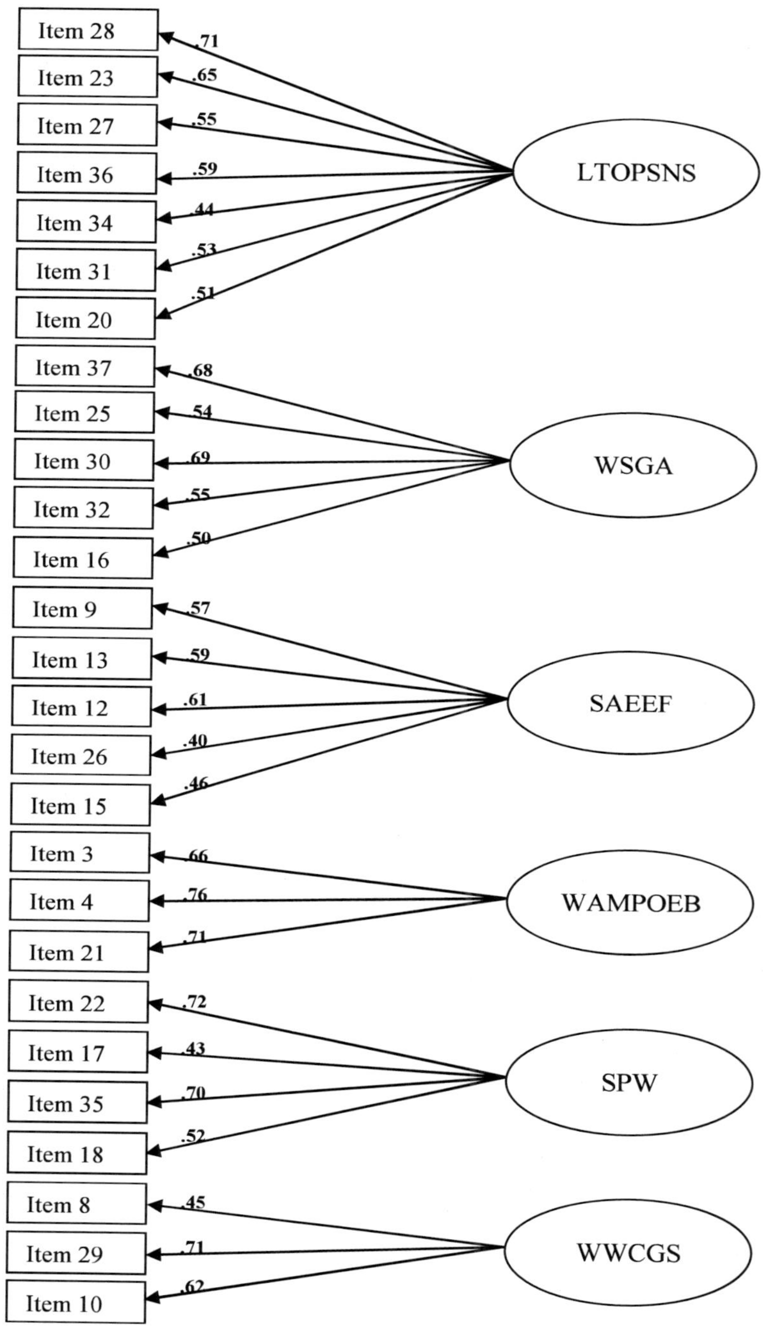

Legend: LTOPSNS = Leisure Time as an Occasion for Personal and Social Needs Satisfaction; WSGA = Work as a Stimulating and Gratifying Activity; WSAEEF = Working and Studying as Activities that Entail Effort and Fatigue; WAMPOEB = Work as an Activity that Makes it Possible to Obtain Economic Benefits; SPW = Studying as Preparation for Work; WWCGS = Work as a Way to Contribute to the Good of Society.

Figure 1. Path Diagram.

Procedure

Procedure was the same of the study 1.

RESULTS (STUDY 3)

Measurement invariance. The initial, freely estimated for all six groups revealed an acceptable fit $\chi^2(618, n = 500) = 1209.42$; $p < .001$; CFI = .91; NNFI = .90; RMSEA =.060 (CI_{90} =.055–.065). We then tested measurement invariance, equating the loadings and the intercepts (30). As shown in Table 2, no significant fit changes based on the RMSEA Model Test emerged (The RMSEA value of the nested model fell within the 90% RMSEA confidence interval of the comparison model). Using the CFIΔ test, CFI changes were less than .01 when cross-group constraints were imposed on the measurement model (31). These tests showed invariance of factors when measured across two groups. Table 1 shows the loading and intercept values for each indicator. Moreover, as shown in Table 2 the variance and covariance homogeneity was established. Conversely, the latent means invariance across the two groups was not observed. Further evaluation demonstrated significant differences in the latent factor means (see Table 2). Specifically, girls scored higher than boys did on Leisure Time as an Occasion for Personal and Social Needs Satisfaction, and Work as a Stimulating and Gratifying Activity. Boys conversely scored higher than girls did on Working and Studying as Activities that Entail Effort and Fatigue.

Discriminant validity. Table 3 shows the score correlations for the WSLT, and the Self-Determination Scale, the My Life as a Student measures.

CONCLUSION (STUDY 3)

With respect to our first aim (ensuring the equivalency of the loadings and intercepts of each of the latent constructs), we were able to assume that the constructs' variance and mean-level differences could be meaningfully compared with quantitative precision, because the constructs were defined in the same operational manner for each group (27). Specifically, no across-group differences in the variances of the constructs were found. Gender differences were observed, with girls more frequently reporting leisure time as an occasion for personal and social needs satisfaction and work as a stimulating and gratifying activity, and boys more frequently reporting work and study as activities that entail effort and fatigue. The second aim of the study was to test the instrument's discriminant validity. As expected, the correlation patterns showed positive and higher correlations between positive aspects of work and study especially, satisfaction with the school experience. Moreover, negative aspects of study and work negatively correlated with self-determination.

GENERAL CONCLUSION

The present study's results suggest that the WSLT is a psychometrically valid measure for collecting data on adolescents' concepts of work, study, and leisure time. The factor analysis results supported a six-factor structure with acceptable reliability. The factors yielded for the concept of work showed it to be mostly characterized by its potential benefits. Our findings of work being viewed as an opportunity to reap economic benefits, a stimulating and gratifying activity, and a way to contribute to the good of society, are in line with results from qualitative studies showing a general tendency for youth to underscore its economic aspects, and to consider its psychological and social facets to a lesser degree (5, 6). Conversely, the concept of study appeared to be characterized in terms of a single dimension: as an opportunity to prepare for the world of work and an activity aimed at acquiring skills and abilities. These are crucial characteristics, given that the ability to manage one's own career development by bettering one's knowledge and skills is ever more frequently in demand in today's work world. Moreover, participation in post-diploma training programs greatly contributes to one's employability (7). Both studying and working were perceived as being activities that entail effort and fatigue. This finding reveals how these constructs can also be framed in negative terms and that, as expected, adolescents' representations of work can frequently include the costs that are linked to that activity. The concept of leisure time was characterized as an occasion for personal and social needs satisfaction. These factors are in line with studies underscoring the usefulness of leisure time as a means for individuals to participate in activities that satisfy their own personal interests, by doing what they enjoy doing and being able to socialize by spending time with their families and friends. It is also perceived as an activity that allows them to dedicate attention and time to themselves (17).

The measurement invariance yielded allowed us to assume that the six-factor structure of the WSLT is invariant and can be meaningfully compared across boys and girls. After establishing measurement equivalence, we were able to evaluate the homogeneity of variance and covariance and latent mean invariance across the two groups. This procedure allowed us to establish that there were no across-group differences in the variances of the constructs. Moreover, the latent means differences between groups represents 'real' differences across gender.

The difference observed between boys and girls supported literature results showing that girls tend to focus more on the psychological and individual aspects of leisure time, and have a positive perception of work as a stimulating and gratifying activity. Conversely, their male peers tend to focus more on negative aspects of study and work, such as the effort and fatigue they entail (6). The instrument's capacity to detect gender differences shows that it has adequate discriminant validity requisites. Moreover, the low correlations observed among different instruments on the domains of self-determination and quality of life show that the instruments investigate different constructs and suggest that school counsellors and vocational psychologists can use the questionnaire to probe further into adolescents' views of work, the meaning(s) they attribute to study, and also to their leisure time.

This study was limited in a number of ways. Firstly, the reliability of the Work as a Way to Contribute to the Good of Society was quite low. We note, in fact, that although some authors (20) consider alpha value of .61 to be low but acceptable, DeVellis (32) and de Vaus (33) suggest that data gathered with factors yielding this value be treated with caution.

Secondly, the purpose of the study was to develop an instrument for high school students; thus, future research should verify whether investigation with different-aged students (e.g., middle school students) or with individuals experiencing different life situations (employed vs. unemployed) would reveal similar factor structures and results differing from those obtained herein. Findings to this effect would make generalizations easier and would allow for the comparison of students attending high school versus those that do not, with the aim of identifying variables associated with career planning vulnerability. Thirdly, the fact that the questionnaire is based on self-reported information should not be underestimated. Despite these limits, the results obtained allow us to state that the instrument can be used with 15 to 19-year-old adolescents for school and vocational guidance purposes. It can be particularly useful for screening adolescents whose ideas of work, study, and leisure time poorly reflect actual employment demands, e.g., for flexibility, knowledge updating, and the optimal management of leisure time. These individuals can be helped through early identification and prevention efforts aimed at modifying the meaning(s) they attribute to work, study, and leisure time. Specifically, high scores on Work as an Activity that Makes it Possible to Obtain Economic Benefits indicate a need for reflection on the idea that high expectations of economic benefits, when planning one's own academic and career pathway, go against the labor market's current situation of uncertainty and non-linear dynamics. Expanding on the concept of work makes it possible to launch a debate on the characteristics of what "decent work" might be, and to stimulate reflection on the historical, social, political, economic, cultural aspects of the work global and local situations, to foster views of work benefits that most closely reflect a given person's life context (4, 19). Low scores on the Work as a Stimulating and Gratifying Activity scale point to a need to highlight the idea that work can also facilitate one's quality of life, especially by considering it an opportunity for personal and professional growth and as a means to achieve personal satisfaction. Guidance activities that point out these psychological aspects and illustrate specific case stories linked to quality of life components can help broaden the range of aspects students consider important and can encourage them to invest more effort and self-reflection in their career planning processes (11). High scores on Working and Studying as Activities that Entail Effort and Fatigue suggest a need to implement job analysis activities that illustrate the ways in which most jobs present tasks that entail exertion and effort in what are frequently repetitive and at times boring actions. Young people should be helped to understand that all jobs— both the ones they like and they ones they do not—intrinsically present goals that involve effort and tasks that are not always gratifying or enjoyable. They should also be helped to examine and develop strategies to help them cope with these challenges thereby. Lastly, low scores on Work as a Way to Contribute to the Good of Society point to the need for guidance counselors to underscore the idea that work can contribute to developing a sense of self as an active member of a community. Indeed, it is through work that people find their role(s) in society and contribute to its betterment. Furthermore, this perspective is in line with the theme of social justice, and allows for the discussion of key topics, such as fairness, equal opportunity, and the relation between individual and collective wellbeing, fostering the development of a greater critical consciousness about these issues thereby (19).

Young people who do not believe that studying is important for their career development should be helped to analyze the risks of leaving school for their future work and extra-work lives. They should be helped to understanding that good school achievement is related to their future employment and life opportunities, also with the aim of stimulating their motivation to study and their career planning. Thus, low scores on Studying as Preparation for Work should create awareness that the employment world demands certain core knowledge and skills, the lack of which leaves little probability of getting a decent job and having a personally gratifying life (7). It should also be underscored how professions evolve over time, and how this process requires life-long learning, training, and flexibility (3). It can therefore be helpful to present and discuss research data demonstrating the benefits enjoyed by individuals with university diplomas, in terms of success and career opportunities (including finding work in times of economic crisis) (6).

With respect to the concept of leisure time, it is important to underscore that it is not only a right and an opportunity to have fun, relax, and do what one best enjoys, but that it also represents a chance to broaden one's social network. This process, in turn, can create more opportunities for job placement as well as more emotional support and richer network relationships (34). Hence, low scores on the Leisure Time as an Occasion for Personal and Social Needs Satisfaction suggest the need to stimulate reflection on the fact that leisure time allows people to cultivate their own interests (18) by participating in activities they find to be gratifying. It also allows them to construct relational support networks that help render their own existence significant and help them tolerate and cope with difficult situations, including ones encountered on the job (4). Guidance counselors should also help students identify the skills they are developing, or could develop, during their leisure time, by highlighting the professional advantages involved, and thus, by promoting the idea that some leisure-time pursuits could be chosen with vocational growth potential in mind.

REFERENCES

[1] Farber HS. Is the company man an anachronism? Trends in long term employment in the US between 1973 and 2005. Network Transitions Adulthood Policy Brief 2006;38:1-2.

[2] Savickas ML, Nota L, Rossier J, Dauwalder JP, Duarte ME, Guichard J, et al. Life designing: A paradigm for career construction in the 21st century. J Vocat Behav 2009;75:239-50.

[3] Blustein DL. The role of work in psychological health and well-being: A conceptual, historical, and public policy perspective. Am Psychol 2008;63(4):228-40.

[4] Blustein DL. A relational theory of working. J Vocat Behav 2011;79:1- 17.

[5] Chaves AP, Diemer MA, Blustein DL, Gallagher LA, DeVoy JE, Casares MT, et al. Conceptions of work: The view from urban youth. J Couns Psychol 2004; 51:275-86.

[6] Ferrari L, Nota L, Soresi S, Blustein DL, Murphy KA, Kenna AC. Constructions of work among adolescents in transition. J Career Assess 2009;17(1):99-115.

[7] Bridgstock R. The graduate attributes we've overlooked: Enhancing graduate employability through career management skills. HERD 2009; 28(1):31-44.

[8] Yazzie-Mintz E. Voices of students on engagement: A report on the 2006 high school survey of student engagement. Bloomington, IN: Center for Evaluation and Education Policy, 2007.

[9] Hull-Blanks E, Kurpius SER, Befort C, Sollenberger S, Nicpon MF, Huser L. Career goals and retention-related factors among college freshmen. J Career Dev 2005;32(1):16-30.

[10] Nota L, Ferrari L, Soresi S. Construction of work and school concepts: The view from Italy. Paper presented at the 117th Annual Convention of the American Psychological Association; Los Angeles 2005 May 29-26.

[11] Snir R, Harpaz I. To work or not to work: Nonfinancial employment commitment and the social desirability bias. J Soc Psychol 2002;142(5):635-44.

[12] Berg JM, Grant AM, Johnson V. When callings are calling: crafting work and leisure in pursuit of unanswered occupational callings. Organ Sci 2010;21:973-94.

[13] Ravenscroft N, Gilchrist P. The Emergent working society of leisure. J Leis Res 2009;41(l):23-39.

[14] Passmore A. The occupation of leisure: Three typologies and their influence on mental health in adolescence. OTJR 2003;23(2):76-83.

[15] Eccles JS, Barber BL, Stone M, Hunt J. Extracurricular activities and adolescent development. J Soc Issues 2004;59:865-89.

[16] Armstrong PI, Rounds JB. Vocational psychology and individual differences. In: Brown SD, Lent RW. Handbook of counseling psychology. Hoboken, NJ: John Wiley, 2008:375-91.

[17] Nota L, Ferrari L, Solberg SV, Soresi S. Career search self-efficacy, family support, and career indecision with Italian youth. J Career Assess 2007;5:181-93.

[18] Savickas ML. The theory and practice of career construction. In: Brown SD, Lent RW. Career development and counseling. Hoboken, NJ: John Wiley, 2005:42-70.

[19] Richardson MS. Counseling for work and relationship. Couns Psychol 2012;40(2):190-242.

[20] Nunnally JC, Bernstein IH. Psychometric theory. New York: McGraw- Hill, 1994.

[21] Kline RB. Principles and practice of structural equation modeling. New York: Guilford, 1998.

[22] Tabachnick BG, Fidell LS. Using multivariate analysis. Boston, MA: Allyn Bacon, 2001.

[23] Horn JL. An empirical comparison of methods for estimating factor scores. Educ Psychol Meas 1965;25(2):313-322.

[24] Pett MA, Lackey NR, Sullivan JJ. Making sense of factor analysis: The use of factor analysis for instrument development in health care research. Thousand Oaks, CA: Sage, 2003.

[25] Jöreskog KD, Sörbom D. Lisrel 8. User's reference guide. Lincolnwood, IL: Scientific Software International, 2004.

[26] Schermelleh-Engel K, Moosbrugger H, Müller H. Evaluating the fit of structural equation models: Tests of significance and descriptive goodness-of-fit measures. MPR 2003;8(2):23-74.

[27] Meredith W. Measurement invariance, factor analysis and factorial invariance. Psychometrika 1993;58:525–43.

[28] Soresi S, Nota L. Portfolio Clipper per l'orientamento dai 15 ai 19 anni - Volume III°: Abilità sociali e qualità della vita [Portfolio Clipper for vocational guidance from 15 to 19 years of age – Vol. III°: Social skills and quality of life]. Firenze: ITER-Organizzazioni Speciali, 2003.

[29] Ferrari L, Nota L, Soresi S. Self-determination and career choice. An instrument for assessment-implications for practice. GIPO 2004;5(2):30-49.

[30] Little TD, Card NA, Slegers DW, Ledford EC. Representing contextual effects in multiple-group MACS models. In: Little TD, Bovaird JA, Card NA, eds. Modeling contextual effects in longitudinal studies. Mahwah, NJ: LEA, 2007:121-147.

[31] Cheung GW, Rensvold RB. Evaluating goodness-of-fit indexes for testing measurement invariance. Struct Equ Modeling 2002;9(2):233- 255.

[32] DeVellis RF. Scale development. Newbury Park, CA: Sage, 1991.

[33] De Vaus D. Analysing social science data. London: Sage, 2002.

[34] Merino R. Pathways from school to work: can the competences acquired in leisure activities improve the construction of pathways? J Educ Work 2007;20(2):139-59.

In: Child and Adolescent Health Issues
Editor: Joav Merrick

ISBN: 978-1-63463-574-5

Chapter 7

CIGARETTE SMOKING, CLOSE FRIENDSHIP, SEXUAL INTERCOURSE AND SCHOOL-GOING ADOLESCENTS

David Mulenga*, BSc, MPH*[1]*,
Mazyanga L Mazaba-Liwewe, BSc*[2,3]*,
***Olusegun Babaniyi, MBBS, MPH, MSc*[3]
***and Seter Siziya, BA(Ed), MSc, PhD*[1]
[1]Copperbelt University, School of Medicine, Ndola, Zambia
[2]University Teaching Hospital, Lusaka, Zambia and
[3]EPI Unit, World Health Organization, Lusaka, Zambia

There are undesirable consequences of early commencement of sexual activity among adolescents which include human immunodeficiency virus infection and unwanted pregnancy. The objective of the chapter was to determine associations of cigarette smoking and close friendships with ever having had sexual intercourse among school-going adolescents in Mauritania. Secondary analysis of 2010 Mauritania Global School-based Health Survey data was conducted. Associations were established using weighted logistic regression analysis. A total of 2,063 students participated in the survey of which 43.5% were males. A third (33.2%) of students reported ever had sexual intercourse. Compared to female adolescents, males were 15% (AOR=1, 15, 95% CI [1.13, 1.17]) more likely to report having had sexual intercourse. Overall, adolescents who smoked cigarettes were more likely (AOR=2.01, 95% CI [1.96, 2.06]) to report having had sexual intercourse compared to non-smokers. Having close friends was negatively associated with sexual intercourse (AOR=0.64, 95% CI [0.62, 0.67]). Future work is needed to develop and employ measures that would prevent early sexual intercourse using the factors identified in the current study.

* Corresponding: David Mulenga, BSc, MPH, Copperbelt University, School of Medicine, POBox 71191, Ndola, Zambia. E-mail: mulengingo@yahoo.co.uk.

INTRODUCTION

Issues of reproductive health and sexuality are very important fundamental aspects of our day to day living (1) and yet not much has been documented on the prevalence and correlates of sexual behaviour among adolescents (2,3). There are undesirable consequences of sexual activity among school going adolescents which include human immunodeficiency virus infection and unwanted pregnancy (4). School going adolescents may also engage in substance use risk behaviours (5), which have an impact on their sexual behaviour, for instance researchers have documented that sexual risk taking and heavy alcohol use coexist in many communities of young people (6,7). Zabin (8) in the study that sought to explore the association between smoking and sexual behaviour among teens in US contraceptive clinics, noted that smoking may be representative of a cluster of behaviours which are especially problematical when initiated outside the normative schedule of such behaviours. Therefore, accurate and up-to-date information on sexual behaviour and its correlates of this particular group is crucially important.

According to Biddlecom et al. (9), parents have an influence on the sexual and reproductive health of adolescents that they can help to develop necessary skills on safe sexual life and good reproductive health. According to Gevers et al. (10) in South Africa, it is illegal for adolescents under age 16 years to engage in any sexual behaviour whether kissing, petting, or penetrative sex, regardless of consent. Feleke et al. (11) also noted that the utilization of reproductive health services is an important component in preventing adolescents from different sexual and reproductive health problems.

Sexual and reproductive health problems among adolescents are not only in African countries like Mauritania, but even developed countries experience similar challenges. It has been reported by Hellerstedt et al. (12) that half of the students in grades 9 to 12 in the United States reported that they had sexual intercourse at least once. They also reported that about 80% of pregnancies among those aged 15 to 19 years which made up to a quarter of all US unintended pregnancies were not planned. In Canada, where reports indicate that while less than 50% of teenagers reported having had sexual intercourse before the age 18, more than two-thirds would have had sexual intercourse by the age of 20 (13).

In most African countries, in-school adolescents engage in sexual activities in their teens. In a study by Oljira et al. (14), it was reported that a significant proportion of in-school adolescents in Eastern Ethiopia were engaged in sexual relationships. In another study done in two major universities of Ethiopia, Wasie et al. (15) observed that a significant number of students had history of sexual intercourse. In Mauritania, sexual behaviour of school going adolescents is not different from many parts of Africa. The 2010 Global School-based Health Survey (Mauritania 2010 fact sheet) reported that among students who ever had sexual intercourse, the percentage that had sexual intercourse for the first time before age 14 years was as high as 73.7%. In another study done by Ndiaye et al. (16) in Nouakchott in the Islamic Republic of Mauritania, it was noted that there was multiplication of sexually-transmitted diseases, including HIV, among the pupils due to insufficient condom use among sexually active students. Therefore, research in this area of study will yield a lot of information to correct the situation by informing preventive strategies. Hence, the objective of the study was to determine associations of cigarette smoking and close friendship with ever had sexual intercourse among school-going adolescents in Mauritania in order to inform interventions to prevent early sexual intercourse.

OUR STUDY

Analysis was based on data obtained from the 2010 Mauritania Global School-based Student Health Survey (GSHS) that is available on a World Health Organization web site (http://www.who.int/chp/gshs/mauritaniadataset/en/). The focus of the GSHS is on students aged 13-15 years, and grades with the majority of students were selected. In Mauritania, the majority of these students were in year 1 to 4 of high school. Drawing of the sample involved sampling schools proportional to their enrolment size. This was followed by randomly selecting classes and all students in the selected classes were requested to participate in the survey. The school response rate was 96% and that of the students was 74%, giving an overall response rate of 70%.

Data collection

A questionnaire found on a web site for Centers for Disease Control and Prevention (http://www.cdc.gov/gshs/countries/africa/mauritania.htm) with many modules among which was on sexual behaviour and Tobacco use was used to collect data. The questionnaire was self-administered by the students. They responded to questions on a computer scannable answer sheet.

Variables

Variables that were considered in this manuscript are those that were significantly associated with ever had sexual intercourse in the literature. The exposure variables were Smoked cigarettes and Had close friend. The variable Smoked cigarettes was obtained from the question: "During the past 30 days, on how many days did you smoke cigarettes? Responses were 0 days, 1 or 2 days, 3 to 5 days, 6 to 9 days, 10 to 19 days, 20 to 29 days and all 30 days. At analysis, the variable was recoded as 1 for having smoked cigarettes for at least 1 day and 0 for not having smoked cigarettes in the past 30 days. The other explanatory variable Had close friends was obtained by asking the question: "How many close friends do you have?" Responses were 0, 1, 2, 3 or more. This variable was recoded as either 0 for having no close friends or 1 if had at least one close friend. The outcome variable: Ever had sexual intercourse was obtained by asking the question: "Have you ever had sexual intercourse?" Responses were Yes or No.

OUR FINDINGS

A total of 2,063 students participated in the survey of which 54.5% were males. Among all students, 17.5% of them (17.9% of males and 16.4% of females) smoked cigarettes. About a third (33.2%) of all students (35.6% of males and 29.3% females) reported ever had sexual intercourse. These results are shown in table 1.

Table 1. Sample description for 2010 Mauritania Global School-based Health Survey

	Total	Males	Females
Factor	n* (%)**	n* (%)**	n* (%)**
Age (years)			
<14	312 (15.6)	157 (16.4)	148 (14.2)
14	410 (20.0)	185 (19.5)	220 (20.5)
15	595 (28.9)	256 (27.3)	334 (31.0)
16+	711 (35.6)	348 (36.8)	356 (34.3)
Gender			
Male	964 (43.5)	-	-
Female	1069 (45.5)		
Smoked cigarettes			
Yes	339 (17.5)	161 (17.9)	167 (16.4)
No	1594 (82.5)	732 (82.1)	845 (83.6)
Had close friends			
Yes	1862 (92.6)	872 (92.9)	967 (92.5)
No	151 (7.4)	71 (7.1)	77 (7.5)
Ever had sexual intercourse			
Yes	550 (33.2)	282 (35.6)	254 (29.3)
No	1134 (66.8)	509 (64.4)	618 (70.7)

n* - unweighted frequency (%)** - weighted percent.
Totals may not all up due to missing data.

Associations between smoking cigarettes and possible confounding factors with having had sexual intercourse are shown in Tables 2 and 3. Age, gender, smoking cigarettes and having close friends were associated with sexual intercourse. In both males and females, adolescents aged less than 14 years were less likely to report having ever had sexual intercourse compared to those aged 16 years or older. While male adolescents aged 14 or 15 years were less likely to have had sexual intercourse compared to males adolescents age 16 years or older, female adolescents aged 14 or 15 years were more likely to have had sexual intercourse compared with females adolescents of age 16 years or older. Compared to female adolescents, male adolescents were 15% (AOR=1,15, 95% CI [1.13, 1.17]) more likely to report having had sexual intercourse. Adolescents who smoked cigarettes were more likely (AOR=2.01, 95% CI [1.96, 2.06]) to report having had sexual intercourse (AOR=2.45, 95% CI [2.36, 2.54] among males and AOR=1.58, 95% CI [1.53, 1.65] among females). Adolescents who had close friends were less likely (AOR=0.64, 95% CI [0.62, 0.67]) to report having had sexual intercourse (AOR=0.68, 95% CI [0.65, 0.72] among males and AOR=0.58, 95% CI [0.55, 0.62] among females).

Table 2. Factors associated with sexual intercourse in bivariate analyses

	Total	Males	Females
Factor	OR* (95% CI**)	OR* (95% CI**)	OR* (95% CI**)
Age (years)			
<14	0.81 (0.78, 0.85)	0.86 (0.81, 0.90)	0.67 (0.62, 0.71)
14	0.86 (0.83, 0.89)	0.80 (0.76, 0.83)	1.02 (0.97, 1.07)
15	1.06 (1.02, 1.09)	1.01 (0.96, 1.05)	1.15 (1.10, 1.20)
16+	1	1	1
Gender			
Male	1.16 (1.14, 1.18)	-	-
Female	1		
Smoked cigarettes			
Yes	2.06 (2.01, 2.11)	2.37 (2.29, 2.45)	1.63 (1.57, 1.69)
No	1	1	1
Had close friends			
Yes	0.65 (0.62, 0.67)	0.72 (0.68, 0.75)	0.59 (0.56, 0.62)
No	1	1	1

OR* - unadjusted odds ratio; CI** - Confidence interval.

Table 3. Factors associated with sexual intercourse in multivariate analyses

	Total	Males	Females
Factor	AOR* (95% CI**)	AOR* (95% CI**)	AOR* (95% CI**)
Age (years)			
<14	0.76 (0.72, 0.79)	0.84 (0.80, 0.89)	0.62 (0.58, 0.67)
14	0.93 (0.89, 0.96)	0.84 (0.80, 0.89)	1.09 (1.03, 1.15)
15	1.00 (0.97, 1.04)	0.91 (0.87, 0.95)	1.14 (1.09, 1.20)
16+	1	1	1
Gender			
Male	1.15 (1.13, 1.17)	-	-
Female			
Smoked cigarettes			
Yes	2.01 (1.96, 2.06)	2.45 (2.36, 2.54)	1.58 (1.53, 1.65)
No	1	1	1
Had close friends			
Yes	0.64 (0.62, 0.67)	0.68 (0.65, 0.72)	0.58 (0.55, 0.62)
No	1	1	1

AOR* - Adjusted odds ratio; CI** - Confidence interval.

DISCUSSION

The current study has established that cigarette smoking and close friendships are related to ever had sexual intercourse among school-going adolescents in Mauritania. Age and gender were also associated with ever had sexual intercourse. While male adolescents aged 14 or 15 years were less likely to have had sexual intercourse compared to male adolescents aged 16 years or older, female adolescents aged 14 or 15 years were more likely to have had sexual intercourse compared with female adolescents of age 16 years or older. This finding suggests that adolescent girls may have been engaging in sexual intercourse with males who were older than themselves. More male adolescents reported ever had sexual intercourse compared to the female counterparts and this may be due to the explorative nature of young males. This finding is common in many other studies looking at sexual behaviour among school going adolescents (17).

The current study has demonstrated the coexistence of sexual risk behaviour and cigarette smoking. Adolescents who smoked cigarettes were more likely to report ever had sexual intercourse compared to those who did not smoke cigarettes. This accords the findings by Zabin (8) which showed that the relationship of smoking and early coitus appeared among both Blacks and Whites despite strong racial differentials. Zabin (8) further noted that the evidence clearly suggested that those who initiated sexual activity in early adolescence demonstrated levels of smoking well beyond the norm not only for their age groups but even for adult populations.

Both male and female adolescents who had close friends were less likely to report having ever had sexual intercourse in the present study. This might be that these adolescents spent more time with their close ordinary friends than with those who might have wanted to engage in sexual intercourse with them.

This study is unique in its attempt to determine associations of cigarette smoking and close friendship with sexual experience among Mauritanian school going adolescents via a population-based survey. However, the study was not designed to examine the specific experiences of Mauritanian School going adolescents and, thus, we were not able to describe the cultural assets or traditional behaviours that are known to positively affect the sexual and reproductive health of Mauritanian school going adolescents. Because family and cultural ties are important to the health of African school going adolescents, further work is needed to specifically identify salient community and family ties that are associated with health-promoting behaviours and attitudes. Future work is needed to develop and employ measures that would prevent early sexual intercourse using the factors identified in the current study.

ACKNOWLEDGMENTS

We thank the World Health Organization for availing the data set in a public domain, and Centers for Disease Control and Prevention for the questionnaire. We extend our gratitude to the students for their participation in the survey.

REFERENCES

[1] Shiferaw K, Getahun F, Asres G. Assessment of adolescents' communication on sexual and reproductive health matters with parents and associated factors among secondary and preparatory schools' students in Debremarkos town, North West Ethiopia. Reprod Health 2014;11(1):2.

[2] Chi X, Yu L, Winter S. Prevalence and correlates of sexual behaviors among university students: a study in Hefei, China. BMC Public Health 2012;12:972.

[3] De Rosa CJ, Ethier KA, Kim DH, Cumberland WG, Afifi AA, Kotlerman J, Loya RV, Kerndt PR. Sexual intercourse and oral sex among public middle school students: prevalence and correlates. Perspect Sex Reprod Health 2010;42(3):197-205.

[4] Ishida K, Stupp P, McDonald O. Prevalence and correlates of sexual risk behaviors among Jamaican adolescents. Int Perspect Sex Reprod Health 2011;37(1):6-15

[5] Kang M, Rochford A, Skinner SR, Mindel A, Webb M, Peat J, Usherwood T. Sexual behaviour, sexually transmitted infections and attitudes to chlamydia testing among a unique national sample of young Australians: baseline data from a randomised controlled trial. BMC Public Health 2014;14:12.

[6] Connor J, Psutka R, Cousins K, Gray A, Kypri K. Risk drinking, risky sex: a national study of New Zealand University students, Alcohol Clin Exp Res 2013;37(11):1971-8.

[7] Siziya S, Muula AS, Kazembe LN, Rudatsikira E. Harmful lifestyles' clustering among sexually active in-school adolescents in Zambia. BMC Pediatr 2008;8:6.

[8] Zabin LS. The Association between smoking and sexual behavior among teens in US contraceptive clinics. Am J Public Health 1984;74(3):261-3.

[9] Biddlecom A, Awusabo-Asare K, Bankole. A Role of parents in adolescent sexual activity and contraceptive use in four African countries. Int Perspect Sex Reprod Health 2009;35(2):72-81.

[10] Gevers A, Mathews C, Cupp P, Russell M, Jewkes R. Illegal yet developmentally normative: a descriptive analysis of young, urban adolescents' dating and sexual behaviour in Cape Town, South Africa. BMC Int Health Hum Rights 2013;13:31.

[11] Feleke SA, Koye DN, Demssie AF, Mengesha ZB. Reproductive health service utilization and associated factors among adolescents (15--19 years old) in Gondar town, Northwest Ethiopia. BMC Health Serv Res 2013;13(1):294.

[12] Hellerstedt WL, Peterson-Hickey M, Rhodes KL, Garwick A. Environmental, social, and personal correlates of having ever had sexual intercourse among American Indian youths. Am J Public Health 2006;96(12):2228–34.

[13] Rotermann, M. Sexual behaviour and condom use of 15- to 24-year-olds in 2003 and 2009/2010. Health Rep 2012;23(1):1-5.

[14] Oljira L, Berhane Y, Worku A. Pre-marital sexual debut and its associated factors among in-school adolescents in Eastern Ethiopia. BMC Public Health 2012;12:375.

[15] Wasie B, Belyhun Y, Moges B, Amare B. Effect of emergency oral contraceptive use on condom utilization and sexual risk taking behaviours among university students, Northwest Ethiopia: a cross-sectional study. BMC Res Notes 2012;5:501.

[16] Ndiaye P, Abdallahi el HO, Diedhiou A, Tal-Dia A, Lemort JP. Evaluation of condom use among students of the El Mina middle school in Nouakchott in the Islamic Republic of Mauritania. Sante 2005;15(3):189-94.

[17] Leigh BC, Morrison DM, Trocki K, Temple MT. Sexual behavior of American adolescents: results from a U.S. national survey. J Adolesc Health 1994;15(2):117-25.

In: Child and Adolescent Health Issues
Editor: Joav Merrick

ISBN: 978-1-63463-574-5

Chapter 8

HOMESCHOOL CHILDREN, PARENTAL INFLUENCE AND CARDIOVASCULAR HEALTH AND BODY COMPOSITION

David A Wachob*[*], *DEd, CAPE, CHES and Robert E Alman, PhD
Department of Health and Physical Education,
Indiana University of Pennsylvania, Indiana, Pennsylvania,
United States of America

It has been well established that parents can influence their children's physical activity levels and health status. These findings often report on public school children and their parents due to the easy access to this population. However, due to the structure of home education, collecting data on this group is often difficult and is underrepresented in the literature. Objective: The purpose of this chapter was to determine the relationship between the cardiovascular health and body composition within homeschooling families. Study group: Homeschooling children and their primary caregiver. Method: 30 children were tested to determine their cardiovascular health (VO2 Max) and body composition (BMI and body fat %). Those results were then compared to their parent-teacher's (n=14) cardiovascular health (VO_2 Max), and body composition (BMI and body fat %). Relationships were determined by comparing mean scores, and by running Pearson's correlation tests when controlling for each family group. RESULTS: General comparisons within each family group revealed moderate correlations between VO_2 levels ($r = .599$, $p < .01$); BMI ($r = .743$, $p < .01$); and body fat ($r = .616$, $p < .01$). Furthermore, when comparing the parents' health status to their children it was determined that moderate relationships were found between the two groups' VO_2 levels ($r = .667$, $p < .01$), BMI ($r = .663$, $p < .01$), and body fat ($r = .451$, $p < .01$). Conclusion: The parent-teacher's health status is a notable variable when determining factors that influence homeschooling children's cardiovascular health and body composition.

[*] Correspondence: David A Wachob, DEd, CAPE, CHES, Assistant Professor, Homeschool Physical Education Program Director, Department of Kinesiology, Health, and Sport Science, 233 Zink Hall, Indiana University of Pennsylvania, Indiana, PA 15705, United States. E-mail: d.wachob@iup.edu.

INTRODUCTION

Cardiovascular health and the weight status of children have received a lot of attention in recent years. This is partly due to the increased rates of obesity and metabolic syndrome in youth (1). With an estimated one in three children being classified as either overweight or obese, it is crucial to determine variables that influence these patterns. Recent literature has established factors that impact the health status of children; including environmental (2) and parental influence (3). These variables often report on public school children and their parents due to the easy access to this population; resulting in homeschooling families being absent in the data.

The environment plays a vital role on the development of a child's health status. It is suggested that the school environment has the potential to improve the cardiovascular health of a child through providing increased opportunities to be physically active (2). Researchers have found that school's who provide their students with adequate time (i.e. recess, physical education class, before/after school programs) and an adequate environment (i.e. play space, equipment, programming) can significantly increase children's physical activity levels (4-6) which directly impacts cardiovascular health and body composition. Though these findings provide reasonable interventions geared towards reducing health issues in children; the results are specific to traditional (e.g. public or private) school settings. Since none of the literature focuses on the homeschool environment, its impact on children's health is significantly understudied, potentially leaving this population at greater risk for inactivity and cardiovascular disease (7).

Homeschool education has seen a steady increase over the past several decades. It is believed that there are over two million children being educated in the home, up about 3% from 2007 (8). These numbers equate to around 2% of the entire school-age population in United States. With the increased number of children being educated in the home, it is imperative to begin investigating the impact that this unique environment has on the children's health.

This study sought to identify potential variables that may influence the cardiovascular health and body composition of this underrepresented group of children. There is a direct connection between parental influence and their children's overall health (9). For instance, parents establish opportunities to be physically active (10), TV and video game time (11), and direct modeling of healthy behavior choices (3). Since the majority of homeschool children are educated by one of the parents (8), also known as the parent-teacher, this results in a large amount of time spent in the parent-influenced environment. Previous studies have examined the influence that teachers have on public school children's healthy behaviors (5,6). This study looked at the impact that the parent-teacher has on their homeschooling children's health status. More specifically, the cardiovascular health (e.g. estimated VO2 levels) and weight status (e.g. body composition and BMI) was compared between the homeschool children and their respective parent-teacher to determine if any relationship exist between the two groups.

OUR STUDY

This study examined the cardiovascular health and body composition of homeschooling children to determine the impact that the parent-teacher has on these health indicators. Variables that were tested include the children's aerobic capacity (VO_2 levels), Body Mass Index (BMI), and body fat percentage. The children's results were then compared to their parent-teacher's estimated VO_2 levels, Body Mass Index (BMI), and body fat percentage. This research study was approved by the Indiana University of Pennsylvania Institutional Review Board for the Protection of Human Subjects. The consent and assent procedures are briefly discussed in the next section.

The sample involved 14 homeschooling families from western Pennsylvania, including 30 children ages 8-16 years, and each of the 14 family's parent-teacher; which in this case were all mothers of the children. All participants were eligible to participate in the study because the children are educated in the home and the primary caregiver is the teacher. The majority of children participants were females (53.3%) and in the 10-11 (36.4%) age group. Both consent and assent forms were obtained from participants, including a consent form for the parent-teachers, a consent form for the parent of each child participant, and an assent form for each of the child participants. Separate assent forms were used to better address the difference in literacy levels of the 8-10 year olds and the 11-16 year olds.

This descriptive, comparative study used a quantitative study design involving two separate data sets; children and parents. Data were collected on the participants' fitness levels and body composition.

Fitness levels were established by calculating the aerobic capacity (estimated VO2 levels) of both the parent and child participants. The tests administered to the two sample groups are discussed in this section.

Children's fitness levels. The 20-meter PACER (Progressive Aerobic Cardiovascular Endurance Run) was administered to measure the children's aerobic capacity levels. This test requires children to run a series of 20-meter laps to a timed cadence with the speed increasing each minute until the child cannot complete the lap in the designated time. A formula that compares the PACER lap results with the student's height and weight was used to calculate aerobic capacity in the form of estimated VO2 levels (12).

Parent's fitness levels. The single-stage treadmill walking test was administered to measure parent's aerobic capacity. It is suitable for low risk, apparently healthy, non-athletic adults 20-59 years of age (13). This test asked participants to walk on a treadmill for a total of 10 minutes, with the following sequence; four minute warm up at zero incline, four minute testing at five percent incline, and two minute cool-down at zero incline. The Ebbeling (14) submaximal treadmill (EbbTM) formula was used to calculate aerobic capacity in the form of estimated VO_2 max levels.

Body composition was determined by calculating height and weight ratios for both the parent and child participants, being reported as body mass index (BMI). Standing height was measured using a wall-fixed stadiometer. Body weight was measured using a calibrated scale. All subjects were measured in light-weight clothing containing no metal and without shoes. Furthermore, body composition was also established by measuring body fat percentage of both the parent and child participants using a handheld bioelectrical impedance method (BIA). Bioelectrical Impedance Analysis (BIA) is a method of measuring body fat percentage by sending a low-level, safe, electrical current through the body. It has been shown to be an accurate method in estimating body fat percentage in both adults (15) and children (16).

Multiple analysis procedures were used to answer the research questions presented in this paper. Descriptive statistics were used to explain the data results for the fitness levels, and body composition. Because some of the family groups enrolled more than one child in the study, linear mixed models were used to compare fitness levels and body composition between the children and their parents; which accounted for correlations in the data of more than one child per family. This intrafamily correlation was determined from Pearson's correlation coefficient after the clustering effect of the family was taken into consideration.

OUR FINDINGS

This study attempted to identify any significant relationships between the cardiovascular health and body composition of homeschooling children and their parent-teachers. In doing so, comparisons were made between aerobic capacity as well as the weight status of the two groups. The results are presented in this section.

Table 1. Participants' estimated VO_2 levels

	Age Group (n)	**VO_2** Mean (SD)	**Healthy Range for VO_2**
Male	8 – 9 (2)	46.15 (.212)	Not established
	10 – 12 (9)	45.26 (5.52)	38-48
	13 – 16 (3)	49.07 (1.02)	35-45
Female	8 – 9 (6)	43.38 (2.61)	Not established
	10 – 12 (4)	41.28 (1.79)	38-48
	13 – 16 (1)	42 (--)	35-45
Parents (females)	26-35 (3)	27.62 (8.59)	35 – 52
	36-45 (9)	33.13 (6.61)	31 – 45
	46-55 (2)	25.41 (2.11)	28 – 40

Note. The healthy range for children was obtained from Meredith and Welk (2010), and the adult ranges were obtained from Heyward's (2008) textbook.

Aerobic capacity

All of the children participants in this study had aerobic capacity (VO_2) levels within the healthy range for their respective age groups (12). As presented in Table 1, it was discovered that the mean VO_2 scores for every female age groups were on the lower side of what is considered to be the acceptable healthy range. In regards to the male participants, all but one of the age groups (12 year olds) were in the upper half of the acceptable healthy range; suggesting that homeschool boys have a higher aerobic threshold than do the girls.

When comparing the parent-teacher's aerobic capacity to their children, a moderate relationship ($r = .667$, $p < .01$) was found (see table 2). This suggests that aerobic capacity of the parent-teacher is casually associated to the aerobic capacity of their children.

Table 2. Comparisons of test item mean scores

	Children (n =30) M (SD)	Parents (n =14) M (SD)	Pearson's Correlation (r)	Significance (p)
BMI	18.76 (3.42)	25.14 (3.48)	.454	.005
BF%	23.56 (8.39)	31.33 (7.09)	.441	.008
VO_2	43.48 (4.75)	32.57 (7.87)	.601	.000

Body composition

Body mass index. As presented in table 3, one-third of the children participants were either considered overweight (16.7%) or obese (16.7%) weight status based on the Centers for Disease Control and Prevention's (CDC) BMI chart for children. Only one child participant was classified as underweight. In regards to the parent-teachers, nearly half (42.9%) were in the normal BMI weight status. Half (50%) of the parent-teachers were in the overweight category, and only one was in the underweight category. None of the parent-teachers studied were in the obese weight status category.

Table 3. Distribution of participant weights Status

	Weight Status	BMI	Body Fat
Children	Underweight	3.3%	3.3%
	Healthy weight	63.3%	40%
	Overweight	16.7%	40%
	Obese	16.7%	16.7%
Parents	Underweight	7%	14.3%
	Healthy weight	43%	43%
	Overweight	50%	35.7%
	Obese	0	7%

Note. Weight status category ranges were obtained from the Centers for Disease Control and Prevention (www.cdc.gov) for both children and parents, controlling for gender.

The relationship between the parent-teachers' BMI and their respective children were moderate (r = .663, p < .01); suggesting that the weight status, or BMI, of the parent-teacher is casually associated with their children's weight status.

Body fat percentage. Around half (56.7%) of the children participants were either in the overweight (40%) or obese (16.7%) category for body fat percentage. Only one child was classified as being lean. In regards to the parent-teachers, nearly half (42.9%) were in the normal range for body fat percentages for women (17). Only one parent participant was classified as being obese based on body fat percentages. The relationship between the parent-teachers' body fat percentages and their respective children was moderate (r = -.451, p = .002), suggesting that a casual association exists between body fat percentage of homeschooling children and their parent-teacher.

DISCUSSION

The results of this study provide comparisons of cardiovascular health and body composition of homeschooling children and their parent-teacher. This study is the first attempt at comparing actual health indicators within homeschooling families. To date, there has been one study that focuses on homeschooling children and their parents (18); however that study only focused on physical activity patterns. Long et al. (18) found that homeschooling children's physical activity patterns (defined as accelerometer activity counts) appeared to be related their parent's activity patterns. The current study supports these findings in that there appears to be a casual relationship between cardiovascular health and body composition within homeschool families.

This study included a relatively small sample size, so the results cannot be generalized. Further another limitation of this study includes the location. This study focused on a group of homeschoolers who participated in a weekly physical education program at a local university. This demonstrates that these families have an established interest in physical activity and health based on their voluntary participation in a program of this nature. Future studies should attempt to study the general homeschool population and not limit it to those already seeking opportunities to be physically active.

In summary, this study did find the primary caregiver, or parent-teacher, to be a moderate variable to predicting homeschool children's health indicators which supports the literature on this relationship (3). Future studies should seek to establish more environmental variables unique to the homeschooling population (i.e. daily schedule, mealtimes, social influence, etc…) that may contribute to the overall health of the children enrolled in this type of education.

REFERENCES

[1] Zimmet P, Alberti KG, Kaufman F, Tajima N, Silink M, et al. The metabolic syndrome in children and adolescents–an IDF consensus report. Pediatr Diabetes 2007;8(5):299-306.

[2] Stanley RM, Ridley K, Dollman J. Correlates of children's time-specific physical activity: A review of the literature. Int J Behav Nutr Phys Act 2012;9:50.

[3] Gustafson SL, Rhodes RE. Parental correlates of physical activity in children and early adolescents. Sports Med 2006;36(1):79-97.

[4] Nichol ME, Pickett W, Janssen I. Associations between school recreational environments and physical activity. J Sch Health 2009; 79(6):247-54.

[5] Ridgers ND, Fairclough SJ, Stratton G. Variables associated with children's physical activity levels during recess: the A-CLASS project. Int J Behav Nutr Phys Act 2010;7(1):74.

[6] Willenberg LJ, Ashbolt R, Holland D, Gibbs L, MacDougall C, Garrard J, et al. Increasing school playground physical activity: a mixed methods study combining environmental measures and children's perspectives. J Sci Med Sport 2010;13(2):210-6.

[7] 7Welk G, Schaben J, Shelley M. Physical activity and physical fitness in children schooled at home and children attending public schools. Pediatr Exerc Sci 2004;16(2):310-23.

[8] Ray BD. 2.04 million homeschool students in the United States in 2010. National Home Education Research Institute, 2011. URL: www.nheri.org/HomeschoolPopulationReport2010.pdf

[9] Hohepa M, Scragg R, Schofield G, Kolt G, Schaaf D. Associations between after-school physical activity, television use, and parental strategies in a sample of New Zealand adolescents. J Phys Act Health 2009;6(3):299.

[10] Adkins S, Sherwood NE, Story M, Davis M. Physical activity among African-American girls: The role of parents and the home environment. Obes Res 2004;12(S9):38S-45S.

[11] Hager RL. Television viewing and physical activity in children. J Adolesc Health 2006;39(5):656-61.

[12] Meredith MD, Welk GJ. Fitnessgram and activitygram: Test administration manual. Dallas, TX: Cooper institute, 2010.

[13] Mitros M, Gabriel K, Ainsworth B, Lee C, Herrmann S, Campbell K, Swan P. Comprehensive evaluation of a single-stage submaximal treadmill walking protocol in healthy, middle-aged women. Eur J Appl Physiol 2011;111(1):47-56.

[14] Ebbeling CB, Ward A, Puleo EM, Widrick J, Rippe JM. Development of a single-stage submaximal treadmill walking test. Med Sci Sports Exerc 1991;23:966–73.

[15] Haas V, Schütz T, Engeli S, Schröder C, Westerterp K, Boschmann M. Comparing single-frequency bioelectrical impedance analysis against deuterium dilution to assess total body water. Eur J Clin Nutr 2012;66: 994-7.

[16] Talma H, Chinapaw M, Bakker B, HiraSing R, Terwee C, Altenburg T. Bioelectrical impedance analysis to estimate body composition in children and adolescents: A systematic review and evidence appraisal of validity, responsiveness, reliability and measurement error. Obes Rev 2013;14(11):895-905.

[17] Heyward VH. Advance fitness assessment & exercise prescription, 3rd ed. Dallas, TX: Cooper Institute Aerobics Research, 2008.

[18] Long DE, Gaetke LM, Perry SD, Abel MG, Clasey JL. The assessment of physical activity and nutrition in home schooled versus public schooled children. Pediatr Exerc Sci 2010;22:44-59.

In: Child and Adolescent Health Issues
Editor: Joav Merrick

ISBN: 978-1-63463-574-5

Chapter 9

HYPERTENSION IN EARLY CHILDHOOD: A CASE OF 11-BETA-HYDROXYLASE DEFICIENCY

Alphonsus N Onyiriuka**, MD
and Nosakhare J Iduoriyekemwen, MD
Endocrine and Metabolic Unit and Nephrology Unit,
Department of Child Health, University of Benin Teaching Hospital,
Benin City, Nigeria

11-beta-hydroxylase deficient congenital adrenal hyperplasia (CAH) is a rare cause of hypertension in infancy. Such hypertension is usually noted in later childhood and adolescence. Objective: To describe a case of an 18-month old girl with glucocorticoid-responsive hypertension followed up for five years. Methods: In this chapter we describe the case of a seven-year old Nigerian girl whose hypertension secondary to 11-beta-hydroxylase-deficient congenital adrenal hyperplasia was diagnosed at the age of 18 months and followed up for five years. Results: The hypertension responded to glucocorticoid therapy, reoccurred on default and resolved on re-starting glucocorticoid. The blood pressure has remained normal over a period of five-and-half years on maintenance prednisolone. Anthropometry at the age of seven years showed weight 24kg (75th percentile), height (50th percentile), body mass index (50 -75th percentile). Sexual maturity rating showed breast Tanner stage 3 and pubic hair stage 2. No further increase in size of the stump of the clitoris. Some of the management challenges encountered in the care of this patient included lack of laboratory facilities for diagnosis and monitoring of therapy, brief period of default, and irregular supply of oral hydrocortisone. Conclusion: Although 11-beta-hydroxylase deficient CAH is a rare cause of hypertension in early childhood, it should be considered in the differential diagnosis of hypertension with virilisation in any prepubercent female.

* Correspondence: Alphonsus N Onyiriuka, MD, Endocrine and Metabolic Unit, Department of Child Health, University of Benin Teaching Hospital, PMB 1111, Benin City, Nigeria. E-mail: alpndiony@yahoo.com;

INTRODUCTION

Hypertension is one of the cardinal features of 11-beta hydroxylase deficiency (11-beta OHD)(1,2).The hypertension is believed to be due to elevated levels of deoxycorticosterone (DOC), a steroid with 3 to 5 percent of the activity of aldosterone's salt retaining property (3). Hypertension is common but not universal in 11-beta-hydroxylase deficiency, usually noted in later childhood or adolescence (1). Newborn infants often manifest transient salt loss (4,5), presumably as a result of the normal newborn resistance to mineralocortocoids. Hypertension, seen in both sexes, is a distinctive clinical feature but is absent in the first few years of life (3). Patients with blood pressure values 5-10 mmHg above the 99th percentile are usually considered to have severe hypertension (6). Other cardiovascular manifestations include left ventricular hypertrophy and retinopathy and death from cerebrovascular accidents has been documented (7). Biochemically, 11-beta OHD is characterized by increased concentrations of deoxycorticosterone, 11 deoxycortisol and delta 4-androstenedione and decreased plasma rennin concentration (7). Clinically, both sexes have normal internal genitalia and experience postnatal virilisation (i.e., growth acceleration, advanced bone age, and early development of secondary sexual characteristics) (7). Approximately 75% of patients with 11-beta hydroxylase deficiency have hypertension of various degrees (8). The hypertension is usually moderate, but can occasionally be sufficiently severe to cause cardiomegaly and eventual cardiac failure (9).

11-beta-hydroxylase deficiency accounts for approximately 5% of all cases of CAH with an estimated incidence of 1 in 100,000 to 250,000 live births (10). In 11-beta-hydroxylase deficient CAH, cortisol and corticosterone are deficient with overproduction of 11-deoxycortisol and 11-deoxycorticosterone. The precursor hormones are shunted into the androgen pathway causing prenatal and postnatal virilisation (8). Glucocorticoid administration (in adequate dose) is effective in reversing all the abnormalities and inducing remission (8). The glucocorticoid administration will not only normalize cortisol function but should also reduce ACTH secretion, resulting in normal serum ACTH level. Thus, removing the drive for oversecretion of deoxycorticosterone (DOC).

In developing countries, laboratory facilities for accurate and specific diagnosis of endocrine disorders are lacking, thereby adversely affecting management (11). Where the facility is available, the cost is prohibitive.

The purpose of this chapter is to report a case of a Nigerian female toddler with glucocorticoid-responsive hypertension and heart failure followed up for five years and to promote its awareness among clinicians.

OUR CASE STUDY

The patient was delivered in a private hospital in Benin City and was discharged home on the second day of life. The health care providers in the private hospital did not mention to the mother that the external genitalia was abnormal. Following discharge from the hospital, the mother also did not notice any abnormality of the external genitalia. At the age of 2 months, the maternal grandmother noticed a protrusion (enlarged clitoris) from the genitals. The patient was then taken to the private hospital where she was born and was referred to another private hospital being managed by a paediatric surgeon. The parents defaulted from follow up in the hope that the clitoris will regress with time. However, the clitoris continued to increase in size and this forced the parents to consult again the paediatric surgeon at his private clinic at the age of 12 months. She had a clitoridectomy at the age of 12 months and was discharged home 2 weeks later, apparently well. She was not placed on steroid. However, six months later, the patient presented again to the paediatric surgeon with facial swelling and difficulty in breathing which prompted referral to Children's Emergency Room (CHER), University of Benin Teaching Hospital (UBTH), Benin City as a case of bronchopneumonia. Evaluation at the CHER, UBTH revealed no history of maternal ingestion of androgens during pregnancy. She is the younger of two children in the family. The older sibling is a boy. There was no maternal history of hirsutism, genital abnormality or menstrual irregularity. Physical examination revealed a toddler with an advanced muscular development, a weight of 11.8 kg (50th percentile) and a length of 70 cm (< 5th percentile). The occipito-frontal circumference was 50 cm (90th percentile). She had facial puffiness, tachypnoea (respiratory rate 72 cycles/min), respiratory distress and fine basal crepitation. Examination of the cardiovascular system revealed tachycardia (pulse rate 168/min), severe hypertension (blood pressure 140/100 mmHg; > 10mmHg above 99th percentile for age, sex and height) and normal heart sounds. There was no cardiac murmur. She had a tender hepatomegaly (palpable 5 cm below the right coastal margin). Genital examination revealed amputated stump of the clitoris with normal labia majora and minora. The urethral meatus was below the amputated clitoris. The vaginal orifice was well formed. There was no inguinal hernia. Laboratory investigation revealed normal serum urea and electrolytes values. The results of other investigations are summarized in table 1.

Table 1. Summary of laboratory results at first presentation

Test	Results	UBTH normal values
Serum Deoxycorticosterone (DOC)	695 nmol/L*	61-576 nmol/L
Serum 11-Deoxycortisol	6.1 nmol/L*	0.6-4.6 nmol/L
Serum 17-Hydroxyprogesterone	3.94 nmol/L*	0.6-3.0 nmol/L
Serum Dehydroepiandrosterone sulfate (DHEAS)	4.0 μmol/L *	0.1 -1.5 μmol/L
Serum cortisol	108 nmol/L (am)	140- 690 nmol/L (am)
Serum testosterone	4.2 ng/ml *	<0.6 ng/ml
Blood glucose	4.6 mmol/L	4.0-6.7 mmol/L
Buccal smear (for Barr bodies)	Barr bodies present	
Abdomino-pelvic ultrasound scan	Normal uterus, fallopian tubes, and ovaries.	
Chest X-ray	Cardiomegaly	
Bone age	Advanced (about 2 years > chronological age)	

* Elevated results.

A diagnosis of Stage 2 hypertension secondary to 11-beta-hydroxylase deficient CAH with heart failure was made. The differential diagnoses considered were 21 α-hydroxylase deficient CAH, 17 α-hydroxylase deficient CAH, and Cushing syndrome. The patient was commenced on intravenous hydrocortisone which was later changed to oral prednisolone (because of difficulty in procuring oral hydrocortisone). Hydrochlorothiazide therapy was also instituted for the first three days of admission because of the oedema. No specific antihypertensive drug was administered. The hypertension and heart failure resolved without specific antihypertensive therapy. The hypertension responded to glucocorticoid therapy, reoccurred on default and resolved on re-starting glucocorticoid. The blood pressure essentially remained within normal limits during the five-year follow-up period. No further increase in size of the stump of the clitoris. As depicted in table 2, the bone age is advanced at the age of 7 years. Informed consent was obtained from the parents for publication of this report.

Table 2. Summary of physical findings at the age of 7 years

Anthropometry	
Weight	24kg (75th percentile)
Height	122cm (50th percentile)
Body mass index	16.1kg/m^2 (50-75th percentile)
Sexual maturity rating	
Breast	Tanner stage 3
Pubic hair	Tanner stage 2
No menarche	Pre-menarcheal
Blood pressure	Average 90/50 mmHg
Bone age	Advanced (about 2 years > chronological age)

DISCUSSION

In this patient, the diagnosis of 11-beta-hydroxylase-deficient CAH was based on the presence of hypertension (which resolved on steroid therapy only) and signs of hyperandrogenism. The presence of a normal internal genitalia and the experience of postnatal virilisation by the patient are in keeping with a diagnosis 11-beta-hydroxylase-deficient CAH in this female patient. This diagnostic approach is reinforced by the report of Griqoresen Sido et al. (12), in which five patients diagnosed clinically as having 11-beta-hydroxylase deficiency on the same clinical basis were later confirmed on molecular studies to have 11-beta-hydroxylase deficiency. The differential diagnoses included 17 α-hydroxylase deficient CAH, 21 α-hydroxylase-deficient CAH and Cushing syndrome. Although hypertension is a feature of 17 α-hydroxylase deficient CAH, sexual infantilism rather than virilisation is usually seen in females with the condition (10). In this patient, there was virilisation making 17 α-hydroxylase deficient CAH less likely. Epidemiologically, 21 α-hydroxylase-deficient CAH accounts for about 90% of all cases of CAH (10) and was therefore, considered one of the differential diagnoses. Hypertension is not a usual clinical feature of 21 α-hydroxylase-deficient CAH, therefore its presence in the index patient negated the diagnosis of 21 α-hydroxylase deficiency. Although Cushing syndrome may be associated with hypertension and virilisation, particularly if it is due to adrenal carcinoma, the good response of the hypertension to steroid therapy negated its diagnosis. In Cushing syndrome, the serum cortisol level is always elevated. The low serum cortisol level found in the index case excluded Cushing syndrome. In addition, there was no evidence of weight gain both historically and on physical examination. The absence of abdominal mass on physical examination (which was confirmed by ultrasonography), normal BMI at the age of 18 months and 7 years respectively, and the elevated serum DHEAS and advanced bone age were all against the diagnosis of Cushing Syndrome.

In this patient, hypertension and heart failure were observed. This is not surprising as similar observation has been documented in previous studies among patients with 11-beta-hydroxylase- deficient CAH [13-15]. Although it has been documented that in 11-beta-hydroxlase deficiency the hypertension is usually noted in later childhood or adolescence, the index case was noted to have hypertension at the age of 18 months, suggesting that it can occur in very early childhood (1).The hypertension is thought to be due to the accumulation of deoxycorticosterone resulting in sodium and water retention, increased plasma volume which in turn, causes hypertension (10). The heart failure may be due to the very severe hypertension, using the criteria suggested by Gulati and Srivastava (6). It is also possible that the heart failure may be due to reversible cardiomyopathy which is known to occur in patients with 11-beta-hydroxylase deficiency (14). As in previous reports (8,14,15) glucocorticoid therapy was effective in reversing all the abnormalities and inducing remission in the index patient. The control of hypertension with glucocorticoid therapy is as a result of the feedback inhibition of the hypothalamus and the pituitary gland, resulting in a reduction in ACTH secretion. As a consequence, the production of deoxycorticosterone as well as androgens are reduced, lowering blood pressure and preventing further virilization. The virilization and advanced muscular development in our patient were as a result of cortisol precursor hormones which were shunted into the androgenic pathway causing prenatal and postnatal virilization (7).

In conclusion, although 11-beta-hydroxylase deficient CAH is a rare cause of hypertension in early childhood, it should be considered in the differential diagnosis of hypertension with virilisation in any prepubercent female to avoid missed diagnosis.

REFERENCES

[1] New MI. Hypertension in congenital adrenal hyperplasia and apparent mineral ocoticoid excess. Ann New York Acad Sci 2002;970:145-54.

[2] Mimouni M, Kaufman H, Roitman A, Morag C, Sadan N. Hypertension in neonate with 11 beta-hydroxylase deficiency. Eur J Pediatr 1985;143:231-3.

[3] Holla RG. Congenital adrenal hyperplasia. In: Sachdev Y, ed. Clinical endocrinology and diabetes mellitus: A comprehensive text. New Delhi, Jaypee Brothers Medical Publishers, 2009:674-82.

[4] Zachmann M, Tassinari D, Prader A. Clinical and biochemical variability in congenital adrenal hyperplasia due to 11β-hydroxylase deficiency. J Clin Endocrinol Metab 1983;56:222-9.

[5] Holcombe JH, Keenan BS, Nichols BL, Kirkland RT, Clayton GW. Neonatal salt loss in the hypertensive form of congenital adrenal hyperplasia. Pediatrics 1980;65:777-81.

[6] Gulati A, Srivastava RN. Hypertension. In: Srivastava RN, Bagga A, eds. Pediatric nephrology, 5th ed. New Delhi, Jaypee Brothers Medical Publishers, 2011:334-59.

[7] Sarafoglou K, Harrington KD, Bockting WO. Congenital adrenal hyperplasia. In: Sarafoglou K, ed. Pediatric endocrinology and inborn errors of metabolism. New York, McGraw Hill, 2009:385-409.

[8] Nimkarn S, New MI. Steroid 11-beta-hydroxylase deficient congenital adrenal hyperplasia. Trends Endocrinol Metab 2008;19(3):96-9.

[9] White PC, Curnow KC, Pascoe L. Disorders of steroid 11-beta- hydroxylase isoenzymes. Endocr Rev 1995;15:421-38.

[10] White PC. Congenital adrenal hyperplasia and related disorders. In: Kliegman RM, Behrman RE, Jenson HB, Stanton BF, eds. Nelson textbook of pediatrics, 18th ed. Philadelphia, PA: Saunders Elsevier, 2007:2360-8.

[11] Famuyiwa OO. Problems and challenges in the practice of endocrinology in a developing country: An overview. Nig Med Pract 1990;20(1):3-6.

[12] Griqoresen Sido A, Weber MM, Griqoresen Sido P, Claumeyers S, Heirich U, Schulze G. 21-hydroxylase and 11-beta- hydroxylase mutations in Romanian patients with classic congenital adrenal hyperplasia. J Clin Endocrinol Metab 2005;90:5769-73.

[13] Cerame BI, New MI. Hormonal hypertension in children: 11 beta- hydroxylase deficiency and apparent mineralocorticoid excess. J Pediatr Endocrinol Metab 2000;13(3):1537-1547

[14] Al Jarallah AS. Reversible cardiomyopathy caused by an uncommon form of congenital adrenal hyperplasia. Pediatr Cardiol 2004;25(6): 675-6.

[15] Isiawe AR, Ekpbegh CO, Fasanmade OA, Ohwovoriole AE. Steroid responsive hypertension secondary to 11-beta-hydroxylase deficiency – a case report. West Afr J Med 2008;27(3):182-5.

In: Child and Adolescent Health Issues
Editor: Joav Merrick

ISBN: 978-1-63463-574-5

Chapter 10

CHILDHOOD ASTHMA IN GEORGIA

Hani M Samawi**, *James H Stephens, Gerald R Ledlow and Ren Chunfeng

Karl E Peace Center for Biostatistics, Jiann-Ping Hsu College Public Health, Georgia Southern University, United States of America

This chapter investigates the childhood asthma in Georgia compared with the combined data of the remaining forty-nine states of the United States based on survey data from the National Survey of Children's Health (NSCH) (2003), provided by the Centers for Disease Control and Prevention in Hyattsville, Maryland. Some risk factors of asthma in Georgia are found to be statistically significant. The comparison with the factors between Georgia and all other states combined is performed to get insight about the problems of childhood asthma in Georgia. Preliminary logistic regression analysis revealed that race, poverty level, weight, and respiratory allergies are significant covariates for childhood asthma in Georgia. However, in the other states, besides those risk factors for Georgia, the analysis revealed that gender, medical preventive care, metropolitan statistical area location, and insurance status are also significant with regards to childhood asthma. Second-hand smoking is beyond the reach of statistical significance as a risk factor for childhood asthma in both Georgia and the combined states.

INTRODUCTION

Asthma has been defined by the National Heart, Lung and Blood Institute as a common chronic disorder of the airway. The disorder is complex and characterized by variable and recurring symptoms, airflow obstruction, bronchial hyperresponsiveness (bronchospasm), and an underlying inflammation amid various acuity levels. Asthma is one of the leading causes of chronic illnesses among children and adolescents in the USA. Childhood asthma can be very disruptive, causing bothersome daily symptoms that interfere with play, sports, school and sleep. In some children, unmanaged asthma can cause serious or even life-threatening

* Correspondence: Hani Samawi, PhD, Jiann-Ping Hsu College of Public Health, Georgia Southern University, POBox 8015, Statesboro, GA 30460-8015, United States. E-mail: hsamawi@georgiasouthern.edu.

acute asthma attacks. Mayo Clinic Staff (1) stated common childhood asthma symptoms are as follows:

- Coughing
- A whistling or wheezing sound when exhaling
- Shortness of breath
- Chest congestion or tightness

Other signs and symptoms of asthma in children include:

- Trouble sleeping caused by shortness of breath, coughing or wheezing
- Bouts of coughing or wheezing that get worse with a respiratory infection such as a cold or the flu
- Delayed recovery or bronchitis after a respiratory infection
- Fatigue or trouble breathing during active play or exercise — signs of exercise-induced asthma

Nationally, asthma prevalence, health service utilization, and mortality (2) have increased among children and adolescents since 1980. The CDC indicated that nationwide, asthma was the third leading cause of hospitalization among children 15 years and younger. The EPA reported that about 23 million people, including 6.8 million children, have asthma in USA. The national economic burden of asthma increased to $14.5 billion by the year 2000 (3). Similarly, a 2008 Georgia health report indicated that approximately 230,000 (10%) children in Georgia have asthma, with approximately 41,000 (11%) middle school students, and approximately 44,000 (10%) high school students. Hospitalization charges related to asthma totaled more than $124 million in 2006. More than 10,000 hospitalizations for asthma occurred in Georgia in 2006. On average, from 2001 to 2006 there were 116 asthma deaths per year.

Thus, investigating factors and disparities in childhood asthma in Georgia is a very important issue to public health and health care delivery organizations. Current knowledge may not draw definitive conclusions about the causes of asthma onset. Better adherence to current recommendations for medical therapy and environmental management of asthma would decrease the burden of this disease. Although asthma is a potentially serious disease, with appropriate medical treatment and environmental measures, most asthma symptoms and associated morbidity can be prevented or managed if risk factors can be identified. Actually, based on the literature, some possible risk factors can be associated with asthma such as metropolitan statistical area (4,5), racial/ethnic minority populations (4,6), gender (7), medical prevention (8,9), insurance (10), family income (6,11), weight (12,13), household secondhand tobacco smoke (14, 15), respiratory allergy (4), and breastfeeding (16,17). Besides the above variables, this project also incorporated age into the study since this variable is biologically important to the response variable.

Our Study

This study investigates childhood asthma risk factors in Georgia and compares these factors against the combined forty-nine states in the United States. The total population of Georgia in 2000 was about 8.2 million as indicated by US Department of Commerce (18) with about 2.2 million children age 17 years or less (see table 1).

The National Survey of Children's Health (19), served as the database for the study. Description of Georgia sample is given in table 2. Table 2 shows that the majority of the sample is white; this may due to that fact that some of the participants did not provide information on their racial/ethnic background, and this subgroup is identified as "Unknown" in the table.

Table 1. 2000 populations

State	Population-All Ages			Under 18 years			Race (Total Population)			
	Total	Male	Female	Total	Male	Female	White	Black	Hispanic	Other
Georgia	8,186,453	4,027,113	4,159340	2,169,234	1,111,589	1,057,645	5,327,281	2,349,542	435,227	74,403

Source: U.S Census Bureau 2000. Total percentage might be over 100% because some people reported more than one race or ethnicity.

Table 2. National Survey of Children's Health sample

	White		African American		Multi-Racial		Other		Unknown		TOTAL	
	♂	♀	♂	♀	♂	♀	♂	♀	♂	♀	♂	♀
GA	629	534	243	228	19	33	28	23	54	55	973	873

Legend: ♂ = Male; ♀ = Female.

In this chapter the focus is on the data that were obtained from the NSCH database, which contains information from all states. To handle and analyze the data SAS Version 9.2 (20)was used. Several statistical techniques were used to achieve the purpose and the aims of our investigation. Those statistical techniques including, the Pearson Chi-square test (21) was used to investigate proportional differences between Georgia (served as the referent state) and the other states combined, involving participants who were diagnosed with asthma, versus those who were not diagnosed with asthma ($\alpha = 0.05$). Also, odds ratios and 95% confidence limits were calculated to assess the magnitude of observed association by racial/ethnic group, age groups and the other risk factors. Finally, to control for the effect of other factors, two multivariate logistic models are used, one for Georgia and one for the other forty-nine states.

Our Findings

There was 12.84% of children in Georgia have ever been advised that they had asthma by a doctor or a health professional, which is higher than 11.93% in the other combined states (see table 3). Thus, investigating the cases of asthma within the state of Georgia is important.

Table 3. Frequency Table for Georgia and the Other States Together

	Childhood Asthma		
States	**No**	**Yes**	**Total**
Georgia	1622 87.16%	239 12.84%	1861 100%
The other states together	88311 88.07%	11963 11.93%	100274 100%
Total	89933 88.05%	12202 11.95%	102135 100 %

A cross-tabulation of childhood's asthma status by potential risk factors for Georgia and the combined other states is presented in Table 4.

Table 4. Cross-tabulation of childhood asthma with potential risk factors of Georgia and other states together

	Georgia				All States			
Covariates	DF	Chi-square test	P-value	Odds ratio	DF	Chi-square test	P-value	Odds ratio
Age group (0-5, 6-10, 11-17)	2	11.22	0.0037		2	936.08	<0.0001	
Gender (male, female)	1	2.44	0.1180	1.24	1	286.42	<0.0001	1.40
Household Smoking (Yes, No)	1	0.52	0.4717	1.12	1	69.87	<0.0001	1.20
Respiratory Allergy (Yes, No)	1	87.59	<0.0001	3.81	1	8235.50	<0.0001	5.88
Metropolitan area (Yes, No)	1	1.23	0.2682	0.85	1	4.21	0.0401	1.06
Weight groups (Overweight, Normal, under weight)	3	17.93	0.0005		3	170.48	<0.0001	
Race (White, black, Hispanic, multi-racial, other)	4	44.30	<0.0001		4	409.42	<0.0001	
Health care coverage (Yes, No)	1	0.68	0.4089	1.25	1	81.16	<0.0001	1.45
Preventive health care (Yes, No)	1	0.76	0.3829	1.26	1	12.97	0.0003	1.14
Breastfed (Yes, No)	1	2.41	0.1203	1.54	1	124.63	<0.0001	0.61
Poverty level (0-99%, 100-199%, 200-399, 400+% FPT)	3	5.17	0.1596		3	121.90	<0.0001	

The data contains mixed types of possible variables, nominal, ordinal, and continuous. We grouped the continuous variables to transform them to categorical variables. Chi-square tests of association are first conducted to search for potential risk factors on childhood asthma in Georgia and in the other combined states (Table 4). At an alpha level of significance of 0.05, we found that age, respiratory allergy, weight level, race, and poverty level are significant factors affecting childhood asthma in Georgia. In the other states, all factors are found to be significant to asthma.

Table 4 indicates that age is a significant factor for childhood asthma without controlling for other factors. It seems that in Georgia and in the other states, the odds of getting asthma at an older age are less than for a child at a younger age.

Multivariate analysis

Multivariate analysis is used to study the effect of the significant factors found in Table 4 on childhood asthma controlling for other factors. The use of 0.25 as the criterion of screening for factors in the multivariate models is based on the work by (22) on linear regression and by (23) on logistic regression. After fitting the multivariate model, the importance of each variable should be verified by first checking the individual Wald test, then log-likelihood ratio test and potential confounder checking. Variables not contributing to the model based on these criteria should be removed from the model and a new model fit. The new model should be compared to the old model using log-likelihood ratio test. This process of deleting, refitting, and verifying continues until all important variables are included in the model and the excluded variables are not either significant or biologically important to the model.

Model assumption checks of the final models are performed to check the validity of our final models (24). Before the logistic regression models for Georgia and the other states combined are used to describe the relationship between asthma and its predictors, the fit of the models should be assessed. The approach usually consists of five steps: multicolinearity diagnostics, interaction check, computation and evaluation of overall measures of fit; and graphical examination of the individual components of the summary statistics.

For Georgia data, all the interaction terms are not significant in the model. However, for the combined states data, there are 5 interaction terms significant to the model. When an explanatory variable is nearly a linear combination of other explanatory variables in the model, the estimates of the coefficients in the regression model are unstable and have high standard errors. This problem is called collinearity. The Collinearity Diagnostics table is calculated using the eigenstructure of the X'X matrix. A collinearity problem exists when a component associated with a high condition index contributes strongly to the variance of two or more variables. Belsley et al. (25) proposed that a condition index of 30 to 100 indicates moderate to strong collinearity. The highest condition number is 15.24 which appear not to support multicolinearity. However, for the other states together, the largest condition index is 57.02 (19.01 for the model without any interaction term), which seems high multicolinearity does exist. After we removed several interaction terms, the highest condition index was 22.29.

Hosmer-Lemeshow Tests are usually used to evaluate overall measures of fit. The value of Lemeshow and Hosmer about goodness-of-fit test statistic computed is 8.88 for Georgia data. The corresponding p-value is 0.3528, indicating the model seems to fit quite well for Georgia data.

Similarly, the value of Lemeshow and Hosmer about goodness-of-fit test statistic computed is 12.83 for the other states together data. The corresponding p-value is 0.1177, indicating the model seems to fit well for the other states together data.

The index plots are useful to identify extreme values. The index plots of the Pearson residuals and the deviance residuals for Georgia indicate that no cases are poorly accounted for by the model. The index plot of the diagonal elements of the hat matrix for Georgia indicates that there are some extreme cases in the data. After removing these observations, the largest coefficient rate change is 94.2%. Thus, from statistical analysis perspective, these observations cannot be removed from the model.

For the combined states, 3 cases are found to be extreme. However, after removing these observations, the largest coefficient rate change is less than 5%. Thus, we can conclude that there are no potential outliers in the other states together model.

CONCLUSION AND FINAL REMARKS

Using univariate analysis for Georgia data, we found that age, respiratory allergy, poverty level, weight level, and race were all factors affecting childhood asthma with 95% odds ratio confidence intervals (0.939, 0.988), (2.84, 5.12), (1.011,1.324), (1.154,1.560), (1.667,2.977) (White versus Black), (1.078, 3.883) (other versus Black), respectively. Similarly, for the combined states, we found that besides the above five variables, second-hand smoking, metropolitan statistical area location, medical preventive care, and insurance status are all significant to childhood asthma.

The final model for Georgia (table 5) revealed that when the other independent variables are controlled, one year increase in age has no significant effect on childhood asthma. From one weight level to another weight level (underweight, normal weight, at risk for overweight, and overweight), the odds of children overweight are higher than the odds of lower weight children to develop an asthma. The odds for blacks to develop asthma is 2.41 (1.679, 3.457) times higher than for whites and 5.58 (1.69, 18.86) times more than other groups. There are no significant differences on asthma based on poverty level. Moreover, the odds of children with respiratory allergy are 4.413 (3.122, 6.229) times higher than children without respiratory allergies to develop asthma.

For the combined states (see table 6), controlling for the other variables in the model, a one year increase in age didn't result in a significant effect on asthma. Similar to the result of Georgia, from one weight level to another weight level (underweight, normal weight, at risk for overweight, and overweight), the odds of overweight children is higher than the odds of lower weight children to develop asthma. Moving from one poverty level to another (0-99% FPL, 100-199% FPL, 200-399% FPL, and 400% FPL or greater), the odds of poorer children to acquire asthma is higher than those with better income. The odds for blacks are 1.555 (1.432,1.687) times higher than whites to develop asthma and 1.19 (1.05, 1.36) times higher than others to develop asthma. The odds for children living in metropolitan statistical areas are 1.161 (1.087,1.241) times higher than those not living in metropolitan statistical areas to develop asthma. Medical preventive care and insurance status are also statistically significant to childhood asthma, whose 95% confidence intervals of odds ratios (No versus Yes) were

(0.718, 0.868) and (0.713, 0.932), respectively. Gender and respiratory allergies were difficult to interpret since there are significant interaction terms expressed in the models.

Table 5. Final model for Georgia (after removing some observations)

Parameter	Estimate	Standard Error	Wald Chi-Square	Odds Ratio		Pr > Chi Sq
				Point estimate	95% CI	
Age groups (0-5, 6-10, 11-17)	0.0197	0.0186	1.1162	1.020	(0.983,1.058)	0.4410
Weight level (Underweight, normal, at risk of overweight, overweight)	0.3083	0.0920	11.2168	1.361	(1.136,1.630)	0.0024
RACER (black vs other)	-1.7377	0.6164	7.9487	0.176	(0.053, 0.589)	0.0028
RACER (black vs white)	-0.8793	0.1843	22.7711	0.415	(0.289,0.596)	<.0001
Poverty level (0-99%, 100-199%, 200-399, 400+% FPT)	-0.1027	0.0867	1.4043	0.902	(0.761,1.069)	0.2375
Respiratory Allergy (Yes, No)	1.4845	0.1759	71.2233	4.413	(3.126,6.229)	<.0001

Table 6. Final Model for the Other States Together

Factors	Estimate	Standard Error	Odds ratio	
			Point Estimate*	95% CI
Age groups (0-5, 6-10, 11-17)	0.00840	0.0101	1.008	(0.989,1.029)
Gender (Male, female)	-0.6724	0.0751	1.234	(0.865,1.258)
			1.043	(0.992,1.097)
Respiratory allergy (Yes, no)	-1.9019	0.0751	0.905	(0.986,1.104)
			1.043	(0.992,1.097
Weight level (Underweight, normal, at risk of overweight, overweight)	0.1489	0.0163	1.121	(1.124,1.198)
Poverty level (0-99%, 100-199%, 200-399, 400+% FPT)	-0.1484	0.0157	0.862	(0.836,0.889)
Insurance (yes, no)	-0.2045	0.0685	0.815	(0.713,0.932)
RACER (black vs white)	0.4412	0.0418	1.555	(1.432,1.687)
Others vs white)	0.2631	0.0555	1.301	(1.167,1.451)
Preventative Medical Care (yes, no)	-0.2364	0.0481	0.789	(0.718,0.868)
Metropolitan Statistical Area	0.1497	0.0339	1.161	(1.087,1.241)
Interaction (age*respiratory allergy)	0.0336	0.00647		
Interaction (age*gender)	-0.0284	0.00653		

* The point estimate of odds ratio for each group of gender and respiratory allergy represents when age changes in 5 years and the other covariates are fixed.

In short, when the other variables were controlled, age was not significantly associated with childhood asthma in both Georgia and the combined states. In Georgia, race, weight level, and respiratory allergies are risk factors for childhood asthma while poverty level is barely significant in the model. However, in the combined states, besides those risk factors, gender, metropolitan statistical area, and poverty level are also found to be risk factors for childhood asthma. Medical preventive care and insurance status were negatively associated with childhood asthma. Compared with the combined states, Georgia had less risk factors associated with childhood asthma; also, there is no significant difference for race.

The data in this project is a representative sample based on National Children Health Survey (NCHS) 2003. Two logistic models were developed to draw meaningful conclusions and comparisons on the basis of purposeful logistic model selection. Insurance status and medical preventive care are negatively associated with asthma. Further analysis should be implemented based on NCHS 2007 survey data to verify this result. If the response variable is "currently, does your child have asthma?" instead of "in the past 12 months, has your child ever been told they have asthma", maybe different results will be found. However, this study agrees with prior findings in the literature.

ACKNOWLEDGMENTS

We are grateful to the Center for Child and Adolescent Health for providing us with the 2003 National Survey of Children's Health. Also, we would like to thank the referees and the associate editor for their valuable comments which improved the manuscript.

REFERENCES

[1] Mayo Clinic Staff. Childhood asthma. Accessed 2009May 5. URL:http://www. mayoclinic. com/health/childhood-asthma/DS00849/DSECTION=symptoms
[2] Gergen PJ. The increasing problem of asthma in the United States. Am Rev Respir Dis 1992; 146:823-4.
[3] Jack E, Boss L, Millington WA. Speakers kit for public health professionals. Atlanta, GA: Centers Disease Control Prevention, 1999.
[4] Noreen MC, Randall WB, Edith PL. Childhood asthma. Environl Health Perspect 1999;107:421-9.
[5] Floyd JM, Sheryl AF. Environmental risk factors of childhood asthma in urban centers. Environ Health Perspect 1995;103(Suppl6):58-62.
[6] Lauren AS, Juliet LH, Richard W, Robert SK. Rethinking race/ethnicity, income, and childhood asthma: Racial/ethnic disparities concentrated among the very poor. Public Health Rep2005;120:109-20.
[7] Bernard A, Carbonnelle S, Burbure CD. Chlorinated pool attendance, atopy, and the risk of asthma during childhood. Environ Health Perspect 2006;114(10):1567-73.
[8] Shahani AK, Korve N, Jones KP, Paynton DJ. Towards an operational model for prevention and treatment of asthma attacks. J Operation Res Soc1994;45(8):916-26.
[9] Yates CE. Prevention and treatment of asthma. Dissertation. South Hampton: Faculty Math Stud, Univ South Hampton, 1989.
[10] Yu C, Martin JB. Helicobacter pylori colonization is inversely associated with childhood asthma. J Infect Dis 2008;198:553-60.
[11] Miller JE. The effects of race/ethnicity and income on early childhood asthma prevalence and health care use. Am J Public Health2000;90:428-30.
[12] Schachtera LM, Salomea CM, Peatb JK. Obesity is a risk for asthma and wheeze but not airway hyperresponsiveness. Thorax2001;56:4-8.
[13] Tim JT, Sutherland JOC, Sarah Y. The association between obesity and asthma-interactions between systemic and airway inflammation. Am J RespirCrit Care Med 2008;178:469-75.
[14] Gilliland FD, Li YF, Peters JM. Effects of maternal smoking during pregnancy and environmental tobacco smoke on asthma and wheezing in children. Am J Respir Crit Care Med 2001;163(2):429-36.
[15] Sturm JJ, Yeatts K, Loomis D. Effects of tobacco smoke exposure on asthma prevalence and medical care use in North Carolina middle school children. Am J Public Health 2004;94(2):308-13.

[16] Yousuke T, Yutaka S, Satoshi H. Relation between breastfeeding and the prevalence of asthma. Am J Epidemiol 2001;154(2):115-9.

[17] Raisler J, Alexander C, O'Campo P. Breast-feeding and infant illness: Adose- response relationship? Am J Public Health1999;89:25–30.

[18] US Department of Commerce. United States Census: 2000 census of population and housing. Washington, DC: US Department of Commerce. Accessed 2009 Jul 09. URL: http://www.census.gov/prod/cen2000/index.html.

[19] Child and Adolescent Health Measurement Initiative 2003. National survey of children with special health care needs: Indicator dataset 6. Data Resource Center for Child and Adoles-cent Health website. Accessed 2009 Jul 9. URL: www.childhealthdata.org.

[20] SAS Institute. SAS/STAT Version 9.1. Cary, NC: SAS Institute, 2010.

[21] Agresti A. Categorical data analysis. New York: John Wiley, 1990.

[22] Bendel, RB, Afifi, AA. Comparison of stopping rules in forward regression. J Am Statistical Assoc1977;72:46-53.

[23] Mickey J, Greenland S. The impact of confounder selection criteria on effect estimation. Am J Epidemiol1989;129:125-37.

[24] Hosmer DW, Lemeshow S. Applied logistic regression. New York: John Wiley, 1989.

[25] Belsley DA, Kuh E, Welsch RE. Regression diagnostics. New York: John Wiley, 1980.

In: Child and Adolescent Health Issues
Editor: Joav Merrick

ISBN: 978-1-63463-574-5

Chapter 11

CHILDREN WITH ASTHMA: WHAT ABOUT THE QUALITY OF LIFE OF THEIR PARENTS?

***Anna Trzcieniecka-Green, MA, PhD*[1], *Kamilla Bargiel-Matusiewicz, MA, PhD*[2], *Agnieszka Wilczyńska, MA, PhD*[3] *and Hatim A Omar, MD*[4*]**

[1]Department of Social Sciences, Katowice School of Economics, Katowice, Poland
[2]Faculty of Psychology, University of Warsaw, Warsaw, Poland
[3]Faculty of Psychology, Silesian University, Katowice, Poland
[4]Division of Adolescent Medicine, Kentucky Children's Hospital, University of Kentucky College of Medicine, Lexington, Kentucky, United States of America

An increased frequency of asthma in children has been lately observed. The course of asthma depends not only on treatment, but also on the actions taken by the parents of a sick child. Design: A non-experimental cross-sectional design. Methods: In this study the Pediatric Asthma Quality of Life Questionnaire (PACQLQ) and Satisfaction with Life Scale (SWLS) were administered to 60 parents of children with asthma. Two groups of parents were compared. The first group consisted of parents of children who had been diagnosed with asthma less than three months before the beginning of the study. The second group consisted of parents of children who had been diagnosed at least one year previously. Results: It was observed that, in the group of parents aged 20-30 years, the level of life satisfaction was significantly higher for parents of children who had suffered from asthma for at least one year than for the parents of children recently diagnosed with asthma. There were no statistically significant differences in the other age groups. There was a positive correlation between the level of satisfaction with life and emotional functioning in the parents of children diagnosed recently. Conclusions: The results of the present study point to a general ability of parents to adapt to the situation of having an ill child. This may be related to the relative ease of access to information that enables parents to understand more about the condition.

---

* Correspondence: Professor Hatim A Omar, MD, Division of Adolescent Medicine and Young Parents Program, KY Clinic, J422, Lexington, KY 40536-0284, United States. E-mail: haomar2@uky.edu

Introduction

An increased prevalence of asthma in children has been reported (1). The course of asthma depends not only on treatment, but also on the actions taken by the parents of a sick child (2,3). Caring for a patient with asthma requires a lot more work than caring for a healthy child (4,5). Accordingly, this study focused on the quality of life and satisfaction with life of those who take care of children with asthma.

Quality of life has become an issue of interest for both academics and practitioners. At the academic level, quality of life is treated as a concept that is largely based, on objective factors, whereas the concept of well-being is more subjective (6). Problems with definition arise from the fact that the quality of life concept has its origins in the medical and economic sciences, whereas the concepts of well-being and satisfaction with life are commonly used in psychology (7).

Background

The authors of this paper applied research tools that made it possible to capture these two perspectives and to analyse the relationships between them.

The World Health Organisation (WHO) distinguishes six basic domains related to quality of life: the physical dimension (pain and discomfort, energy and fatigue, sleep and rest, sex and sensory functions); the psychological domain (positive and negative feelings, body image and cognitive processes, and self-esteem); independence (mobility, activities of daily living, working capacity, lack of dependence on medication); social relationships (practical social support, personal relationships, behaviours that support others); environment (freedom and physical safety and security, home environment, satisfaction with work, financial resources, recreation and leisure, access to health and social care) and spiritual domain.

In order to reduce errors and to conduct a deep analysis of a patient's mental and physical state, standard surveys are used to study quality of life. There are general, specific, and mixed surveys. General surveys are used to assess the quality of life of healthy and sick people, and are intended for use with those with a number of conditions, irrespective of their nature. Specific surveys assess quality of life in patients with a specific condition or a group of conditions, and include questions on the course of an illness and its symptoms.

In patients with allergies, quality of life means not only a lack of symptoms but it also refers to the emotional, social, and professional domains, as well as activity and the possibility of self-fulfilment. In the case of asthma, an important role is played by the fear related to their expected occurrence, which is often the reason that patients feel less comfortable and have the sense that their life is in danger even if the symptoms do not occur. The satisfaction with life concept is based primarily on mood, the balance of emotional experience, and the emotional attitude to one's life (6).

A chronic disease is connected with a particularly strong emotional involvement, especially for the parents of the patient. It may become a factor that threatens family integrity or, conversely, it may improve the functioning of the entire family (8).

The behaviour and emotional state of such parents of children with chronic illnesses often display negative changes, involving fear and feelings of hopelessness and helplessness. Some studies have indicated the possibility of finding a deeper sense of a difficult situation, and experiencing satisfaction and joy in connection with performing activities related, among others, to providing care for an ill person (9,10). The parents' attitudes and emotions have a considerable influence on the psychological comfort of an ill child. They may either be a source of support and provide a sense of security, or be a source of fear and provide a sense of helplessness.

OUR STUDY

The authors obtained approval from the Ethics Committee at University of Warsaw to perform the study. The Polish version of the Satisfaction with Life Scale SWLS (11) was used to measure satisfaction with life, as expressed through a sense of satisfaction with one's achievements and conditions. The scale has five items, and the answers are based on a seven-point scale. The Pediatric Asthma Caregiver's Quality of Life Questionnaire PACQLQ (12) was used to measure the parents' quality of life. The PACQLQ tool comprises 13 questions, four of which are related to restrictions in functioning, with the remaining nine describing emotional factors. The answers are given on the basis of a seven-point scale.

The study involved 60 parents of children treated in the pediatric ward and the allergy clinic of the John Paul II Pediatric Centre in Sosnowiec, Katowice urban area in Poland. The study group included 30 parents of children who had just been diagnosed with asthma, and 30 parents of children who had been ill for at least one year. The parents ranged in age from 20-47 years, with the average age being approximately 32 years. Most of the participants in the study were married (91.7%), and most of the parents were employed (78.3%). The analysis covered three age groups (20-30, 31-40 and 41-47 years), and was based on the Kruskal-Wallis test, which is a non-parametric equivalent of the one-way analysis of variance.

Statistical analysis of correlation between the two measures used in the study was based on Spearman correlation coefficient R.

OUR FINDINGS

The analysis of differences in the quality of life between a group of parents whose children had been diagnosed with asthma during the last three months and those whose children had been sick for at least a year did not show statistically significant differences. This was true of both aspects of the quality of life studied using PACQLQ. Put differently, the time that had elapsed since the time of diagnosis had no significant effect on parents' sense of having limited possibilities for action or their emotional functioning.

The analysis of differences in satisfaction with life (measured with SWLS) between the two groups of parents showed that the differences occurred only for people aged 20-30 years.

It was observed that in 20-30 year-olds, the level of satisfaction with life was significantly higher (chi-square (1)=5.17; $p<0.05$) for parents of children who had been suffering from asthma for at least a year than in parents of children recently diagnosed with asthma (see figure 1).

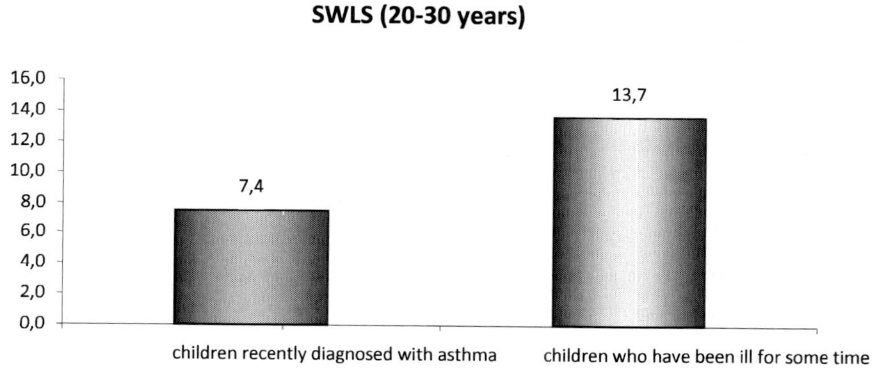

Figure 1. Differences in satisfaction with life between parents of children recently diagnosed with asthma and those whose children had been diagnosed at least one year previously.

The correlation between satisfaction with life (measured with SWLS) and emotional functioning (measured with PACQLQ) of parents of children who had recently been diagnosed with asthma was statistically significant (R=0.42: p<0.005). There was no such correlation for parents whose children had been ill for at least a year (R= 0.05 p=0.392).

DISCUSSION

As mentioned above, parents' emotions and attitude have a considerable impact on the psychological and physical comfort of children suffering from asthma. The purpose of the study was to investigate whether the quality of life and satisfaction with life of the parents depend on the stage of the child's illness.

Two groups of parents were compared: those whose children had recently been diagnosed with asthma and those whose children had been ill for at least a year. Differences in the quality of life reported by these two groups were not statistically significant.

The areas studied within the concept of the quality of life included activity limitation and emotional problems parents experience as a result of their child's asthma. Thus it may be concluded that these areas do not show large changes related to the time that has passed since a child was diagnosed with asthma. However, although the differences recorded were not statistically significant, the general tendency showed that slightly higher scores for the quality of life were recorded by parents whose children had been ill for at least a year. It might demonstrate the ability of parents to adapt to an existing situation.

With regard to satisfaction with life, it was observed that, in the age group comprising 20 - 30 year olds, the level of satisfaction was significantly higher in parents whose children had been suffering from asthma for at least a year when compared with those whose children had been recently diagnosed with asthma. No statistically significant differences were observed in other age groups. Thus, younger parents might have a greater capacity to adapt to coping with chronic disease in their child.

The adaptation to the new situation immediately after receiving the diagnosis requires the family to reorganize family life and resign from current habits. This poses a considerable challenge for parents. At the same time the parents might suffer anxiety and uncertainty as to whether they will be able to face the challenge. A study conducted by Trojanowska and Emeryk (8) showed that the diagnosis of children with bronchial asthma affects their parents' emotional functioning. Furthermore, it can be observed that there is a positive dependence among the seriousness of the condition, side effects of the therapy, financial burden and the quality of life of parents whose children suffer from asthma.

Everyday life is often more stable in families that have dealt with a child's illness for a relatively long period of time. The parents are experienced and can cope with asthma attacks and treatment-related inconvenience. Callery and Milnes (13) suggest that relationships between parents and nurses are especially important as far as adaptation to the situation is concerned.

The significant difference in satisfaction with life between the two subsets within the group of 20-30-year-old parents may mean that younger parents adapt most easily to a child's illness and they tend to be optimistic. Therefore after a period of anxiety and experiencing difficulties with the introduction of activities related to providing care for the child, their satisfaction with life grows. Equally it is possible that a factor correlated with the age of the parents, not the age alone, might account for the differences observed.

However, although the results of the present study point to a general ability of parents to adapt to the situation of having an ill child, no significant differences were found in the quality of life between the parents of children who had just been diagnosed with asthma, and the parents of children who had been ill for at least one year.

This may result from the fact that, with current medical care, anxiety related to the diagnosis, and uncertainty in relation to the character of the illness and the prognosis, can be reduced much more quickly than in the past. This is related to the relative ease of access to information that enables parents to understand more about the condition.

In addition, support groups, including those active on internet forums, allow parents with greater experience to help those who have just received a diagnosis of their child's illness. Parents can thus obtain additional information and receive emotional support.

The results of this study also showed that, in the group of parents whose children had recently been diagnosed with asthma, there was a positive correlation between the sense of satisfaction with life and emotional functioning related directly to the child's illness. No such effect was observed in the more experienced group of parents.

An interpretation of this finding may be based on the “Onion” theory of happiness developed by Czapiński (14), who proposed that the sense of happiness is made up of three layers. The outer-most part, which is most vulnerable to changes, covers current affective experience and partial satisfaction related to a number of life aspects - e.g. professional work, place of residence, close interpersonal relations and current health condition.

The middle part combines affective balance with a sense of the purpose and meaning of life. The inner-most - and most stable - layer is the will to live, which is to a large extent determined genetically.

The results of the current study show that, following an initial period characterised by a clear relationship between a child's illness and general satisfaction with life, these variables are no longer significantly linked to each other.

In the parents of children who had been ill for at least a year, no correlation was noticed between these two variables. Thus it may be assumed that emotions related to a child's illness in this group of parents are mostly connected with the outer-most layer of the sense of happiness, and have no impact on the general satisfaction with life, which is related more closely to the deeper layers.

The relationship could be seen only in parents whose children had recently been diagnosed with asthma. It has been confirmed by numerous scientific studies that difficult situations reduce well-being only for limited period. An internal mechanism of affective regulation, called the hedonic treadmill, makes it possible to return to the previous level of satisfaction with life (15).

Conclusion

The results of the present study point to a general ability of parents to adapt to the situation of having an ill child. This may be related to the relative ease of access to information that enables parents to understand more about the condition. Based on these results, parents of children ill with bronchial asthma need the support from medical staff and psychological help especially during the first year after diagnosis. The results also indicated that cooperation between nurses and psychologists was especially important as far as patients' quality of life is concerned.

Acknowledgments

The paper was financed with educational funds for the year 2012 as a research project no. BST 164645/2012. There are no conflicts of interest.

References

[1] Asher MJ, Weiland SK. The international study of asthma and allergies in childhood (ISAAC). Clin Exp Allergy 1998;28(Suppl):52-66.

[2] Ritz T, Steptoe A, DeWilde S, Costa M. Emotions and stress increase respiratory resistance in asthma. Psychosom Med 2000;62:401-12.

[3] Lehrer P, Feldman J, Giardino N, Song H, Schmaling K. Psychological aspects of asthma. J Consult Clin Psychol 2002;70:691-711.

[4] Milton B, Whitehead M, Holland P, Hamilton V. The social and economic consequences of childhood asthma cross the life course: a systematic review. Child Care Hlth Dev 2004;30:711-28.

[5] Tzeng LF, Chiang LC, Hsueh KC, Ma WF, Fu LS. A preliminary study to evaluate a patient-centred asthma education programme on parental control of home environment and asthma signs and symptoms in children with moderate-to- severe asthma. J Clin Nurs 2010;19:1424-33.

[6] Diener E, Lucas RE. Personality and subjective well-being. In: Kahneman D, Diener E, Schwarz N. Well-being: The foundations of hedonic psychology. New York: Russell Sage Foundation, 1999:213-29.

[7] Trzebińska E. Positive psychology. Warszawa: Wydawnictwa Akademickie i Profesjonalne, 2008. [Polish]

[8] Trojanowska A, Emeryk A. Selected aspects of quality of life in parents of children with bronchial asthma. Public Health 2009;119:399-402.

[9] Folkman S, Moskowitz JT. Stress, positive emotion and coping. Curr Dir Psychol Sci 2000;9:115-8.

[10] Folkman S, Moskowitz JT. Coping: Pitfalls and promise. Annu Rev Psychol 2004;55:745–74.

[11] Pavot W, Diener E. The Satisfaction with life scale and the emerging construct of life satisfaction. J Positive Psychol 2008;3:137-52.

[12] Juniper EF, Guyatt GH, Ferrie DH, Ferrie PJ, Griffith LE, Townsed M. Measuring quality of life in the parents of children with asthma. Qual Life Res 1996;5:27-34.

[13] Callery P, Milnes L. Communication between nurses, children and their parents in asthma review consultations. J Clin Nurs 2012;21:1641-50.

[14] Czapinski J. Positive psychology. Warszawa: Wyd Nauk PWN, 2005. [Polish]

[15] Diener E, Lukas RE, Napa Scolon C. Beyond the hedonic treademill. Revising the adaptation theory of well-being. Am Psychol 2006;5:305-14.

In: Child and Adolescent Health Issues
Editor: Joav Merrick

ISBN: 978-1-63463-574-5

Chapter 12

BIBLIOTHERAPY'S EFFECT ON ANXIETY IN CHILDREN WITH CANCER

Nicole M Schneider, PsyD*, Mary Peterson, PhD, Kathleen A Gathercoal, PhD and Elizabeth Hamilton, PhD

Graduate Department of Clinical Psychology, George Fox University, Newberg, Oregon, United States of America

Children who have cancer and undergo various treatment procedures tend to have higher levels of emotional distress than their peers. Although traditional therapy can be effective in decreasing such distress, bibliotherapy has been found to be a convenient, inexpensive, effective psychological intervention. This study examined how reading a disease-relevant story, embedded with literature-supported coping strategies, influenced a child's chronic illness-related distress. It was expected that children who read this book would experience a decrease in their perceived distress compared to their pre-intervention level distress. Twenty-one children ages 4 to 12 with various cancers, primarily hematological diagnoses, were recruited for this study and asked to rate their functioning across several domains utilizing the Child Outcome Rating Scale and a supplemental form targeting perceived physiological arousal. Participants were read an illustrated bibliotherapy intervention and subsequently asked to rate themselves utilizing the same scale both immediately after and several months later. Results indicate that perceptions of intrapersonal functioning improved and physiological arousal decreased immediately after the initial book reading. Significant improvements were found several months after the initial intervention when books were left with participants. This study demonstrates the value of a low-investment intervention.

INTRODUCTION

Anxiety is the most common mental health problem in children, with 13% of children aged 9 to 17 in the United States experiencing it (1). Anxiety is paired with physiological arousal,

* Correspondence: Nicole Schneider, PsyD, George Fox University, Graduate Department of Clinical Psychology. 422 N. Meridian St. V277, Newberg, OR 97132 United States. E-mail: nik.m.schneider@gmail.com

including a more rapid heart rate and increased blood pressure in individuals experiencing such extreme stress (2). A child's constant worry may result in numerous somatic issues, including headaches, stomachaches, nausea, dizziness, and respiration (3). In up to half of those individuals who experience anxiety, co-occurring mental health problems also exist; usually the co-occurring problem is another anxiety disorder or a mood disorder, like depression (1).

Sub-clinical levels of anxiety are even more common and may occur in up to 25% of the general population of children. These symptoms may develop or become further exacerbated by stressful life events, which include a myriad of traumatic family situations or major life changes, like the death of a loved one, divorce of parents, birth of a sibling, or sudden or major illness or accident (3). While sub-clinical anxiety may later diminish, depending on a variety of factors and circumstances, it can also progress into clinically significant anxiety. As such, early intervention in sub-clinical levels of anxiety may prevent the development of future mental health problems.

Anxiety and cancer

While anxiety is quite common among children in the general population, its prevalence is particularly high in children who have serious health conditions and who are undergoing ongoing medical procedures, as in the case of cancer. Children with cancer have trouble managing their stressors, especially those related to their medical care, which increases their overall anxiety (4). In one study examining this population, 27% of children who were recently diagnosed with acute lymphoblastic leukemia (ALL) in the month prior were found to be at risk for clinically significant anxiety (5).

The ALL study indicates that children with cancer experience a rate of anxiety that is twice as common as that in the general population. This is of concern because with anxiety often comes a decrease in quality of life; individuals who are anxious may be in a constant state of worry and even feel the physical burden of these emotions.

Predictors of increased stress and anxiety

There are several factors that have been demonstrated to be related to the level of anxiety that children with cancer experience. One predictor of emotional stress is the age at which a child is diagnosed with cancer, as it is inversely related to his or her level of anxiety; those diagnosed at a younger age tend to have more anxiety than those diagnosed at an older age (6). Presumably, this difference is due to a lack of development of cognitive skills that coping strategies hinge upon (7). Therefore, although cancer is unarguably traumatic for nearly any individual, it is even more so challenging for young children, which contributes to high levels of anxiety.

Another contributor to one's anxiety level is gender. In a comprehensive study of child survivors conducted in 2009, females were found to endorse anxiety symptoms one and a half times more often than males (8). While there are likely a number of contributing factors, many attribute this phenomenon to gender role socialization. For example, females' externalization of anxiety and worry tend to be reinforced more so than males, who are often socialized to "get over it" (9).

Anxiety levels are also related to pain levels. Anticipatory anxiety often co-occurs with pain, which is especially concerning since cancer medical procedures are often physically demanding. Bone-marrow biopsies, blood tests, and central line surgeries are all common cancer-related procedures that children are faced with experiencing during and following diagnosis (10). Not surprisingly, research has shown that children who have cancer are forced to employ coping strategies that are far beyond what a typical, healthy child would normally utilize (7).

Treatments for anxiety in children

Recently, research efforts have been devoted to studying symptoms of anxiety and emotional distress in children and discovering the most effective treatment methods. Treatment interventions for anxious children most often include traditional cognitive-behavioral therapy with a counselor or psychologist once per week over the course of several months (11). In working to diminishing anxiety, relaxation training is often utilized, in which individuals learn to be attuned to their breathing and their body's physical tension (12). Successful treatment occurs when patients are able to regulate their breathing and reduce muscle tension, which in turn reduces symptoms of anxiety, because stress and relaxation are mutually exclusive. Additionally, self-monitoring can be utilized, in which children rate how anxiety provoking a specific situation or event is, and how it affects them emotionally and physically (3). In such therapy sessions, the mental health professional focuses on helping the child recognize, understand, and learn appropriate coping skills to manage symptoms of anxiety.

Reducing anxiety in children with cancer

For children with cancer, there are a variety of attempts to manage treatment-related anxiety. Avoidant coping, which involves denying or evading the ongoing stressor, has been correlated with children's increased depression and anxiety (6). In contrast, acknowledging and working to emotionally cope with or adapt to the stressor is inversely related to anxiety (13). Further, encouraging self-statements by both parents and children has been associated with a more effective and less stressful adjustment to cancer with decreased levels of hopelessness (14).

Distraction is a coping strategy that is associated with less fear and distress when used during a medical procedure (15). When this strategy was encouraged with imagery and relaxation during physically demanding procedures, children reported having, on average, no additional fear after the intervention than they had originally.

One notable change, however, was their perceived level of pain, which was *reduced* following the distraction, visualization, and relaxation tactics (16). Other effective strategies to lessen anxiety include helping children learn more about their illness and teaching them to be inquisitive about their disease (6).

An adjunctive method to reduce anxiety is bibliotherapy, in which books are utilized as a form of therapy. These books provide the individual with tools needed to better cope with their current life situation. Although not as effective as traditional psychotherapy, bibliotherapy has been found to be more effective than no therapy at all; giving non-cancer patients with mild to moderate anxiety psychoeducational literature about relaxation techniques and stress management diminished overall anxiety (17-18). Bibliotherapy interventions eliminated anxiety disorders in 15% of the sample children. In addition, this intervention can also be helpful in improving the problem-solving abilities of individuals (19).

Practically, bibliotherapy is far less expensive and much more accessible than traditional therapy, with an intervention book costing as little as $10. Psychotherapy, in contrast, is a far more financially-laden venture; a single counseling session by a mental health professional typically ranges from about $100 to $200 per 50-minute session and also requires one to navigate the logistics of scheduling an appropriate referral. Furthermore, psychotherapy is time-intensive, lasting several months at minimum, and labor-intensive, requiring the child's parents to schedule and attend sessions when their schedules are likely crowded with other medical appointments. Taken together, psychotherapy is quite costly when compared to bibliotherapy interventions (11). Although bibliotherapy may not be as effective as traditional psychotherapy, this economically and time efficient intervention holds a great deal of merit.

Bibliotherapy can be very helpful for children with cancer because it teaches individuals how to deal effectively with problems that are out of one's control and that cannot necessarily be eradicated (20). When bibliotherapy books have a character who the child can relate to, then children have a "powerful tool" to help them develop coping strategies (21; p. 19). Discussing the contents of the book is a crucial element of bibliotherapy, because the opportunity to generalize and apply the coping strategies allows the information to become an individualized intervention, thus increasing its effectiveness as a psychological tool (20). In addition, a bibliotherapy text can be read by a parent, allowing the natural parent-child relationship to further develop (22).

Not surprisingly, being diagnosed and subsequently receiving treatment for cancer presents a major, stressful change in both the life of the ill child and the life of his or her family. Though cancer treatment regimens vary depending on type and stage of cancer, among a myriad of other factors, the ensuing distress can last for months or even years. For children who are undergoing cancer treatments, therapeutic interventions can help them learn to cope with the psychological side effects of their disease.

Bibiotherapy is an accessible, relatively inexpensive, and yet still effective psychological tool for reducing anxiety. It is hypothesized that reading a children's book that describes what a character undergoes when he or she has cancer, along with coping strategies employed, will improve a child's subjective perception of functioning and decrease their perceived emotional distress.

OUR STUDY

Participants were English-speaking male and female children aged 4 to 12 years (M = 9.1, SD = 2.1) who had been diagnosed with cancer and undergoing or had recently completed treatment. Approximately 57% of participants were Caucasian (n = 12), 29% were Hispanic (n = 6), and 14% were African-American (n = 3). Fifty-seven percent were male (n = 12) and

43% were female (*n* = 9). Most participants had acute lymphoblastic leukemia (ALL) diagnoses (*n* = 14). Table 1 highlights the demographic distribution of the participants.

Table 1. Demographic data

	n	%
Gender		
Male	12	57.1
Female	9	49.2
Ethnicity		
Caucasian	12	57.1
African-American	3	14.3
Hispanic	6	28.6
Diagnosis*		
Acute Lymphoblastic Leukemia (ALL)	14	66.7
Other leukemia	1	4.8
Lymphoma	2	9.5
Neuroblastoma	1	4.8
Kidney cancer	1	4.8
Osteosarcoma	1	4.8
Hepatoblastoma	1	4.8
Unknown	1	4.8
Treatment Type**		
Chemotherapy	17	81.0
Radiation	2	9.5
Surgery	9	42.9
Oral medication only	1	4.8
Unknown	3	14.3
Treatment Clinic Type		
Inpatient	2	9.5
Outpatient	9	42.9
Both	7	33.3
Unknown	3	14.3
Primary Caregiver's Marital Status		
Married/Partnered	7	33.3
Divorced	3	14.3
Single/Widowed	7	33.3
Unknown	4	19.0

*Percentages do not add up to 100; one child had dual cancer diagnoses.

**Percentages do not add up to 100; many children received more than one treatment during their illness.

Procedure

As part of the informed consent process, patients and their caregivers were shown the intervention book, *Nikki's Day at Chemo*. The book was developed for this study and was embedded with coping strategies for a child diagnosed with cancer including the emotional implications of diagnosis and treatment. This bound book was written in English, illustrated with color pictures, and independently published. The intervention was provided in the patients' home by masters-level caseworkers who had been assigned to specific patients by the non-profit cancer foundation which provides psychosocial support to cancer patients and families.

Caseworkers provided participants (time 1) with a demographic questionnaire and a measure of general functioning, Child Outcome Rating Scale (CORS; 22). The CORS asks children to report their functioning across four domains: intrapersonal, family, school and global functioning. The CORS is designed as a 10-point visual analog scale with a frowning face on one end of the Likert-type scale and a smiling face on the other end of the scale. In addition to the standardized questions on the CORS, two symptom-specific items were included to assess physiological arousal.

The caseworker then read the book to the patient. Following the reading, the child was asked several questions about the book and its story line to gauge their comprehension level. Next, the child was asked how he or she would generalize or apply the coping strategies that were used by the character in the book in their own lives. For example, the book explained how Nikki used her imagination to "fly to the park" when she was nervous; in the intervention component of this protocol, the child was asked how he or she might use his or her imagination to feel better. Following the reading of the book and the discussion questions, which lasted approximately 15 minutes, the CORS and supplemental questions were repeated along with the participant's report of satisfaction with the book (time 2).

As an incentive to participate, patients were given a copy of *Nikki's Day at Chemo* after the caseworker visit was completed with the child's answers to his or her comprehension and coping strategy questions recorded inside. Caseworkers were paid for the home visit by the cancer foundation, which was reimbursed by the grant that supported this study.

Approximately one month after the initial visit patients' caregivers were contacted via the telephone number they provided on the initial questionnaire. Follow-up assessment packets were then mailed to patients' homes; the follow-up packets included a third and final administration of the CORS, a second satisfaction survey, a questionnaire regarding frequency of reading the book, and an updated demographic form to record any significant changes in treatment or disease status. Participants were asked the return the surveys as soon as possible.

Instruments

The Child Outcome Rating Scale (CORS) is a self-administered tool available in English (23). This measure is highly effective in measuring quality of life and self-esteem in children ages 6 to 12, as well as quantifying depression and anxiety as a whole. Its simplicity is likely to be appreciated by children, who are constantly undergoing extensive and draining procedures, as well as by their caregivers.

OUR FINDINGS

This study examined whether a bibliotherapy intervention affected a child's subjective perception of functioning and level of emotional distress. It was hypothesized that reading a book describing coping strategies used by a child undergoing treatment for cancer would increase subjective perception of functioning as measured by the four domains (intrapersonal, family, school, and global) of the Child Outcome Rating Scale (CORS) as well as reduce perceived levels of physiological arousal.

Differences between time 1 and time 2

In order to compare participants' perception of functioning and emotional distress from immediately before and after the book reading (n = 21), a paired samples t-test was conducted. On the item targeting children's perceived ability to manage their nervousness, there was not a significant difference in the scores prior to the book reading (M = 7.26, SD = 3.82) and immediately after the book reading (M = 7.82, SD = 3.17); $t(20) = -0.93$, p = 0.363, but there was a small effect size (0.20). The results suggest that although statistical significance was not reached, the reading may lessen overall arousal; with a larger sample size, significance would have been reached. Other constructs tested yielded similar results; for example, paired-samples t-tests used to compare participants' intrapersonal functioning initially (M = 8.08, SD = 2.41) and following the book reading (M = 8.72, SD = 1.65); $t(20)$ = -1.1, p = 0.286. This data failed to show significance but yielded a small effect size (0.24). Table 2 shows the means for all outcome measures at T1 and T2. All other comparisons showed no effect (ES < 0.2).

Table 2. Outcome measure means across time (T1 & T2)

	T1 Mean *(SD)*	T2 Mean *(SD)*
Intrapersonal: How am I doing?	8.08 (2.41)	8.72 (1.65)
Family: How are things in my family?	8.13 (1.74)	8.47 (2.58)
School: How am I doing at school?	8.07 (2.58)	8.41 (2.07)
Global: How is everything going?	8.7 (1.72)	8.52 (2.14)
Physiological Arousal:		
Perceived ability to relax	7.86 (2.71)	8.31 (2.24)
Perceived ability to manage nervousness	7.26 (3.82)	7.82 (3.17)
Child's Satisfaction with Book	-	8.48 (2.32)

Participants were also asked how *Nikki's Day at Chemo* compares to other books they have read, based on a 1 to 10 scale (n = 21). As a whole, participants indicated a general sentiment that they enjoyed the book, with higher scores indicating greater satisfaction (M = 7.8, SD = 2.48). All participants accurately answered basic comprehension questions following the initial book reading, suggesting that children sustained attention throughout.

This comprehension check also served as a validity measure, ensuring that participants comprehended the material.

Differences between time 1 and time 3

Twenty-nine percent of participants responded to follow-up surveys, which were collected one to three months after the intervention. No significant patterns were found between participants who responded in time 3 compared to those who did not respond. Paired-samples *t*-tests were conducted to determine the change across the intrapersonal measure of the CORS from immediately before the initial book reading and from several months later ($n = 6$). With no reported differences in additional treatment or prognosis between T1 and T3, there was a significant improvement in scores reporting perception of intrapersonal functioning prior to the book reading ($M = 8.47$, $SD = 1.28$) and several months later ($M = 9.51$, $SD = 0.68$); $t(5) = -2.64$, $p = 0.046$. Table 3 presents the mean paired samples outcome measures at T1 and T3.

Table 3. Outcome measure means across time (T1 & T3)

	T1 Mean *(SD)*	T3 Mean *(SD)*
Intrapersonal: How am I doing?	8.47 (1.28)**	9.52 (0.68)**
Family: How are things in my family?	9.10 (1.06)	9.57 (0.78)
School: How am I doing at school?	9.32 (0.86)	9.93 (0.10)
Global: How is everything going?	8.82 (1.66)	9.93 (0.10)
Physiological Arousal:		
Perceived ability to relax	7.68 (3.00)	9.72 (0.44)
Perceived ability to manage nervousness	5.98 (5.19)	7.52 (3.85)
Child's Satisfaction with Book	-	8.95 (2.10)
Parent's Satisfaction with Book*	-	96 (8.94)
Frequency of Book Reading	-	1.40 (2.61)

*Parents rated the book on a 1 to 100 scale, with higher numbers indicating greater satisfaction.

**Significant differences ($p < .05$ for mean score comparison of intrapersonal functioning at T1 vs. T3). No other *t*-test comparisons yielded significant differences.

It is clear that children's sentiments about the book were relatively positive throughout the duration of this study. Using a scale ranging from 1 to 100, parents were asked to rate their perception of how much their child liked the book, with higher numbers indicating more satisfaction. Children ($n = 5$) appeared to be very satisfied with the book ($M = 94$, $SD = 13.4$). Parents ($n = 5$) appeared to have similar positive opinions about the book, as they were also asked to evaluate how much they liked it using the same 1 to 100 scale ($M = 96$, $SD = 8.94$).

Analysis of qualitative data

Post-intervention questions at Time 2 encouraged the child to apply the book character's coping strategies (e.g., talking to a trusted adult, using their imagination) to their own situation. Children were asked to identify someone they could turn to when they felt worried. When encouraged to think about how they might use their own imagination to feel better, the children responded with a range of adaptive coping strategies including "I could go to outer space to jump around freely and collect rocks," as well as go to "California" or to "the park, running, which I can't do right now." In the open-ended questions, several children expressed their desire to ask questions and share their feelings, just as the character in the book had done. One child told the caseworker "having you read this book to me makes me want to write my own story that everyone can read."

Parents generally agreed that the book was "appreciated" and "covers everything," with different individuals stating that "this is the first time I've seen a book like this where it explains everything so well" and it "captured everything a child needs to know or can feel in the book." Other parents noted that they "love the book" and that, along with their child, they "read it all the time." One of the parents further stated that reading the book has prompted her child to be more forward with asking his doctor questions, which has in turn allowed him to gain confidence to speak freely about his disease, with both peers at school and with the general public at a fundraising event.

Discussion

This study attempted to determine if a brief bibliotherapy intervention could affect a child's subjective perception of functioning and decrease his or her perceived emotional distress. Although a small pilot study, the findings supported the hypothesis that positive results that may emerge by providing children with a book that not only details a realistic portrayal of what one faces during a cancer experience, but also includes questions to activate coping strategies. Quantitative data suggested that the intervention might have improved the perception of intrapersonal functioning while decreasing physiological arousal on a self-report measure. For participants remaining in the study, the perception of improvement remained stable or increased during the three months following the intervention. Qualitatively, participants consistently recalled the specifics of the coping strategies employed in the book. Many children were able to custom-fit the strategies used by the main character to their own lives. During follow-up contact, qualitative responses indicated several children had continued to use the coping strategies that they learned from the book.

As previous literature on the subject suggests, bibliotherapy is an effective intervention, for reducing symptoms of anxiety and emotional distress (18). The study's positive results extend the literature by suggesting that bibliotherapy may also be an effective intervention for children who show sub-clinical levels of anxiety.

In recent decades, pediatric cancer survivor rates have drastically improved. Compared to 50 years ago when a child's diagnosis was often synonymous with a death sentence, advances in treatments have vastly improved children's cancer prognoses. Statistics now show that approximately four out of five pediatric cancer patients survive at least five years past their diagnosis (24). Therefore, learning evidence-based strategies may continue to help patients when dealing with stress and anxiety throughout their lives, far beyond coping with their illness.

Aside from the positive outcome that children experienced, parents also appeared to benefit from the intervention. Many voiced their appreciation for this type of therapeutic tool aimed to help their children; several of them described positive effects that the book had on their children. Overall, participants' and parents' interest and enjoyment in the intervention highlight a demand for such products, yet a paucity of books targeted for children dealing with serious chronic illness exists.

Unlike other studies, this research focused on identifying and affecting a child's subjective perception of global functioning as well as reducing physiological arousal. This represents a unique contribution to the literature by looking at patients' perceptions across these domains, rather than using objective anxiety and biofeedback measures with a specific clinically diagnosed population. As sub-clinical anxiety is even more common than clinically significant anxiety, this is a relevant population for evidenced-based interventions (3).

Implications

This research demonstrates the effectiveness of a brief intervention that yields meaningful results in improving intrapersonal functioning as well as reducing physiological arousal. After participants had several months with the book, their improvements were even more evident, suggesting that the positive effects are likely to continue with increased exposure to the intervention. The bibliotherapy tool employed in this study is easy to use and portable, two qualities that are vital for patients and families with demanding and time-consuming medical treatment schedules. *Nikki's Day at Chemo* is further effective as it empowers both the parent and child to cope with cancer together. As a whole, this book represents a tool that is a low investment and has a high yield for an incredibly vulnerable population.

Limitations

This study has several limitations. With a greater participant pool, a randomized-control design could have been employed, allowing the participants to be parsed into two groups, one of which would be assigned *Nikki's Day at Chemo* and one of which would be assigned a non-cancer related control book of a similar length. This would have strengthened the validity of the study, as the change could then have been attributed to the specific intervention book, rather than reading in general. Another limitation was the varying times between participants' diagnoses; more stringent selection criteria would have been helpful so that, for example, newly diagnosed individuals could have been compared to their counterparts. Children who have dealt with their illness for several years compared to those who have recently been diagnosed undoubtedly have different levels of knowledge about their disease, treatment, and how to cope.

Directions for future research

Future research examining this specific book would be valuable. Based on qualitative responses from participants' parents, a future study identifying caregiver anxiety would be valuable, particularly in determining how a bibliotherapy tool like *Nikki's Day at Chemo* affects it. Finally, as the study was conducted in a single geographical region, it would be valuable to expand the study to include a wider, more diverse range of individuals in different geographical regions. As the bibliotherapy tool is currently written solely in English, a Spanish translation would be valuable in order to expand eligibility criteria to include Spanish-speaking children in the United States.

ACKNOWLEDGMENTS

This study was made possible by a generous grant from the Paul K. Richter Memorial Fund and the Evalyn E. C. Richter Memorial Fund. The study would also not have been possible without the participation of the Emmanuel Cancer Foundation in Scotch Plains, NJ or the children and their families who participated in this study.

REFERENCES

[1] Substance Abuse and Mental Health Services Administration 2009. Accessed 2010 April 18. URL: http://www.samhsa.gov/data/

[2] Lang PJ, Davis M, Öhman A. Fear and anxiety: Animal models and human cognitive psychophysiology. J Affect Disord 2000;61:137-59.

[3] Last CG. Help for worried kids. New York, NY: Guilford, 2006.

[4] McCaffrey CN. Major stressors and their effects on the well-being of children with cancer. J Pediatr Nurs 2006;21:59-66.

[5] Buchanan N, Maloney K, Tsang S, Stork LC, Neglia JP, Kadan-Lottick NS. Risk of depression, anxiety, and somatization one month after diagnosis in children with standard risk ALL on COG AALL0331. [Abstract] J Clin Oncol 2008; 26(15), np.

[6] Frank NC, Blount RL, Brown RT. Attributions, coping, and adjustment in children with cancer. J Pediatr Psychol 1997;22:563-76.

[7] Dcrevensky JL, Tsanos AP, Handman M. Children with cancer: An examination of their coping and adaptive behavior. J Psychosoc Oncol 1998;16:37-61.

[8] Zeltzer LK, Recklitis C, Buchbinder D, Zebrack B, Casillas J, Tsao JC, et al. Psychological status in childhood cancer survivors: A report from the Childhood Cancer Survivor Study. J Clin Oncol 2009;27:2396-2404.

[9] Stewart SH, Taylor S, Baker JM. Gender differences in dimensions of anxiety sensitivity. J Anxiety Disord 1997;11:179-200.

[10] Kuttner L, Bowman M, Teasdale M. Psychological treatment of distress, pain, and anxiety for young children with cancer. J Dev Behav Pediatr 1988;9:374-81.

[11] Kendall PC, Hudson JL, Gosch E, Flannery-Schroeder E, Suveg C. Cognitive-behavioral therapy for anxiety disordered youth: A randomized clinical trial evaluation child and family modalities. J Consult Clin Psychol 2008;76:282-297.

[12] Friedberg RD, McClure JM. Clinical practice of cognitive therapy with children and adolescents: The nuts and bolts. New York, NY: Guilford, 2002.

[13] Miller KS, Vannatta K, Compas BE, Vasey M, McGoron KD, Salley CG, et al. The role of coping and temperament in the adjustment of children with cancer. J Pediatr Psychol 2009;34:1135-43.

[14] Coletti DJ. Stressful medical procedures in the context of cancer: Patterns of parent and child coping strategies and psychological adaptation. Dissertation. Nashville, TN: Vanderbilt Univ, 1997.

[15] Windich-Biermeier A, Sjoberg I, Dale JC, Eshelman D, Guzzetta CE. Effects of distraction on pain, fear, and distress during venous port access and venipuncture in children and adolescents with cancer. J Pediatr Oncol Nurs 2007;24:8-19.
[16] Broome, ME, Lillis PP, McGahee TW, Bates T. The use of distraction and imagery with children during painful procedures. Eur J Cancer Care 2007;3:26-30.
[17] Parslow R, Morgan AJ, Allen NB, Jorm AF, O'Donnell CP, Purcell R. Effectiveness of complementary and self-help treatments for anxiety in children and adolescents. Med J Aust 2008;188:355-9.
[18] Rappee RM, Abbott MJ, Lyneham HJ. Bibliotherapy for children with anxiety disorders using written materials for parents: A randomized controlled trial. J Consult Clin Psychol 2006;74:436-44.
[19] Forgan JW. Using bibliotherapy to teach problem solving. Interv Sch Clin 2002;38:75-82.
[20] Rokke K. Bibliotherapy: A place for childrens' literature in dealing with cancer. J Pediatr Oncol Nurs 1993;10:57.
[21] Nicholson JI, Pearson QM. Helping children cope with fears: Using children's literature in classroom guidance. Prof School Couns 2003;7:15-19.
[22] Fosson A, Husband E. Bibliotherapy for hospitalized children. South Med J 1984;77:342-6.
[23] Duncan BL, Miller SD, Sparks JA. The Child Outcome Rating Scale. Fort Lauderdale, FL: Authors, 2003.
[24] Childhood cancer survivors: Healthy living. AICR Science Now 2010;31:1-2.

In: Child and Adolescent Health Issues
Editor: Joav Merrick

ISBN: 978-1-63463-574-5

Chapter 13

ASYMPTOMATIC BACTERIURIA IN CHILDREN AND ADOLESCENTS WITH TYPE 1 DIABETES MELLITUS

Alphonsus N Onyiriuka, MD* and Edirin O Yusuf, MD
Department of Child Health and Department of Medical Microbiology,
University of Benin Teaching Hospital, Benin City, Nigeria

It is commonly believed that patients with diabetes mellitus are at increased risk of urinary tract infection compared with non-diabetic patients. Methods: Bacteriuria was screened for in 34 patients (17 with type 1 diabetes mellitus and 17 with non-diabetic endocrine disorders) at their regular follow-up visits. Mid-stream urine sample was collected every three months for 12 months and cultured. The subjects were matched for age and sex. Results: Among the 34 patients screened, only two (one (5.9%) out of 17 diabetic and one (5.9%) out of 17 non-diabetic) had asymptomatic bacteriuria and the urine culture of each of them yielded a growth of Escherichia coli sensitive to gentamycin. The duration of diabetes in the girl with asymptomatic bacteriuria (ASB) was 7 years. She had a poor glycaemic control and some psychosocial challenges. Her pubertal maturation was delayed (Tanner Stage II at the age of 15 years and has not attained menarche). She weighed 29 Kg, with BMI of 16.0 kg/m^2. In addition, she had vaginal candidiasis for which she was appropriately treated, using ketconazole. The other patient with ASB was a 7-year-old girl with precocious puberty due to congenital adrenal hyperplasia diagnosed at the age of 18 months. The two patients with ASB did not progress to symptomatic bacteriuria after a follow-up period of one year. Conclusion: The prevalence and incidence of asymptomatic bacteriuria in diabetic children and adolescents do not differ from those of their non-diabetic counterparts.

INTRODUCTION

Asymptomatic bacteriuria refers to the presence of a positive urine culture in an asymptomatic person (1). It is commonly believed that individuals with diabetes mellitus are at increased risk of infection, particularly urinary tract infection (UTI) (2-4). Such an

* Correspondence: Alphonsus N Onyiriuka, MD, Department of Child Health, University of Benin Teaching Hospital, PMB 1111, Benin City, Nigeria. E-mail: alpndiony@yahoo.com or didiruka@gmail.com

infection in diabetic patients may result in severe complications and death more frequently than would be anticipated among non-diabetics (2, 4). Most UTI in diabetic patients are relatively asymptomatic (4). Among diabetic patients, factors presumed to predispose to UTI include age, neurogenic bladder, duration of diabetes and degree of glycaemic control (2,5). Some clinicians consider asymptomatic patients being screened for bacteriuria to be at risk of UTI if two or three consecutive cultures of freshly voided urine reveal more than 10^5 organisms/ml (6). Whether or not individuals with asymptomatic bacteriuria (ASB) should be treated with antibiotics remains debatable (4). It is recommended that ASB should be treated with antibiotics in pregnant women, children aged 5-6 years and prior to invasive genitourinary procedures (7).

It is not known with certainty whether individuals with diabetes mellitus are at a higher risk of bacteriuria than non-diabetics. Studies on this subject have yielded mixed results. For instance, Lindberg et al. (8) reported that three out of 304 (0.99%) girls and zero out of 337 boys with type 1 diabetes mellitus screened for bacteriuria were positive. They, therefore, concluded that the prevalence of ASB in diabetic children and adolescents did not differ from that of their non-diabetic peers. In contrast, a meta-analysis of published data involving 22 studies revealed that the prevalence of ASB was 12.2% in diabetic children compared with 4.5% in healthy controls (9). Point prevalence was also higher in children and adolescents with diabetes (12.9%) compared with their non-diabetic (2.7%) counterparts (9). A similar increased risk among diabetic children and adolescents was reported from Egypt (10). Some studies have concluded that screening for ASB in diabetic patients is warranted because it has been found to be a risk factor for developing symptomatic urinary tract infection (11). In a survey in Port Harcourt, Nigeria of secondary school students aged 10-17 years the prevalence of ASB was 6.5% and 4.5% in girls and boys respectively (12).

Despite the recognized potential of ASB in diabetic patients to cause renal damage and ultimately, chronic kidney disease, there is a general paucity of information in the literature on its incidence, particularly in developing countries. Besides, it is not known how often ASB progresses to symptomatic bacteriuria. In addition, infection itself can lead to poor diabetic control by increased secretion of counterregulatory hormones (glucagon, cortisol, growth hormone, catecholamines), inhibition of insulin secretion, and insulin resistance of peripheral tissues/increased cytokine secretion (13,14).

The purpose of the present study is to determine the incidence of ASB among children and adolescents with T1DM attending the Paediatric Endocrine-Metabolic Clinic, UBTH and compare the result with those of their non-diabetic peers.

OUR STUDY

The study was conducted in the Paediatric Endocrine-Metabolic Clinic of the University of Benin Teaching Hospital (UBTH), Benin City, Nigeria over a 12-month period for each of the subjects. The study was approved by UBTH Ethical Committee. Consent was obtained from both the patient and their parents. Information sought from the subjects included age, sex, parents' educational attainment, parents' occupation, antibiotic use and duration of type 1 diabetes mellitus (T1DM). Patients with complaints suggestive of symptomatic urinary tract infection (such as dysuria, frequent micturiction, urgency, pain in the loin or suprapubic region) were excluded from the study. The socio-economic status of the parents of the subjects was determined using the classification suggested by Ogunlesi et al. (15). This was analyzed via combining the highest educational attainment, occupation and income of the parents (based on the mean income of each educational qualification and occupation). In this Social Classification System, classes I and II represent high social class, class III represents middle social class while classes IV and V represent low social class. In this way, the subjects were categorized into high, middle and low socio-economic groups.

A clean catch mid-stream urine specimen was obtained from each of the subjects every three months, over a total period of 12 months, amounting to four urine specimens per subject. In all the subjects, appropriate care was taken before collection of the urine specimen to avoid contamination. Each urine specimen was transported to the Research Laboratory, Department of Child Health, UBTH, where it was refrigerated immediately and cultured within two hours of collection. All the urine samples were cultured on Blood and MacConkey agar plates. The plates were incubated at 37 degree Celcius aerobically for 48 hours. Standard procedure was applied in the handling, staining, microscopy and culture of all the urine specimens (16). Full clinical examination was conducted on each of the patients at every visit. The presence of bacterial growth of 10^5 colony-forming units/ml was accepted as significant bacteriuria (17). Descriptive statistics such as frequencies, means, ratios, standard deviations, confidence intervals, percentages were used to describe all the variables.

OUR FINDINGS

Two (one diabetic and one non-diabetic) out of the 34 patients screened for asymptomatic bacteriuria (ASB) had positive urine culture, giving a prevalence of 5.9% for diabetic and non-diabetic patients respectively. The urine culture of each case with significant asymptomatic bacteriuria yielded a growth of Escherichia coli sensitive to gentamycin. The diabetic patient was a 15-year-old girl diagnosed of type 1 diabetes mellitus 7 years ago. She had a poor glycaemic control and some psychosocial challenges. Her pubertal maturation was delayed (Tanner Stage II at the age of 15 years and has not attained menarche). She weighed 29 Kg, with BMI of 16.0 kg/m^2.

In addition, she had vaginal candidiasis for which she was appropriately treated, using ketconazole. During the follow-up, appropriate urine samples were collected and screened every 3 months for 12 months for each of the patients but no other patient had significant asymptomatic bacteriuria. Neither of the two patients with significant asymptomatic bacteriuria progressed to symptomatic bacteriuria after two years of follow up. The mean age at presentation of the patients with diabetes was 11.0±4.2 years (95% Confidence Interval, CI=7.7-14.7) for boys; 13.5±1.6 years (95% CI=12.6-14.4) for girls; 12.8±2.9 years (95% CI=11.4-14.1) for both sexes combined. Mean age at presentation: boys versus girls $t= 1.28$ $p>0.05$. The age and gender distribution of the subjects is depicted in Table 1.The mean body mass index (BMI) was 18.6±2.5 kg/m^2 (95% CI=17.4-19.8) with 6 (35.3%) having a BMI below 19.0 kg/m^2. None of the subjects had BMI > 25 kg/m^2. Over half of the families (52.9%) of the subjects were in the middle social class. Eleven point eight percent and 35.3% of the families of the subjects were in the high and low social classes respectively.

Table 1. Age and gender distribution of patients with diabetes mellitus

Age group at presentation	Gender		
	Male	Female	Both sexes
	No(%)	No(%)	No(%)
Below 10 years	2(33.3)	0(0)	2(11.8)
10-12 years	0(0)	3(27.3)	3(17.6)
13-15 years	3(50.0)	8(72.7)	11(64.7)
Above 15 years	1(16.7)	0(0)	1(5.9)
Total	6(100.0)	11(100.0)	17(100.0)

DISCUSSION

The prevalence (5.9%) of asymptomatic bacteriuria (ASB) found in the present study is two- and 5-fold lower than the 12.2% and 30.0% respectively reported from two different studies, one a meta-analysis of 22 studies and the other among diabetic Egyptian children and adolescents (9,10). Prevalence rates lower than that observed in the present study have been reported (8). All reflecting the mixed results of prevalence of ASB in children and adolescents, suggesting that some unidentified socio-demographic factors might influence the prevalence of ASB in these subjects. For instance, age, sex, glycaemic control, duration of diabetes and presence of long-term complications have all been variously reported as risk factors (2-4). The method of collection and processing of the urine specimens might have also influenced the different prevalence rates observed. The lower prevalence rate observed in the present study compared to the Egyptian study may partly be because of the differences in the age of the two study populations. Most of the subjects in the Egyptian study were older than 15 years while most the patient in the present study were below 15 years of age. This view is supported by the reports of two studies in Egypt and Hungary which separately showed the prevalence of ASB was higher in girls aged 15 years or older (10,17). In consonance, the only diabetic patient with ASB in the present study was 15 years old. However, the prevalence from our data was within the range (4.5-6.5%) reported from Port Harcourt, Nigeria among non-diabetic secondary school students aged 6 to 15 years(11), suggesting that ASB is not commoner in diabetic compared to non-diabetic children and adolescents. This conclusion is reinforced by the results of the present study which showed that of the two patients with ASB one was diabetic and the other was non-diabetic. Furthermore, as reported by Rozsai et al. (14), the urinary cytokine response to pathogens in both diabetic and non-diabetic children with bacteriuria was comparable.

Consistent with previous reports, the most common bacterial agent in the present study was Escherichia coli (4,10,18). This finding is partly explained by the report of Geerlings et al. (19) which indicated that E. coli expressing type 1 fimbrae adhere better to the uroepithelial cells of women with diabetes mellitus compared to the cells of women without diabetes mellitus. The girl with type 1 diabetes and ASB also had vaginal candidiasis which responded satisfactorily to treatment with ketoconazole. The finding of candidial infection in this adolescent with diabetes mellitus is not surprising as other investigators have reported a similar finding (20). The increased frequency of vaginal candidiasis in patients with diabetes mellitus is believed to be due to increase in ambient vaginal glycogen stores in them (20).

In conclusion, prevalence and incidence of asymptomatic bacteriuria do not differ between diabetic and non-diabetic children and adolescents.

REFERENCES

[1] Ooi S, Frazee LA, Gardner WG. Management of asymptomatic bacteriuria in patients with diabetes mellitus. Ann Pharmacotherapy 2004;38(3):490-3.

[2] Guillausseau PJ, Farah R, Laloi-Michelin M, Tielmans A, Rymer R, Warnet R. Urinary tract infections and diabetes mellitus. Rev Prat 2003;53(16):1790-6.

[3] Funftuck R, Nicolle LE, Hanefeld M, Naser KG. Urinary tract infection in patients with diabetes mellitus. Clin Nephrol 2012;77(1):40-8.

[4] Balachandar MS, Pavkovic P, Metelko Z. Kidney infections in diabetes mellitus. Diabetologia Croatica 2002;31(2):95-103.

[5] Keane EH, Boyko EJ, Reller LB, Hamman RF. Prevalence of asymptomatic bacteriuria in subjects with NIDDM in San Luis Valley of Colorado. Diabetes Care 1988;11:708-12.

[6] Rifkin RH. Urinary tract infection in childhood. Pediatrics 1977;60:508.

[7] Raz R. Asymptomatic bacteriuria: Clinical significance and management. Int J Antimicrob Agents 2003;22(Suppl 2):45-7.

[8] Lindberg U, Bergstrom AL, Carlsson E, Dahlquist G, Hermansson G, Larsson Y, et al. Urinary tract infection in children with type 1 diabetes. Acta Pediatr Scand 1985;74:85-8.

[9] Renko M, Tapaainen P, Tossavainen P, Pokka T, Uhari M. Meta-analysis of the significance of asymptomatic bacteriuria in diabetes. Diabetes Care 2011;34(1):230-5.

[10] Salem MA, Matler RM, Abdelmaksond AA, El Masry SA. Prevalence of asymptomatic bacteriuria in Egyptian children and adolescents with type 1 diabetes mellitus. J Egypt Soc Parasitol 2009;39(3):951-62.

[11] Ribera MC, Pascual R, Barbar PC, Pederera V, Gil V. Incidence and risk factors associated with urinary tract infection in diabetic patients with or without asymptomatic bacteriuria. Eur J Clin Microbiol Infect Dis 2006;25:389-93.

[12] Frank-Peterside N, Wokoma EC. Prevalence of asymptomatic bacteriuria in students of University of Port Harcourt Demonstration Secondary School. JASEM 2009;13:55-8.

[13] Leibovici L, Yehehzkelli Y, Porter A et al. Influence of diabetes mellitus and glycaemic control on the characteristics and outcome of common infections. Diabet Med 1996;13:457-463.

[14] Rozsai B, Lanyi E, Berki T, Soltesz G. Urinary cytokine response to asymptomatic bacteriuria in type 1 diabetic children and young adults. Pediatr Diabetes. 2006;7(3):153-8.

[15] Ogunlesi TA, Dedeke IOF, Kuponiyi OT. Socio-economic classification of children attending Specialist Paediatric Centres in Ogun State, Nigeria. Nig Med Pract 2008; 54(1):21-5.

[16] Collee JG, Duguid JP, Frasar AG. Laboratory strategy in the diagnosis of infective syndromes. In: Collee JG, Duguid JP, Frasar AG, Marmion DP, Simmon A eds. Mackie and McCarteney practical medical microbiology, 13 ed. Edinburgh: Churchill Livingstone, 1989:601-49.

[17] Rozsai B, Lanyi E, Soltesz G. Asymptomatic bacteriuria and leucocytouria in type 1 diabetes children and young adults. Diabetes Care 2003;26(7):2209-10.

[18] Makuyana D, Mhlabi D, Chipfupa M, Munyombwe T, Gwanzura L. Asymptomatic bacteriuria among outpatients with diabetes mellitus in urban black population. Cent Afr J Med 2002;48(7-8):78-82.

[19] Geerlings SE, Meiland R, Hoepelman AI. Pathogenesis of bacteriuria in women with diabetes mellitus. Int J Antimicrob Agents 2002;19(6):539-45.

[20] Rein MF, Holmes KK. Non-specific vaginitis, vulvovaginal candidiasis and trichomoniasis. Curr Clin Topics Infect Dis 1983;4:281.

In: Child and Adolescent Health Issues
Editor: Joav Merrick

ISBN: 978-1-63463-574-5

Chapter 14

EVALUATION OF AN HIV ANTI-STIGMA CAMPAIGN

Sara A Millimet[1], Beau Miller[2], Michael W Ross*[3], Pahl Samson[2] and Chaitanya Churi[3]

[1]School of Health Sciences and Kinesiology, Rice University, Houston, Texas
[2]LIVE Consortium, Houston, Texas and [3]School of Public Health, University of Texas, Houston, United States of America

We evaluated an HIV anti-stigma campaign at a large liberal arts university in the southern United States using a modified version of the Bogardus and Ross & Hunter Social Distance scale. Data on pre- and post-campaign cross-sectional samples with nearly 50% overlap indicated that the campaign (which included lectures, slogans, t-shirt distribution and chocolates containing slogans) significantly decreased the social distance from (willingness to interact with) people with HIV. Time between pre-test (n=685) and post-test (n=515) was 1 month. Decrease in social distance was uneven, with males changing more than females and white and Hispanic students changing the most. Data suggest that this social distance measure is an effective instrument for measuring a decrease in HIV-associated stigma and that brief anti-stigma campaigns of this nature have an impact short-term on expressed HIV-stigma.

INTRODUCTION

Stigma against HIV/AIDS has been identified as a barrier to effective diagnosis and treatment of the disease (1). The nature and modes of transmission of HIV/AIDS are taboo in most societies. The unfortunate association of homosexuality with this disease early on additionally attached the stigma that came along with homophobia (2) and has led to a further isolation of patients of this disease, irrespective of sexual orientation. Thus, the disease lends itself to particular scrutiny and discrimination among members of society, as well as health care professionals. It is this stigma, and the opposition borne from it, that prevents many efforts to control and combat the spread of HIV/AIDS from being successful (3).

* Correspondence: Professor Michael W Ross, School of Public Health, University of Texas, 7000 Fannin #2622, Houston TX 77030, United States of America., E-mail: Michael.W.Ross@uth.tmc.edu

Researchers have shown the adverse effect of stigma against individuals infected with HIV has on testing, prevention and treatment activities. That stigma prevents and delays individuals from accessing timely diagnostic tests as well as counseling are well documented, especially among those forming the so called "high-risk" groups (4). Further, some have shown that anti-retroviral treatment programs which do not address the issues of stigma, affect treatment seeking behavior (5).

The impact of stigma however, extends beyond these avenues. Stigma against adolescents orphaned by HIV/AIDS has been shown to be associated with fewer positive activities and poorer psychological outcomes (6). Stigma associated with HIV/AIDS creates hostile environments at places of employment, and has been proposed as a predictor of unemployment in people affected with HIV/AIDS (7). In some parts of the world, this stigma even extends to those healthcare providers engaged in caring for HIV/AIDS patients. It may lead to some leaving work related to HIV/AIDS care (8) or burnout (9). It has been noted that even though HIV-related stigma declined from 1991-1999, in 1999, one-third of a population sample in the US still expressed discomfort and negative feelings towards people with AIDS (PWA)(10). In 2009, 87% of US college students did not perceive themselves to be at risk and only 29% had ever been tested for HIV (11).

In this scenario, campaigns looking to address stigma against those affected by HIV/AIDS assume special importance. Experts contend that in order to be successful, campaigns to reduce HIV/AIDS stigma need to be evidence based, and designed after extensive needs-assessment (12). Numerous such campaigns have been developed that look to reduce the stigma around HIV/AIDS in developed as well as developing countries. The WHO developed an international campaign called "Live and Let Live" that looked to eradicate AIDS related stigma through the use of various educational activities including poster campaigns (13).

There is however, a dearth of scientific evidence that examines the impact of such campaigns. It is important to evaluate whether interventions designed to reduce stigma are in fact working. Researchers under the Horizons Program have collated and examined programs regarding stigma prevention. Their report looked at 22 studies on stigma campaigns and their success in reducing stigma and discrimination related to HIV. They found that most studies were lacking in a rigorous evaluation of trends and data. Further, they found that samples were often small and convenience based, and measures of stigma weren't clearly defined. Finally, it was noted that most studies did not look at the long term effects of these campaigns, and whether changes in attitude, if any, persisted for a long duration after the intervention (14).

With this background in mind, in this study, we looked to conduct an educational intervention regarding HIV/AIDS and the stigma attached to it in adolescents (undergraduate college students in a large southern US liberal arts university, Rice University in Houston, Texas), and examine its impact on the study population.

The intervention

In student focus groups, students crafted interventions based on focus groups which asked the question about HIV/AIDS "what do you and your peers need to hear?" The main message from these groups was that this is a US issue at home and not just an African problem. The campaign took place in Spring 2011 and consisted of: a month long HIV and stigma education marketing campaign in the Rice University student newspaper, the "Thresher"; weekly announcements and emails sent out by the Rice Health Advisors to their respective residential colleges; and Anti-Stigma Day, a day proclaimed by the Mayor of the City of Houston, which included a one thousand t-shirt giveaway (these t-shirts were still being worn a year later on campus) and a lunchtime lecture on stigma, HIV, and homophobia. Fortune chocolates (with a relevant message in the chocolate) were given in return for the student filling out a questionnaire. Business-size cards were handed out across campus with HIV and stigma-related messages (Figure 1) and there was a "viral" campaign in the campus newspaper with black squares containing the same messages, which spread from week to week until they covered almost an entire page. Broad (This is our problem) plus specific(One Houstonian is diagnosed every eight hours with HIV)messages. Each week focused on a particular aspect of the problem, starting with the problem of HIV stigma, what it means to you, what can be done about it, and implementing local and personal solutions. The intervention was focused on the residential colleges as the effective "communities" of the University, which function much as fraternities or sororities. Illustrations of the intervention messages and media are at www.liveconsortium.org.

OUR STUDY

The pre-and post surveys were distributed and collected by the Rice Health Advisors (RHAs). The RHAs are a student run organization at Rice University which seeks to educate and promote both physical and mental well-being among fellow students. They are on hand in the residential colleges to discuss problems, mediate issues, and also provide basic medical supplies such as band-aids, ibuprofen, condoms, and cough drops. Rice has 11 residential colleges on campus, each with a varying number of Rice Health Advisors. The advisors at each residential college were given 100 pre and 100 post surveys per college. The surveys were collected primarily at meal time. Some RHAs took surveys door to door around the college were people were living as well. The pre survey was completed in return for chocolates containing anti-stigma slogans provided by LIVE and the post-surveys were completed in return for an Anti-Stigma Day t-shirt. The surveys were attempted to be collected in a 2-5 day period.685 surveys were collected for the pre-test (62.3% of those provided) and 515 (46.8% of those provided)for the post-test. Once gathered, the data were entered and analyses analyzed using SPSS (version 19). The data were summed for knowledge and for social distance.

The social distance scale items were derived from the Bogardus measure (15) as modified for HIV/AIDS by Hunter and Ross (16). For HIV knowledge, the total number of questions each student got correct was averaged to develop a single mean score and standard deviation for the pre- and post-survey. The questions measuring social distance were scored on a Likert scale of 1 to 7, seven being the most willing to engage in the situation, and scores for each student were summed for all thirteen questions. The increase in the means of social distance implies an increase in willingness to engage in social situations and a consequential decrease in social distance. Questions on sympathy for people with HIV, how much HIV is on one's radar, and how personally one was affected by HIV were also measured on a Likert scale of 1 to 7, and these numbers were averaged individually. Two-sided *t*-tests were run on the on the means from the pre- and post- tests to determine whether changes were statistically significant. Pre-post differences were also run by gender and race/ethnicity. A *p*-value of ≤.05 was considered to be statistically significant.

At the start of the survey, students were asked for demographic information, including age, gender and race/ethnicity. The distribution was split fairly equally between male and female students for both the pre- and post-surveys, while race and ethnicity was more distributed predominantly in the White and Asian categories. This is representative of the overall Rice University population. The study was not longitudinal, in that both the pre- and post-surveys were anonymous, so the surveys could not be linked to individual people before and after. Nearly 50% of the respondents who took the pre-survey also completed the post-survey. The study was approved by the appropriate university committee for the protection of human subjects.

OUR FINDINGS

Demographic data appear in table 1. All participants were undergraduates, with a modal age of 21. Pre-and post-differences for HIV/AIDS salience, social distance, sympathy for people with HIV, the amount HIV was on the student's radar, how personally affected the student felt towards HIV, and how many people a student knew with HIV.

These data appear in table 2. Pre-and post-test differences were significant only for the social distance measure. The *p*-value for the pre- and pre-test results was significant ($p<.008$), indicating an increase in willingness to engage in certain situations with someone who is HIV+ statistically. Measures of HIV/AIDS salience, sympathy for people with HIV, the amount HIV was on the student's radar, how personally affected the student felt toward HIV, and how many people a student knew with HIV were all statistically insignificant.

In order to examine the difference in the social distance measure in more detail, *t*-tests were run on the pre- and post-test differences in social distance according to gender and race/ethnicity.

Table 1. Demographics of sample

	Pre-test	Post-test	Statistic	*p*
Gender: Male	47.5%	48.1%		
Female	52.2%	51.9%	χ^2 =1.77, df=2	.41
Race/ethnicity: White	51.3%	46.0%		
African American	5.9%	4.5%		
Hispanic	13.3%	15.7%		
Asian/Pacific Isl.	25.9%	29.4%		
Other	3.7%	4.5%	χ^2 =5.64, df=4	.23

*Post-test respondents who had done pre-test: 49.9%.
All tests 2-tailed.

Table 2. Pre- and Post-test Differences, LIVE HIV anti-stigma Campaign

	Pre-test*	Post-test*	Statistic	p
HIV/AIDS knowledge	5.31±1.26	5.30±1.25	*t*=0.27, df=1200	.79
Social Distance	**71.76±15.68**	**73.96±14.74**	***t*=2.65, df=1181**	**.008**
Sympathy for people with HIV	5.95±1.28	5.93±1.20	*t*=0.31, df=1158	.75
HIV "on radar"	3.51±1.69	3.39±1.68	*t*=1.19, df=1157	.23
Feel personally affected	2.00±1.39	2.02±1.36	*t*=0.26, df=1159	.79
People with HIV known personally†	0: 86.0%	0: 85.2%	χ^2 =7.10, df=5	.21
Close friends/family with HIV†	0: 94.5%	0: 93.9%	χ^2 =4.37, df=4	.36
Recognized LIVE logo:		39.1%		
Recognized pseudologo:		14.9%		

*Mean±SD.
†Modal category (0, 1, 2, 3, 4, 5+).
All tests 2-tailed.

Complete data can be found in Tables 1-3, and Figures 1 and 2. When analyzing the social distance means for males, the social distance means increased in a manner that was statistically significant. The difference in social distance means for females who took the survey showed a similar trend (*p*=.056). Therefore, the decrease in social distance demonstrated by the male students likely contributed greatly to the decrease in social distance displayed by the entire student body.

Table 3.

	Pre-test*	**Post-test***	**Statistic**	***p***
Social Distance	69.46±17.35	72.41±14.92	t=2.16, df=551	.031
Pre- and Post-test Differences in Social Distance by Gender: FEMALE				
	Pre-test*	**Post-test***	**Statistic**	***p***
Social Distance	73.62±13.46	75.73±13.51	t=1.92, df=557	.056
Pre- and Post-test Differences in Social Distance by Race/Ethnicity				
	Pre-test*	**Post-test***	**Statistic**	***p***
Caucasian	74.0±14.4	76.6±13.3	t=2.25, df=521.6	p=.03
African American	72.6±11.9	71.5±11.6	t=0.35, df=44.4	p=.74
Hispanic	71.7±15.0	76.7±14.0	t=2.21, df=165	p=.03
Asian	66.7±17.9	70.0±15.4	t=1.78, df=321	p=.06
Social Distance based on Recognition of LIVE Logo				
	YES: Recognition	**NO: Recognition**	**Statistic**	***p***
Social Distance	77.16±12.15	71.85±15.74	t=4.22, df=474	.0001

*Mean±SD.
All tests 2-tailed.

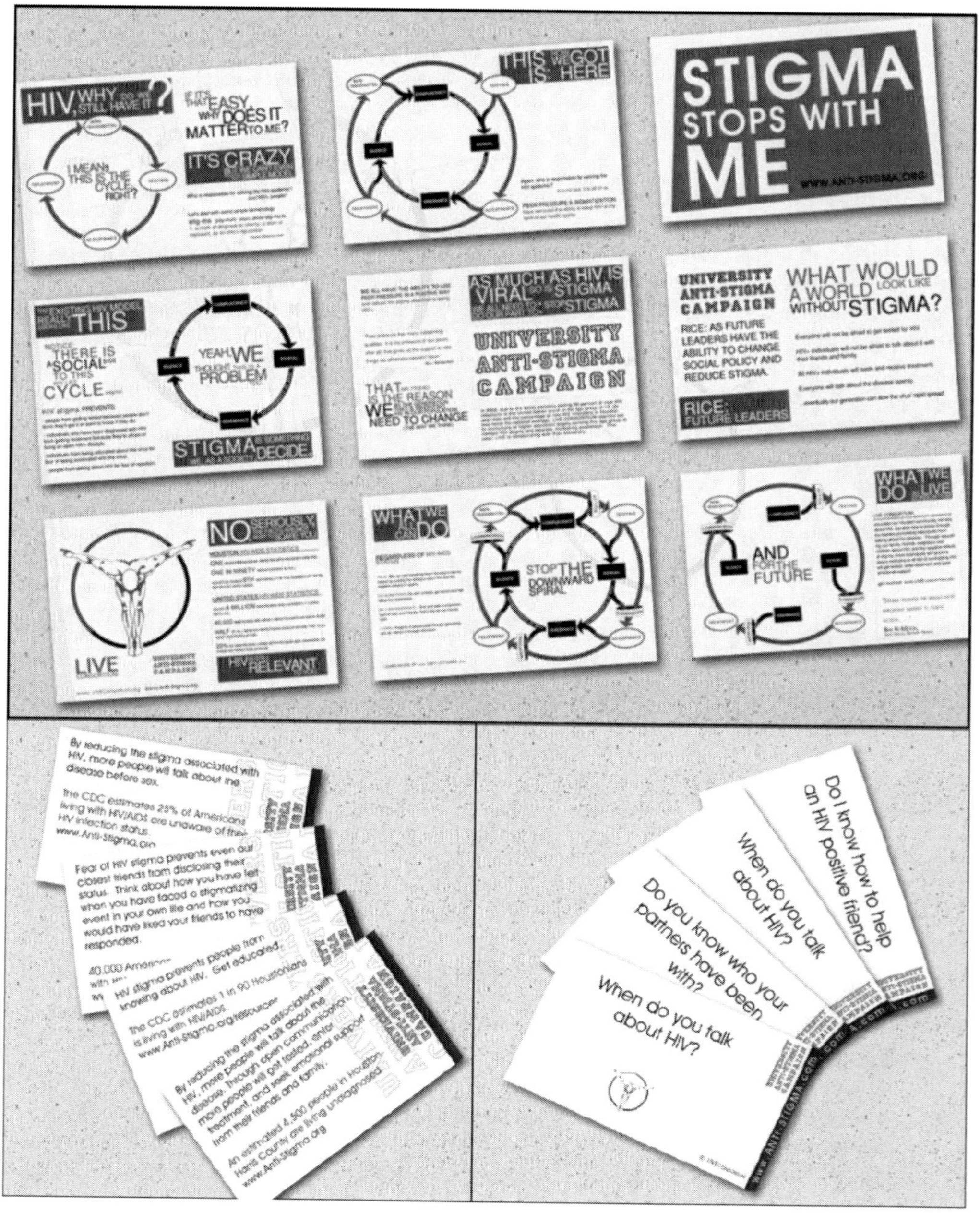
STIGMA STOPS WITH ME
WWW.ANTI-STIGMA.ORG
IT'S CRAZY
UNIVERSITY ANTI-STIGMA CAMPAIGN
WHAT WOULD A WORLD LOOK LIKE WITHOUT STIGMA?
RICE: AS FUTURE LEADERS HAVE THE ABILITY TO CHANGE SOCIAL POLICY AND REDUCE STIGMA.
RICE: FUTURE LEADERS
AS MUCH AS HIV IS VIRAL
STIGMA
STOP THE DOWNWARD SPIRAL
AND FOR THE FUTURE
LIVE
HIV RELEVANT
By reducing the stigma associated with HIV, more people will talk about the disease before sex.
The CDC estimates 25% of Americans living with HIV/AIDS are unaware of their HIV infection status.
www.Anti-Stigma.org
Fear of HIV stigma prevents even our closest friends from disclosing their status. Think about how you have felt when you have faced a stigmatizing event in your own life and how you would have liked your friends to have responded.
HIV stigma prevents people from knowing about HIV. Get educated.
The CDC estimates 1 in 90 Houstonians is living with HIV/AIDS
By reducing the stigma associated with HIV, more people will talk about the disease. Through open communication, more people will get tested, enter treatment, and seek emotional support from their friends and family.
Do I know how to help an HIV positive friend?
When do you talk about HIV?
Do you know who your partners have been with?
When do you talk about HIV?

Figure 1. Intervention materials.

All race/ethnicities experienced a decreased social distance, aside from the African Americans, who experienced a slight (non-significant) increase in social distance. The most drastic increase was among Caucasian and Hispanic students, and likely contributed to the overall decrease in social distance among the entire student body. Both these increases in willingness were statistically significant. There was a trend toward decrease in social distance among Asian students, however, it was only borderline statistically significant (p=.06).

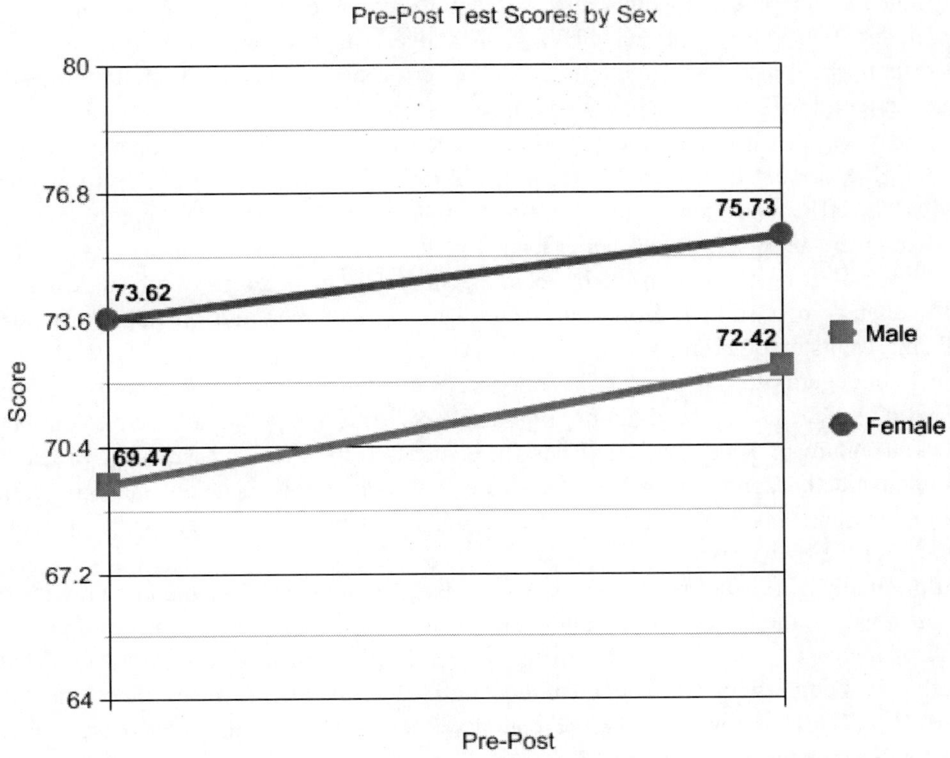

Figure 2. Pre-Post-test scores by Sex.

Finally, a *t*-test was run on only the post-survey data to examine the social distance compared to recognition of the LIVE Consortium logo of a diver, which branded all the stigma week materials, compared with a bogus logo from an unrelated campaign in the northeast US. A total of 39.1% students reported on the post-survey that they recognized the LIVE Consortium logo. Those students who responded that they did recognize the LIVE Consortium logo on the survey had a significantly higher willingness to engage in situations with HIV+ persons, compared to those who did not recognize the logo.

DISCUSSION

These data, while limited by the lack of a longitudinal design and lower power with subsample analyses, indicate that there was a significant decrease in social distance (willingness to interact) with HIV positive individuals on a modification of the Bogardus social distance scale (15). The differences were however uneven, with males changing more than females, and White and Hispanic students changing the most, followed by Asian students. These data suggest that one of the best indicators of an anti-stigma campaign is a measure of social distance from persons with HIV such as that used in the present study.

Breakdown of the data by those who recognized the LIVE logo, while a crude measure of the attention paid to the material, also suggests that those who recognized it (and presumably had recalled more of the content) also had significantly decreased social distance scores toward interaction with people with HIV. This suggests that recognition of the logo meant those respondents paid more attention to LIVE Consortium's educational material, resulting in their increased willingness to interact with people with HIV.

In analyzing the differences in HIV/AIDS salience, social distance, sympathy for people with HIV, the amount HIV was on the student's radar, how personally affected the student felt towards HIV, and how many people a student knew with HIV, before and after differences were only statistically significant for the social distance measure. As explained later, the social distance measure is the most essential data gathered from the survey, as it is directly related to a stigma. However, there were several potential barriers to obtaining significant results on other measures.

First, in regards to students' HIV salience, Rice students' HIV/AIDS knowledge was initially high (students averaged 5.3 out of 7 answers correct), a possible tribute to the highly intellectual nature of Rice students. Therefore, successfully educating students in order to yield a statistically significant increase is difficult to achieve. Nonetheless, in observations made on campus, many students actually complained about never receiving the correct answers after the first survey was distributed.

Additionally, it was not necessarily expected that the number of people known with HIV would increase, as the intervention did not address that issue in particular. There were also no significant increases in the sympathy for people with HIV yet, like HIV/AIDS knowledge, sympathy for people with HIV started rather high, at an average of nearly 6 on the Likert scale of 1 to 7. Therefore, due to the ceiling effect, it is difficult to increase students' sympathy in a manner that would yield statistically significant results.

The most important result from the surveys was the significant difference in students' social distance after the intervention's implementation. The results demonstrate that the University Anti-Stigma Day campaign had a significant impact on the social distance measure indicating Rice students had a greater comfort with people with HIV/AIDS. The social distance scale was the heart of the survey and was the most critical evaluation of whether the campaign effectively reduced stigma.

As there is no generally accepted quantitative instrument to measure stigma, stigma reduction is best measured by a reduction in social distance people feel between themselves and others. In his book defining the study of stigma, Goffman (17) described stigma as "an attribute that is deeply discrediting" in social situations and explains that "an attribute that stigmatizes one type of possessor can confirm the usualness for another" (17, page 3-4). Thus, stigma operates by making one less like oneself and creates a social distance between oneself and the other.

A greater stigma implies a greater social distance, due to the unwillingness to engage in social situations. Therefore, demonstrating a decrease in social distance likely implies a decrease in stigma towards a person as well. Consequently, the significant reduction in social distance to HIV demonstrates that the University Anti-Stigma campaign was successful in reducing HIV-associated stigma. This university-based campaign indicates that, in terms of short-term impact, the campaign was effective, although it is not possible to know, in this study, whether the difference was maintained in the longer term.

APPENDIX: HIV SOCIAL DISTANCE SCALE ITEMS

Please consider how willing would you be to partake in the following scenarios with an HIV+ person. Rank your willingness on a scale of 1-7 (1=Not at all 4=Moderately 7=Very much)

1.	Interact with him/her at a party or function	1 2 3 4 5 6 7
2.	Have him/her as a near neighbor	1 2 3 4 5 6 7
3.	Become close friends with her/him	1 2 3 4 5 6 7
4.	Become friends with him/her if he was male	1 2 3 4 5 6 7
5.	Become friends with him/her if she was female	1 2 3 4 5 6 7
6.	Become friends with him/her if he/she was transgender	1 2 3 4 5 6 7
7.	Become intimately and romantically involved with him/her.	1 2 3 4 5 6 7
8.	Accept him/her as a visitor to the United States.	1 2 3 4 5 6 7
9.	Allow him/her to become a roommate/suitemate.	1 2 3 4 5 6 7
10.	Allow him/her to be a member of your club or team	1 2 3 4 5 6 7
11.	Allow him/her to become a student at Rice University	1 2 3 4 5 6 7
12.	Allow him/her to become employed in your place of work	1 2 3 4 5 6 7
13.	Accept him/her as a member of your family as a partner of a Sibling	1 2 3 4 5 6 7

REFERENCES

[1] Machine EM, Ross MW, McCurdy SA. Issues of expressed stigma of HIV/AIDS among professionals in Southern Sudan. Qual Health Res 2011;21:1041-50.

[2] Flowers P, Langdridge D. Offending the other: Deconstructing narratives of deviance and pathology. Br J Soc Psychol 2007;46:679-90.

[3] Miller RL, Reed SJ, Francisco VT, Ellen JM. Conflict Transformation, stigma, and HIV-preventive structural change. Am J Commun Psychol 2011.doi: 10.1007/s10464-011-9465-7.

[4] Dowson L, Kober C, Perry N, Fisher M, Richardson D. Why some MSM present late for HIV testing: a qualitative analysis. AIDS Care 2012;24(2):204-9.

[5] Nattabi B, Li J, Thompson SC, Orach CG, Earnest J. Factors associated with perceived stigma among people living with HIV/AIDS in post-conflict Northern Uganda. AIDS Educ Prev 2011;23:193-205.

[6] Cluver LD, Gardner F, Operario D. Effects of stigma on the mental health of adolescents orphaned by AIDS. J Adolesc Health 2008;42:410-7.

[7] Liu Y, Canada K, Shi K, Corrigan P. HIV-related stigma acting as predictors of unemployment of people living with HIV/AIDS. AIDS Care 2012;21(1):129-35.

[8] Haber DB, Roby JL, High-George LD. Stigma by association: the effects of caring for HIV/AIDS patients in South Africa. Health Soc Care Commun 2011;19:541-9.

[9] Bennett L, Miller D, Ross MW. Health workers and AIDS. Research, intervention and current issues in burnout and response. Chur, Switzerland: Harwood Academic, 1995.

[10] Herek GM, Capitanio JP, Widaman KF. HIV-related stigma and knowledge in the United States: Prevalence and trends, 1991-1999. Am J Public Health 2002;92:371-7.

[11] Inungu J, Mumford V, Younis M, Langford S. HIV knowledge, attitudes and practices among college students in the United States. J Health Hum Serv Adm 2009;32:259-77.

[12] Bos AE, Schaalma HP, Pryor JB. Reducing AIDS-related stigma in developing countries: the importance of theory- and evidence-based interventions. Psychol Health Med 2008; 13:450-60.

[13] Johnny L, Mitchell C. "Live and let live": An analysis of HIV/AIDS-related stigma and discrimination in international campaign posters. J Health Commun 2006;11:755-67.
[14] Brown L, Macintyre K, Trujillo L. Interventions to reduce HIV/AIDS stigma: what have we learned? AIDS Educ Prev 2003;15:49-69.
[15] Bogardus ES. A social distance scale. Sociol Soc Res 1933;17:265-71.
[16] Hunter CE, Ross MW. Determinants of health care workers' attitudes toward people with AIDS. J Appl Soc Psychol 1991;21:947-56.
[17] Goffman E. Stigma. London: Penguin, 1963.

SECTION THREE: INJURY, ABUSE AND SAFETY

In: Child and Adolescent Health Issues
Editor: Joav Merrick

ISBN: 978-1-63463-574-5

Chapter 15

MUNCHAUSEN SYNDROME BY PROXY

Eunice Grace and Nithya Jagannathan*
Department of Oral Pathology, Saveetha Dental College,
Chennai, India

Munchausen syndrome by proxy was first described by a pediatric professor, Sir Samuel Roy Meadow, in the year 1977. The typical form involves inducing illness in the child by a parent or other caregiver, and fooling the clinician with fabricated stories. It involves the parents exaggerating symptoms of illness of their child, thereby resulting in overly aggressive medical evaluations and interventions. Usually in such cases the mother is more frequently involved than the father. A common scenario is that sometimes even the physician plays a role in inflicting abuse in the child. It is imperative that the physician recognizes this because failure in diagnosing leads to repeated abuse of the child, sometimes even resulting in death. Hence diagnosing Munchausen syndrome by proxy with increased self-awareness reduces the morbidity and mortality rates amongst the children. The article reviews Munchausen syndrome by proxy, particularly as it relates to the diagnosis and its management to bring about an increase in the awareness of this syndrome. This article aims at bringing about that awareness thereby helping in its management and being beneficial to the child.

INTRODUCTION

Munchausen syndrome by proxy (MSBP), a common form of child abuse, involves fabrication of illness by the caretaker on the child by subjecting them to immense levels of trauma, both physically and emotionally (1). The syndrome is characterized by repeated fabrications of physical illness that are usually acute, dramatic and convincing. It was initially recognized in adults, who made-up symptoms for the purpose of adopting a sick role and subjecting themselves to medical investigations (2).

* Correspondence: Nithya Jagannathan, Department of Oral Pathology, Saveetha Dental College, Saveetha University, 162 Poonamalle High Road, Chennai, 600077 India. E-mail: dr.nithya@ymail.com

History

Munchausen syndrome is named after an extravagant raconteur, Hieronymus Carl Friedrich Baron van Münchausen (1720-1797), a German nobleman and famous recounter of fairy tales. His famous and fanciful narrations of his imagined exploits in the form of fictions made his name in the literature. The syndrome was likened to be called when a parent or a care taker of the child fabricates symptoms on a dependent individual about child's illness or when the perpetrator directors induces illness to the child by harming them (3).

The syndrome was used in 1952 by Richard Asher (1912-1969), an eminent Britis endocrinologist and hematologist, to describe adults who fabricated medical illness to gain medical attention (4). In 1977, the terminology was coined by a British pediatrician Sir Samuel Roy Meadow to describe two cases of mothers, who induced symptoms in their own children resulting in severe physical assault to their body and death. In this relevance, Munchausen syndrome by proxy gained importance and recognition due to the seriousness of these consequences (5).

In 1994, the Diagnostic and Statistical Manual of Mental Disorders, Fourth Edition (DSM-IV) stated the terminology "facetious disorder by proxy (FDP)" to describe psychiatric illness of the perpetrator who fabricated illness on their victims (3).

There has been some confusion in the terminology regarding the use of Munchausen syndrome by proxy, because some experts insist that the term be used only, when the parent is seeking medical care due to personal compulsion in relation to the medical care system (6,7), whereas others commented that it is not the parent's motivation, which is important (8,9). Further, a few authors insisted that the term has to be extended to those cases, where medical neglect or noncompliance resulted in physical or mental assault (10-12). To alleviate these queries the American Professional Society on the Abuse of Children (APSAC) instead suggested the term "pediatric condition falsification" (PCF) in order to describe more precisely this condition in the abused child. PCF may or may not be associated with FDP. However, the APSAC requires the presence of both FDP and PCF to diagnose Munchausen syndrome by proxy (13).

The term medical child abuse (MCA) was proposed recently by Roesler and Jenny (6) to describe the excessive, unnecessary and harmful medical or surgical treatments unknowingly imposed on the child at the instigation of a caregiver.

Munchausen Syndrome by Proxy

The terminology applies to a child receiving excessive medical care, which is unwarranted due to the parent misinterpreting the symptom. Sometimes the parents also purposefully harm the child and manipulate the laboratory tests to create symptoms (14). It is important to determine this because ignorance of the physician/ dentist to diagnose this condition may result in harm and death to the child.

Incidence

More than 700 cases from 52 different countries have been reported of this syndrome so far with an equal incidence of both boys and girls affected (15). The incidence of MSBP is reported to be 0.4 in 100,000 children less than 16 years of age and 2 per 100,000 in children younger than 1 year of age. Studies by different groups suggested that at least 1% of children with asthma and 16-30% of children with allergy have been subjected to MSBP (16,17). In an English town, about 39 cases out of 20,000 had reports of intentional suffocation (18). A survey by the British Paediatric Association Surveillance Unit found 128 cases in the UK and Ireland over a two year period with 2.8 cases per 100,000 children younger than 1 year and 0.5 cases per 100,000 younger than 16 years are affected (19).

Perpetrators

In more than 95% of the cases of MSBP the mother acts as a perpetrator of the child's illness. In a review by Sheridan et al. (20) mothers were the perpetrators in 76.5% and fathers were the perpetrators in 6.7% of the 450 cases. Studies reported by Feldman et al. (21) suggested that mothers were the perpetrators in all the cases. This is completely in contrast to the parental hypothesis theory, which suggests that mothers are more interested in the wellbeing of their children. Saad et al. (22) proposed that in some female patients their motherly instincts are subverted by narcissistic attributed which increased the need for attention. Often many of the abusing mothers have a history of psychiatric illness.

EFFECTS ON CHILD

MSBP is characterized by four important features (i) fabrication of illness by caretaker or giver, (ii) child subjected to multiple diagnostic procedures and characterized by persistent illness, (iii) the perpetrator denies the cause of child illness and (iv) the separation of the child from the perpetrator stops the symptoms and signs presented by the child (23). The effect of MSBP on a child includes physical, emotional and psychological harm. The child often experiences a deterioration of existing medical health condition due to non-adherence to the medical treatment towards a genuine illness or he/she may acquire medical problems due to invasive diagnostic procedures and surgeries ordered by unwitting physicians. The child victims may undergo an acute or chronic harm resulting in death (24). Emotional and psychological effect in this illness is even more devastating, as the trust in parent child relationship is violated. Recent studies suggest that child victims of MSBP have a high chance of getting affected by this syndrome (25).

The most common symptoms of MSBP includes recurrent sepsis due to injection of fluids, chronic diarrhea due to laxative abuse, false renal stones by placing peppbles in the urine, apparent fever from heating a thermometer, rashes from trauma and false laboratory reports by placing blood or sugar in the urine (23). Other symptoms include apnea, CNS depression, seizures, bleeding, vomiting, diarrhea, fever, rash, allergies and psychiatric symptoms (26).

Morbidity and Mortality

The incidence of deaths and medical complications are vaguely understood as most of the cases go unreported. The mortality rate ranges between 9-31% in index cases. Based on a study, Sheridon (20) reported a mortality rate of 6% and long term injuries in7.3% of the index cases.

Morbidity can result either due to the direct result of the abuse or due to the various unnecessary invasive diagnostic and surgical procedures done by the physician. Mclure et al. (27) reported that 122 children out of 128 admitted in the hospital for physical abuse of which 93% received unnecessary interventions, 45 had major medical illness and 31 had minor physical illness and died.

Bools et al. (28) based on evaluation of 54 children aged between 1-14 years concluded that several had behavioral issues, achievement problems, emotional and conduct disorder, sleep disorders and post-traumatic stress disorder (PTSD). Adult survivors who were child victims also seem to be suffering from PTSD.

Diagnosis

The inconsistent signs and symptoms are undetectable and this makes the diagnosis of this fabricated disease difficult. The exaggeration and fabrication of the symptoms can often be differentiated by the researchers. The role of a clinician is very important and should be based on the amount of potential harm to the child. Physicians are often attracted in these scenarios to make making unnecessary diagnostic tests and treatments which could be injurious. The harmful medical care in these instances can range from a range of diagnostic search that supports the fabrications of the symptoms given by the parent (29).

When a clinician doubts that an illness could have been fabricated, it becomes pivotal for him to make a diagnosis to protect the child from any further harm. To find whether the signs and symptoms have been fabricated the clinician should collect information from the people involved and discuss the event with the concerns. It is imperative to know that fabrication of medical illness in these situations is a medical diagnosis. Although opinions from professionals such as psychologists and social workers are helpful in making a diagnosis, the confirmatory diagnosis is often difficult to make (29-31).

Management

To recognize MSBP as a form of child abuse occurring in medical practice, a multidisciplinary protocol must be established to protect the children (30). Child protective agencies have been mandated to handle the abused child safety regardless of whether the abuse occurs at home or in the hospital. The basic principles to be considered in child abuse are to make sure the child is safe, the child's future safety is assured and to allow treatment to occur in the least restrictive setting as possible.

If the parent or caretaker persists in harming the child, child abuse in this form should be reported in the same way as physical or sexual child abuse. When a dependent child is being hurt by an adult's action the child protective services should be involved. The interventions includes the application of individual and family therapy by a multidisciplinary team in order to monitor the ongoing medical care and monitor the signs and symptoms in a hospital setting. The primary care should also place the child in a safe setting, prosecute the offending family members and eliminate their access to the child if possible (1).

CONCLUSION

The detection and management of Munchausen syndrome by proxy is a challenging task by itself due to fabricated results. MSBP requires an effective multidiciplinary management, as it is a serious form of child abuse with a considerable rate of mortality.

ACKNOWLEDGMENTS

The authors thank the Department of Oral Pathology, Saveetha University for their support and contribution in preparation of the manuscript.

REFERENCES

[1] Stirling J. Beyond Munchausen syndrome by proxy: Identification and treatment of child abuse in a medical setting. Pediatrics 2007;119:1026-30.

[2] Hettler J. Munchausen syndrome by proxy. Pediatr Emerg Care 2002;18:371-4.

[3] American Psychiatric Association. Diagnostic and statistical manual of mental disorders, 4th ed, Text rev. Washington, DC: American Psychiatric Association, 2000:513.

[4] Asher R. Munchausen's syndrome. Lancet 1951;257:339-41.

[5] Meadow R. Munchausen syndrome by proxy: The hinterlands of child abuse. Lancet 1977;310:343–5.

[6] Meadow SR. Different interpretations of Munchausen syndrome by proxy. Child Abuse Negl 2002;26:501-8.

[7] Fisher GC. Etiological speculations. In: Levin AV, Sheridan MS, eds. Munchausen syndrome by proxy: Issues in diagnosis and treatment. New York: Lexington Books, 1995:39–57.

[8] Rand DC. Munchausen syndrome by proxy: integration of classic and contemporary type. Issues Child Abuse Accusations 1990;2:83-9.

[9] Wilson RG. Fabricated or induced illness in children: Munchausen by proxy comes of age. BMJ 2001;323:296-7.

[10] Ernst TN, Philp M. Severe iron deficiency anemia: an example of covert child abuse (Munchausen by proxy). West J Med 1986;144:358-9.

[11] Godding V, Kruth M. Compliance with treatment in asthma and Munchausen syndrome by proxy. Arch Dis Child 1991;66:956-60.

[12] Ayoub CC, Schreier HA, Keller C. Munchausen by proxy: presentations in special education. Child Maltreat 2002;7:149-59.

[13] Schreier H. Munchausen by proxy defined. Pediatrics 2002;110:985-8.

[14] Meadow SR. Different interpretations of Munchausen syndrome by proxy. Child Abuse Neglect 2002;26:501-8.

[15] Bodegård G. [Munchausen by proxy syndrome. When a parent who seems to engaged falsifies symptoms of his child]. Läkartidningen 2001;98(19):2294-6.

[16] Godding V, Kruth M. Compliance with treatment in asthma and Munchausen syndrome by proxy. Arch Dis Child 1991;66:956-60.
[17] Warner JO, Hathaway MJ. Allergic form of Meadow's syndrome (Munchausen by proxy). Arch Dis Child 1984;59:151-6.
[18] Oliver JE. Successive generations of child maltreatment: social and medical disorders in the parents. Br J Psychiatry 1985;147:484-90.
[19] McClure RJ, Davis PM, Meadow SR, Sibert JR. Epidemiology of Munchausen syndrome by proxy, non-accidental poisoning, and non-accidental suffocation. Arch Dis Child 1996;75:57-61.
[20] Sheridan MS. The deceit continues: an updated literature review of Munchausen syndrome by proxy. Child Abuse Negl 2003;27:431-51.
[21] Feldman KW, Feldman MD, Grady R, Burns MW, McDonald R. Renal and urologic manifestations of pediatric condition falsification/Munchausen by proxy. Pediatr Nephrol 2007;22:849-56.
[22] Saad G. Munchausen by proxy: the dark side of parental investment theory? Med Hypotheses 2010;75:479-81.
[23] Brown P, Tierney C. Munchausen syndrome by proxy. Pediatr Rev 2009;30(10:414-5.
[24] Sheridan M. The deceit continues: An update literature review of Munchausen syndrome by proxy. Child Abuse Negl 2003;27:431-51.
[25] Parnell TF. Defining Munchausen by proxy syndrome. In: Parnell TF, Day DO, eds. Munchausen by proxy syndrome: Misunderstood child abuse. Thousand Oaks, CA: Sage, 1998:9-46.
[26] Trejo-Hernandez J, Loredo-Abdala A, Orozco-Garibay JM. Munchausen syndrome by proxy in Mexican children. Rev Invest Clin 2011;63(3): 253-62.
[27] McClure RJ, Davis PM, Meadow SR, Sibert JR. Epidemiology of Munchausen syndrome by proxy, non-accidental poisoning, and non-accidental suffocation. Arch Dis Child 1996;75:57-61.
[28] Bools CN, Neale BA, Meadow SR. Follow up of victims of fabricated illness (Munchausen syndrome by proxy). Arch Dis Child 1993;69:625-30.
[29] Southall DP, Plunkett MC, Banks MW, Falkov AF, Samuels MP. Covert video recording of life-threatening child abuse: Lessons for child protection. Pediatrics 1997;100:735-60.
[30] Sanders M. Hospital protocol for the evaluation of Munchausen by proxy. Clin Child Psychol Psychiatry 1999;4:379-91.
[31] Hall DE, Eubanks L, Meyyazhagen LS, Kenney RD, Johnson SC. Evaluation of covert video surveillance in the diagnosis of Munchausen syndrome by proxy: Lessons from 41 cases. Pediatrics 2000;105:1305–12.

In: Child and Adolescent Health Issues
Editor: Joav Merrick

ISBN: 978-1-63463-574-5

Chapter 16

ACCIDENTAL BURN INJURIES IN CHILDREN TWELVE YEARS AND YOUNGER

Theodora M Chikwanha*, BScHOT, MPH,
Tamisayi Chinhengo, BScHOT, MPH
and Addmore Chadambuka, BScEHS, MPH
Departments of Rehabilitation and Community Medicine,
University of Zimbabwe, Harare, Zimbabwe

Chitungwiza and Harare Central hospitals experienced increases in paediatric burn injuries occurring at home from 35% and 31% in 2008 to 41% and 38% in 2009 respectively. A study was carried out to determine factors associated with these accidental burn injuries occurring at home. Methods: A matched 1:1 case control study was carried out at Chitungwiza and Harare Central Hospitals. A case was a child twelve years and below admitted with accidental burn injuries occurring at home between 1st May 2010 and 31st July 2010 residing in Chitungwiza and Harare. A control was a child twelve years and below admitted for other medical conditions at the two institutions during the same period and residing in the same neighbourhood as the case. Interviewer-administered questionnaires were administered to consenting caregivers of cases and controls within the wards. Results: 131 cases and 131 controls were interviewed. Independent risk factors for accidental burn injuries were child unattended at home AOR=2.88 (1.10-7.55), using same room for cooking and sleeping AOR= 5.08 (2.29-11.27), not taking precaution when cooking AOR =4.86 (1.73-13.65) and not taking precautions when serving food AOR =7.85 (2.18 -28.25). Previous health education on burn prevention AOR =0.39 (0.26-0.71) was protective. Conclusion: Most of the identified risk factors for burn injuries were within the home environment yet most caregivers reported taking precautions. There is need to educate the community on methods of modifying the home environment in order to reduce occurrence of burn injuries at home.

* Correspondence: Theodora M Chikwanha, Department of Rehabilitation, University of Zimbabwe, POBox A178, Harare, Zimbabwe. E-mail: middychiky@yahoo.co.uk or tchikwanha@medsch.uz.ac.zw

INTRODUCTION

Burn injuries are emerging as an important largely preventable, growing public health problem in developing countries, gradually climbing the ranking list of causes of mortality and morbidity. Every year over 300 000 people die from burns. In addition, millions of people are disabled and disfigured by severe burns (1).

Globally, paediatric burn injuries occurring within the home are the third most frequent cause of injury and death among all children from birth up to the age of nineteen years. Statistics on burn injuries are often fragmented when available as many burn injuries often go unreported if they are considered minor. This underestimates the severity of the problem. Despite global acknowledgement of burn injuries as a major public health problem, many countries have given it limited attention. This is due to limited resources and co-existence of other competing health problems e.g. HIV/AIDS (2, 3).

Thousands of survivors have to live with permanent disabilities. This is experienced even more by children as they grow into adolescents and adults with permanent physical and sometimes psychological scarring caused by an accident that occurred in childhood (4).

In Africa approximately 99% of the burn injuries in children occur within the home (4). In Zimbabwe, burn injuries account for an estimated 37.5% of hospital admissions and contribute 15% of the total deaths annually in children fourteen years and under (5). However, relatively little policy formulation and intervention work on burn injuries has been reported (6,7). Much of the intervention strategies on burn prevention in Zimbabwe have been on provision of health information and education material to public health institutions.

Since 2005 paediatric burns continued to account for over a quarter of accidents occurring at home, leading to hospital admissions at Harare and Chitungwiza Central Hospitals (see table 1). In 2008 burn injuries accounted for 35% of injuries occurring at home leading to hospital admissions in the paediatric ward at Chitungwiza Hospital and 31% at Harare Central Hospital. In 2009 paediatric burn injuries accounted for 41% of injuries occurring at home leading to hospital admissions at Chitungwiza Hospital and 38% at Harare Central Hospital.

A study was carried out to determine factors associated with burn injuries in children aged 12 years old and below. Specific Objectives were to describe occurrence of burns by time, place and person, to determine causes of burns among admitted children, to assess severity of paediatric burns, to assess burn prevention measures taken within the home, to determine risk factors for burn injuries.

Table 1. Paediatric Burns Admissions at Chitungwiza and Harare Central Hospitals 2005-2009

Year	Total Paediatric burns admissions Chitungwiza Central Hospital	Total paediatric admissions Harare Central Hospital
2005	194(29%)	469(30%)
2006	157(26%)	693(39%)
2007	295(37%)	572(28%)
2008	308(35%)	740(31%)
2009	306(41%)	807(38%)

OUR STUDY

A matched 1:1 case control study was conducted at Chitungwiza and Harare Central Hospitals. Cases and controls were frequency matched for place of residence. A case was a child twelve years and below admitted with burn injuries occurring at home between 1st May 2010 and 31st July 2010 at Harare and Chitungwiza Central Hospitals residing in Chitungwiza and Harare. A control was a child twelve years and below admitted for other medical conditions at the same institutions during the study period residing in the same neighbourhood as the case.

Assuming overcrowding was the most significant risk factor in burn injuries occurring in children twelve years and below with an odds ratio of 2.2 (8) and that 61% of burns in Zimbabwe occur in children twelve years and below (9), using a case to control ratio of 1:1 at the 95% confidence interval and 80% power, a sample 134 cases and 134 controls was computed.

Cases were recruited prospectively upon consent as they reported to the paediatric wards at Chitungwiza and Harare Central Hospitals for treatment. Controls were selected prospectively from children twelve years and below admitted for other medical conditions and staying in the same neighbourhood as the cases.

An interviewer-administered questionnaire was administered to consenting caregivers of cases. Patient case files were reviewed to obtain demographic information, diagnosis and severity of injury. The same questionnaire was administered to caregivers of controls within the wards at the two institutions.

Data was entered, cleaned and analysed using Epi Info statistical software. Odds ratios were calculated as measures of associations between identified risk factors. Logistic regression was performed to identify independent risk factors and simultaneously control for various confounding factors.

Approval to conduct study was sought from the Clinical Directors of Harare Central Hospital and Chitungwiza Central Hospital and from the Health studies office.

Ethical approval was sought and obtained from the Medical Research Council of Zimbabwe. Confidentiality was maintained and information obtained from participants was only used to identify risk factors for burn injuries. Purpose and benefits of the study were explained to participants and informed consent was sought from all caregivers.

OUR FINDINGS

A sample size of 134 cases and 134 controls had been calculated for the study; however 131cases and 131 controls were enrolled during the study period. Eighty one (62%) of the cases were males, fifty (38%) were females. Seventy of the controls (54%) were males, 61 (46%) were females. Five (4%) of the cases and one (1%) of the controls had epilepsy. Three of the cases (2%) and four of the controls (3%) had previous burn injuries. Median age of cases was 3 years (Q1=1, Q3=6) and for controls was 3 years (Q_1=1, Q_3=5).

Causes and time of occurrence of burn injuries

Eighty one (62%) of the burn injuries were caused by hot liquid, twenty two (17%) by hot porridge, seven (5%) by hot oil. The rest were caused by candles, hot ash, electricity, paraffin and hot plastic. Fifty eight (44%) of the burn injuries occurred in the evening, forty one (32%) in the morning and thirty two (24%) in the afternoon.

Place of burn occurrence

Fifty three (41%) of the injuries occurred in the kitchen, thirty (24%) occurred outdoors. Twenty seven (21%) occurred in a room used both as a kitchen and bedroom, thirteen (10%) occurred in the other tenants rooms as some households had two or more tenants sharing the same house and five (4%) in the bathroom.

Severity of burn injuries

Forty (31%) of the children had less than 5% total body surface area injured, Fifty four (41%) had between 5% and 9% total body surface area injured and 37 (28%) had 10% and more body surface area injured. One hundred and fifteen children (87%) had first degree burns and sixteen (13%) second degree burns.

Socio-demographic characteristics for caregivers

One hundred and twenty nine (98%) of caregivers for the cases were female and two (2%) were males. All the caregivers for the controls were female. One hundred and ten (84%) of the cases and one hundred and fifteen (88%) of the controls were cared for by their parents. Ninety percent of the caregivers for the cases and 87% of the caregivers for controls had secondary education. Eighty eight (67%) of the caregivers for the case and one hundred (76%) of the caregivers for the controls were unemployed.

Socio-economic factors associated with burn injuries

Median number of rooms used by the family for cases was 2 (Q_1=1, Q_3=3) and for controls was 3 (Q_1=1, Q_3=3). Average number of people per household for both cases and controls was 4 people. Forty four (34%) of the cases families and seventeen (13%) of the controls families had average monthly incomes of equal to or less than US$100. Ninety four (72%) of the cases and eighty nine (68%) of the controls cooked indoors when there was no electricity. Ninety (69%) of the cases used paraffin, thirty three (25%) used open fire and the rest used gas and gel for cooking when there was no electricity. Seventy three (56%) of the controls used paraffin, thirty seven (28%) used open fire, sixteen (12%) used gel and five (4%) used gas when there was a power cut.

Burn prevention measures practised by caregivers

Seventy eight (60%) of the caregivers for cases and ninety nine (75%) of the caregivers for controls took burn prevention precautions within their homes. Precautions taken by caregivers for both cases and controls included not leaving children unattended near the cooking area (68%), putting pot handles away from children's reach when cooking (6%), sitting children away from cooker (28%), not leaving children with hot beverages (20%) and hot food (62%), putting cold water first when bathing (54%), not boiling bathing water (13%) and not leaving children unattended in the bathroom (10%).

Table 2a. Factors associated with burn injuries burns in children twelve years and below admitted at Chitungwiza and Harare Central hospitals 2010

Factor	Cases n=131	Controls n=131	mOR	95% CI
Child unattended at home				
Y	25	9	3.20*	1.43-7.15
N	106	122		
Using Same room for cooking and sleeping				
Y	68	19	6.36*	3.51-11.54
N	63	112		
Average monthly income (US$)				
<100	44	17	3.39*	1.82-6.34
>100	87	114		
>4 people Per room				
Y	36	14	2.82*	1.45-5.47
N	95	117		
Taking precautions when cooking				
Y	27	6	5.41*	2.15-13.60
N	104	125		
Taking precautions when serving food				
Y	32	3	13.79*	4.10-46.35
N	99	128		
Indoor use of paraffin stove				
Y	94	89	1.20	0.71-2.03
N	37	42		

Factors associated with sustaining burn injuries

Risk factors for burn injuries (Table 2a,2b) were child remaining unattended at home [mOR 3.20 CI 1.43-7.15] ,using the same room for cooking and sleeping [mOR 6.36 CI 3.51-11.54], crowding [mOR 2.82 CI 1.45-5.47] ,having a monthly income of less than or equal to US$100 [mOR 3.39 CI 1.82-6.34] having a caregiver who is less than 18 years old [mOR 1.79 CI 1.05-3.05], not taking precautions when cooking [mOR 5.41 CI 2.15-13.60] and no precautions when serving food [mOR 13.79 CI 4.10-46.35]. Other risk factors not statistically significant were indoor use of a paraffin stove [mOR 1.92 CI 0.71-2.03] and being cared for by a caregiver who had only completed primary school (grade 7) [mOR 1.31 CI 0.42-3.62].

The only statistically significant protective factor was having had health education on burn prevention [mOR 0.39 CI 0.26-0.71]. Health education was given in form of lectures at some clinics in Harare and Chitungwiza.

Table 2b. Risk factors associated with burn injuries in children twelve years and below admitted at Chitungwiza Central Hospital, 2010

Factor	Cases	Controls	mOR	95%CI
Precaution when bathing child				
Y	63	89	1.75	0.93-3.30
N	68	42		
Health education on burns				
Y	21	43	0.39*	0.22-0.71
N	110	88		
Previous burn injury requiring medical care?				
Y	3	8	0.36	0.09-1.39
N	128	127		
Child's Sex				
F	50	61	0.71	0.43-1.16
M	81	70		
Staying with parent				
Y	110	115	0.729	0.362-1.469
N	21	16		

Independent risk factors for burn injuries

Independent risk factors identified using logistic regression (see table 3) were caregivers age less than 18 years [AOR 2.27 CI 1.18-4.35], child remaining unattended at home [AOR 2.88 CI 1.10-7.55], using same room for cooking and sleeping [AOR 5.08 CI 2.29-11.27], not taking precaution when cooking [AOR 4.86 CI 1.73-13.65] and not taking precautions when saving food [AOR 7.85 CI 2.18- 28.25].

Table 3. Independent risk factors associated with burn injuries in children admitted at Chitungwiza and Harare Central Hospitals 2010

Term	AOR	95%CI	Coeff	SE	Z-stats	P-Value
Caregiver age LR	2.27	1.18-4.44	0.82	0.33	2.46	0.01
Child unattended	2.88	1.10-7.55	1.06	0.49	2.15	0.03
Same room cooking and sleeping	5.08	2.29-11.27	1.63	0.41	3.10	0.001
No precautions when cooking	4.86	1.73-13.65	1.58	0.52	3.01	0.03
No precautions when serving food	7.85	2.18-28.25	2.06	0.65	3.16	0.002

DISCUSSION

Low income affected the type of accommodation that the children and their families stayed. Staying in a single room that was used for both cooking and sleeping put the children at a greater risk of sustaining a burn injury. Given that the average size of a room in the high density suburbs were most participants stayed was six square metres, a single room used for cooking and sleeping was more likely to have been overcrowded. Arrangement of furniture and other possessions within this room might not have left enough room for both children and adults to walk freely far away from the cooking area and hence the increased risk for children to sustain burn injuries as they are less likely to always remember to take necessary precautions .

Leaving a child alone at home was a risk factor for burn injuries. While this was consistent with findings in Ghana (10) and Brazil (11) where risk of burns was higher for children who were sometimes left unattended, reasons why children were often left unattended in this study were different. Children were left alone as parents mostly mothers went to their informal work places, to the market, or as parents visited friends in the neighbourhood. Some children were left just for a few minutes as their mothers hurried to the nearest shop (tuckshop) to buy bread for breakfast. In Zimbabwe these are common practices as most mothers who either unemployed or not formally employed cannot afford baby minders even for short periods of time or on a part time basis.

It is important to note that when children are left alone, regardless of the time period that they are left unattended, they are always at risk of having an accidental injury either through playing or as they try to prepare a meal for themselves. Therefore caregiver education should be clear on the risks associated with leaving children alone at home and how accidental injuries occur even when children are left for short periods of time.

Indoor use of paraffin stoves though not statistically significant cannot be ignored as a risk factor for burn injuries. Study results show that most of the burn injuries occur when there are power cuts and many people resort to using paraffin stoves within their homes for cooking. Currently there are frequent power cuts in most parts of Zimbabwe and as such there is likely to be an increased use of alternative sources of cooking energy with paraffin being the mostly used. There is need therefore to educate the communities of the dangers of using paraffin stoves and the necessary precautions they can take to prevent burn injuries.

Having previous health education on burn injuries was found to be protective against burn injuries. This was consistent with findings by Delgado et al. (8) who found that history of previous accident and health education on burn injuries had a significant protective effect among children who lived in good environmental conditions. However health education was only being given at a few clinics in both Harare and Chitungwiza and not all mothers visit these health care facilities. Health education messages should disseminated in such a way that even those who do not visit the health care facilities access the information.

The majority of injuries occurred in the kitchen and were caused by hot liquids. Peak time for burn occurrence was during the evening when evening meals were being prepared. Unlike other meal times when children can play and wait to be called when the meal is ready, during evening meal times most children will be indoors and depending with the available space within the home they might go near the cooking area as they play or move within the room hence occurrence of more burns during this time.

Some of the injuries occurred in the neighbours' house. In Zimbabwe it is common practice to have more than three families sharing the same house with each family occupying one or two rooms. Therefore even if the caregivers of children take precautions within their own homes burn injuries may still occur because the neighbours might not take any precautions possibly because they might not have younger children in their homes. Those without young children in their homes must also be targeted when educating the communities about burn prevention within the homes.

Two thirds of the admissions for burn injuries were children less than five years with more boys being affected than girls. These findings were consistent with those by Mzezewa et al. (9) and Muguti et al. (12). Younger children are less likely to understand and follow burn prevention measures in the home than older ones hence more children less than five years being admitted for burn injuries. Boys are also naturally likely to be more adventurous and engage in play that would result in them sustaining more injuries than girls.

While majority of caregivers reported that they took precautions within their homes to prevent occurrence of burn injuries, not taking burn prevention precaution within the home when cooking and serving food wer seen to increase the likelihood of a child getting a burn injury. Also most of the injuries occurred during meal preparation times. It is essential to look at other precautions that the caregivers may take in the homes during meal preparations apart from the ones they are already taking as several measures may actually be required during meal preparation times to prevent burn injuries.

In conclusion, most burn injuries occurred in low income households. Burn injuries in children were associated with inadequate accommodation, leaving children unattended and not taking precautions when cooking and serving food. Children less than five years were mostly admitted for burn injuries.

RECOMMENDATIONS

Non communicable diseases and health education and promotion departments

- To develop burn prevention programmes focusing on community education on:
  - how burn injuries occur within the homes
  - burn injury prevention methods that can be taken within homes

Health education and promotion department

- To involve the Media in broadcasting burn prevention programmes on local television and radio

Public health officers

- Public Health officers should periodically evaluate the effectiveness of burn prevention strategies in use so that they remain relevant to the communities.

Actions to date

- Study findings and recommendations submitted to Non communicable diseases and health education and promotion departments within the Ministry of Health and Child welfare (Zimbabwe) for use in future development of burn prevention programmes.

ACKNOWLEDGMENTS

Mrs T Chinhengo – Field supervisor, Mr A Chadambuka - Academic supervisor, Department of Community Medicine University of Zimbabwe, Zimbabwe Field Epidemiology and Training Programme, Chitungwiza Central Hospital, Harare Central Hospital, Statisticians. Sponsors: Mr M A Muchengi, Mrs AN Mudondo,

Dr E Chikwanha and Dr IT Chikwanha

REFERENCES

[1] Mock C. World Health Organisation joins forces with international society for burn injuries to confront global burden of burns. Inj Prev 2007; 13(5):303.

[2] Dissanaike S. Epidemiology of burns injuries: Highlighting cultural and sociodemographic aspects. Int Rev Psychiatr 2009;21(6):505-11.

[3] World Health Organization. The injury chart book. A graphical overview of the global burden of injuries. Geneva: WHO, 2009.

[4] Celko AM, Grivna M, Barss P. Severe childhood burns in Czech Republic: risk factors and prevention. Bull World Health Organ 2009;87:384-381.

[5] Ministry of health and child welfare Zimbabwe. Disability and rehabilitation report. Accessed 2009 November 13. URL: www.mohcw.gov.zw/index.php/disability-and-rehabilitation.

[6] Forjour SN, Zwi B, Mock N. Injury control in Africa, getting governments to do more. Trop Med Int Health 1998;3(5):349-56.

[7] Atiyer BS, Rubeiz M, Ghananimeh G, Nassor AN, Al Amm CA. Management of paediatric burns. Euro-Mediterranean Council Burns Fire Disasters 2000;13(3):1-3.

[8] Delgado J, Ramirez-Cardich M, Gilman R, Lavareilo R, Dahodavala N, Bazou A. Risk factors for burns in children: crowding, poverty and poor maternal education. Inj Prev 2000;8(11):38-41.

[9] Muzezewa SN, Johnsson K, Aberg M, Salemark L. A prospective study on the epidemiology of burns in patients admitted to the Harare burns units. Burns 1999;25(6):499-504.

[10] Fourjor SN, Guyer B, Smith GS. Childhood burns in Ghana. Epidemiological characteristics and home based treatment. Burns 1995;21(1):24-8.

[11] Werneck GL, Reichenhem ME. Paediatric burns and associated risk factors in Rio de Janeiro, Brazil. Burns 1997;23(6):478-83.

[12] Muguti GI, Mazabane BN. An analysis of factors contributing to mortality rates in burns patient's treatment at Mpilo Central Hospital, Zimbabwe. J R Coll Surg Edinb 1997;42(4):259-61.

In: Child and Adolescent Health Issues
Editor: Joav Merrick

ISBN: 978-1-63463-574-5

Chapter 17

CHILD AND ADOLESCENT INJURY PREVENTION

Adnan A Hyder*, MD, MPH, PhD[1], Nhan T Tran, PhD, MHS[1], Abdulgafoor M Bachani, PhD, MHS[1], David Bishai, MD, MPH, PhD[1] and Margie Peden, PhD[2]

[1]International Injury Research Unit, Department of International Health, Johns Hopkins Bloomberg School of Public Health, Baltimore, Maryland, United States of America and

[2]Department of Violence and Injury Prevention and Disability, World Health Organization, Geneva, Switzerland

More than 875,000 children die from preventable injuries annually. Developing effective interventions to prevent child and adolescent injuries remains a major challenge for the field. A number of intervention strategies such as the use of helmets, seat-belts, and pool fences, have been shown to be effective at preventing injury-related deaths in children. The objective of this study was to estimate the potential reductions in injury-related child mortality that can be achieved through the implementation of a select group of existing interventions. A review of the literature on intervention strategies applicable to childhood unintentional injuries was conducted. Data on intervention effectiveness were then extracted from the literature identified and applied to current estimates of injury-related child mortality. This study assumed equality of intervention effectiveness across world regions. 80 papers and reports were reviewed from which effectiveness data on twelve intervention strategies applicable to the prevention of injury among children were identified. If each of these twelve intervention strategies were implemented globally, the result may be the prevention of between 8,000 to 80,000 child deaths for each type of injury. While the urgent need to research and identify new intervention strategies for preventing injury deaths in children remains, this analysis has demonstrated that there might be tremendous benefits—up to 1,000 child lives a day, that may be realized through enhanced coverage of existing interventions which have already been tried and tested.

---

* Correspondence: Adnan A Hyder, MD, MPH, PhD, International Injury Research Unit, The Johns Hopkins Bloomberg School of Public Health, 615 North Wolfe Street, Suite E8132, Baltimore, MD 21205, United States. E-mail: ahyder1@jhu.edu

INTRODUCTION

Unintentional injuries continue to be a major cause of death and disability worldwide, especially among children. Each year, more than 875,000 children die from preventable injuries; millions more are injured and permanently disabled (1-3). Road traffic injuries and drowning are the leading cause of death among young people 0-17 years (4, 5). Injuries afflict children everywhere – homes, streets, playgrounds, schools – and occur throughout childhood years; they also disproportionately affect children in low and middle income countries (LMIC) (1-3).

In the last several decades, significant progress has been made in understanding the epidemiology of injuries in children (2). Developing effective interventions to prevent injuries among children, however, remains a global challenge (6). For some types of injuries, such as those related to road traffic crashes, there are numerous interventions that have been demonstrated to be effective in high-income country (HIC) settings, and the challenge is to transfer that technology to LMIC settings (4,7). For other injuries such as drowning, there have been few interventions that have been proven effective anywhere in the world, despite the huge burden of drowning deaths among children (8-11).

As part of the second Disease Control Priorities project (DCP2), the effectiveness of existing intervention strategies for injury prevention were examined (12). The DCP2 work was of great significance as it demonstrated the cost effectiveness of injury prevention interventions compared with other public health interventions globally; injury prevention strategies were among the most cost effective public health interventions currently available between $5 and $556 per disability adjusted life year (DALY) gained. Similarly, Miller and colleagues carried out cost-benefit analyses for various interventions for injury prevention in the United States and found that a $10 bicycle helmet could result in benefits valued at $440 while a $50 child safety seat could result in a potential savings of $1,500 (13).

This study builds upon previous work by providing an overview of available data on intervention strategies applicable to the prevention of childhood injuries globally. The specific objectives of this study are: 1) to conduct a review of the literature on the effectiveness of interventions aimed at the prevention of unintentional injuries among children; and 2) to estimate the total number of children's lives that could be saved worldwide through the implementation of interventions that have been shown to be effective.

OUR STUDY

A review of the literature was conducted to identify efficacy and/or effectiveness data for intervention strategies for unintentional injuries among children. This included a review of the following electronic databases using standardized keyword searches: Scholar Google, Medline, Embase, Current Contents, and the Cochrane Review. Types of keywords used in the search included: unintentional injury, child injury, intervention effectiveness, motorcycle helmets, bicycle helmets, seatbelt, speed control, legislation, speed bumps, child seats, daytime running lights, falls, burns, drowning and poisoning. Additional literature on effectiveness was identified through internet searches, review of organizational websites, review of references of selected papers, and contacts with selected injury researchers recommended by WHO. The review was performed by two members of the study team independently and later reconciled. Studies that described interventions but did not report their effectiveness were excluded from the review, while all those that reported estimates on intervention effectiveness (irrespective of their location), and systematic reviews of child injury intervention effectiveness were included.

Data on the intervention effectiveness, injury related fatalities, study design, and population under study were extracted from the literature and tabulated (see tables 1-2). Effectiveness data obtained through a research study—including non-randomized studies and reported in peer reviewed journals were included in this analysis; estimates of intervention effectiveness reported in the grey literature were not included in this analysis. Due to the limited data on non-fatal injuries among children, this analysis only addresses the potential reductions in mortality; the effectiveness data included is specific to mortality reductions. Lower and upper bounds were then constructed to provide a range of plausible intervention effectiveness. In instances where there were different reports of effectiveness for a given intervention, the lowest reported estimate was used as the lower bound and highest estimate was used as the upper bound. For those interventions where only one effectiveness rate was identified, the lower bound estimate was 90% of the reported effectiveness and the upper bound was 110% of the reported effectiveness. These effectiveness rates were then applied to the number of child deaths that could be prevented by the intervention strategies.

For each intervention strategy included in this analysis, the injury specific death rate for children and number of children unprotected by the intervention were approximated using existing estimates of the injury incidence rates in each of the WHO regions from the Global Burden of Disease 2002 data (14). First, the total number of child deaths resulting from a given injury was determined from information on the age distribution of deaths, type of event/injury, exposure categories, presence of existing interventions as well as the level of intervention coverage, from the current literature. These data were then extracted and applied to WHO population estimates to generate estimates of injury-specific death rates in each region (1,6,7,15-23). Using these estimates the number of children who are unprotected by existing interventions was estimated by identifying from the literature the proportion of children that are impacted by an intervention. In the case of bicycle helmets for example, the proportion of children impacted by the intervention would be those children currently riding bicycles. Next, using current rates of intervention coverage if currently in place, the number of children unprotected was calculated by deducting the number of children already receiving or using the intervention from the total number of child deaths that could be prevented by the intervention (see figure 1).

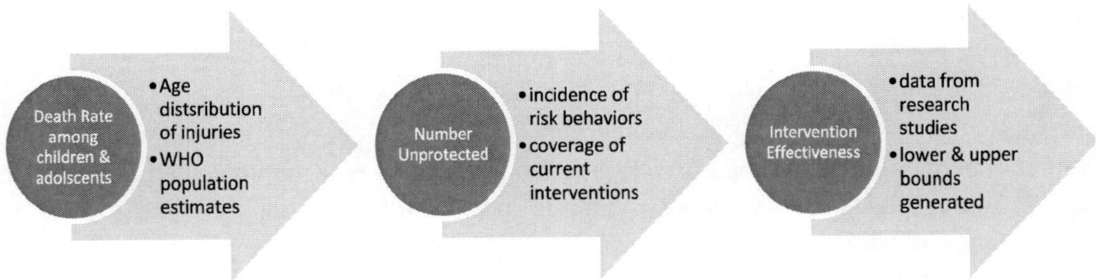

Figure 1. Schematic of the process used to obtain estimates.

Some studies, such as those which measured the impact of bicycle helmets, were carried out using a case control design and reported relative risk reductions among the sample of riders included in the study. In such instances, an "estimated intervention coverage level" was applied to the reported intervention effectiveness in order to approximate the impact of the intervention in non-controlled settings. When possible, actual data on intervention coverage from published studies were generalized to other country settings as the estimated intervention coverage. The estimates of intervention effectiveness were then applied to the population of children (defined as all persons younger than 18 years) impacted by the type of injury addressed by the intervention who were unprotected the intervention (1).

These figures were then used as the baseline against which the new intervention effects were applied in order to yield the projected reduction in child deaths. For interventions targeting road traffic injuries, the intervention effectiveness statistics were only applied to the category of road user that could be prevented from dying as a result of the intervention. For example, motorcycle helmets will only protect child pillion riders who are helmeted. Due to lack of evaluation studies for interventions in many regions, the same effectiveness ratewas used in all regions. In some cases this assumption will underestimate the benefit of the intervention; in other cases it might overestimate the benefit. Ex ante there is no way to predict the overall direction of the bias.

Using the approach outlined above the number of lives saved by each intervention and then by all interventions were estimated. The formula used to estimate the number of lives saved was as follows:

[1] *Lives Saved by intervention k=*
$$\Sigma_i \text{ Number Unprotected}_k \times \text{Effectiveness}_k \times \text{Death Rate}_{ik}$$

[2] *Total Lives Saved in regions 1..i..I=*
$$\Sigma_i \Sigma_k \text{ Number Unprotected}_k \times \text{Effectiveness}_k \times \text{Death Rate}_{ik}$$

Where *Number Unprotected* is an estimate of the number of children who currently do not receive intervention but can benefit from *"k"*; $Effectiveness_k$ is an estimate of the relative risk of those exposed to an intervention vs. those unexposed to *intervention k*; and $Death\ Rate_{ik}$ is the death rate in the *i-th* region from injuries preventable by *intervention k*. This analysis was applied globally by age and also using WHO regions. All of the data on intervention effectiveness thus apply only to the reductions in risk for mortality.

The authors are aware that multiple interventions implemented together might result in a differential impact. While the interaction between interventions may not always result in a simple additive effect (total effect of all the interventions is the sum of each intervention effect singly), there are currently no models available to predict the combined effect of injury prevention strategies. Moreover, no published studies have assessed the impact of risk homeostasis and its effect on the concurrent implementation of interventions, such as motorcycle helmet legislation and drivers licensing programs both implemented at the same time. Therefore, this analysis does not attempt to model the overall impact of the concurrent implementation of all interventions; rather, it models the number of lives that can be saved from the application of single interventions.

Excluded from this analysis were those interventions strategies that only had relevance in North America and Europe such as graduated licensing programs. Moreover, as the purpose of this analysis is to document the potential gains of targeted interventions for preventing childhood injuries, advancements in medical care such as acute burn management strategies that can result in higher survival rates for victims have also been excluded from this analysis. The authors do not intend to devalue the importance of these improvements and have excluded them from this analysis as they are longer term enhancements that should be considered as part of improving the quality of medical care and strengthening of health systems.

OUR FINDINGS

80 papers and reports were reviewed from which 46 interventions for child unintentional injury were identified. As shown in table 1, these ranged from measures to limit alcohol consumption for the prevention of road traffic deaths, to the use of window guards to prevent falls. Fourteen intervention strategies were excluded from the analysis due to the lack of applicability (relevance) to LMICs. These included interventions that had a low predicted probability of being successfully implemented and enforced in the near future in a LMIC such as the regulation of playground standards, establishment of poison centers, graduated driver licensing, and lifeguards. Of the remaining 32 that could be applied globally, effectiveness data was available for only twelve intervention strategies. These intervention strategies addressed the following categories of childhood unintentional injuries: road traffic, poisoning, drowning, and burns (table 2). It should be noted that exclusion from this analysis is not an indication of an intervention's lack of effectiveness; it only indicates that no estimate of the interventions' effectiveness was available. The estimated benefits of implementing these twelve interventions are presented in table 3.

Table 1. Available Interventions for the Prevention of Unintentional Child Injuries

Intervention	Type of injury addressed	Effectiveness data available?	Applicable in LMIC settings?	Included in analysis
1. Motorcycle helmets	Road Traffic	Yes	Yes	Yes
2. Bicycle helmet	Road Traffic	Yes	Yes	Yes
3. Stricter traffic codes	Road Traffic	Yes	Yes	Yes
4. Restraint mechanisms (car seat/ safety belts)	Road Traffic	Yes	Yes	Yes
5. Daytime running lights (motorcycles)	Road Traffic	Yes	Yes	Yes
6. Daytime running lights (cars & lorries)	Road Traffic	Yes	No	No
7. Speed enforcement detection devices	Road Traffic	Yes	Yes	Yes
8. Exclusive motorcycle lanes	Road Traffic	Yes	Yes	Yes
9. Graduated driver licensing	Road Traffic	Yes	No	No
10. Zero tolerance alcohol laws	Road Traffic	Yes	Yes	Yes

Table 1. (Continued)

Intervention	Type of injury addressed	Effectiveness data available?	Applicable in LMIC settings?	Included in analysis
11. Minimum legal drinking age laws	Road Traffic	No	No	No
12. Mass medial publicity on drinking and driving	Road Traffic	No	Yes	No
13. Server intervention training	Road Traffic	No	Yes	No
14. School-based education	Road Traffic	No	Yes	No
15. Rear seating position	Road Traffic	No	Yes	No
16. Rumble strips/speed bumps	Road Traffic	Yes	Yes	Yes
17. Childproof kerosene containers	Poisoning	Yes	Yes	Yes
18. Home visits	Poisoning/Burns/Falls	No	Yes	No
19. Removal of toxic agents in home	Poisoning	No	No	No
20. Non-lethal doses of chemicals in packaging	Poisoning	No	Yes	No
21. Poison control centers	Poisoning	No	Yes	No
22. Fences/barriers around pools and bodies of water	Drowning	Yes	Yes	Yes
23. Lifeguards	Drowning	No	No	No
24. Swimming lessons	Drowning	No	Yes	No
25. Covering water hazard	Drowning	No	No	No
26. Personal floatation devices	Drowning	No	No	No
27. Immediate resuscitation	Drowning	No	Yes	No
28. Drowning awareness education	Drowning	No	Yes	No
29. Standards for baby walkers	Falls	No	Yes	No
30. Multi-faceted programs: "Children can't fly"	Falls	No	No	No
31. Window guards/stops	Falls	No	Yes	No
32. Playground equipment standards	Falls	No	No	No
33. Maintenance of playground equipment	Falls	No	No	No
34. Redesigning nursery furniture	Falls	No	No	No
35. Stair gates	Falls	No	Yes	No
36. Reduced spacing between railings & balusters	Falls	No	Yes	No
37. Protective sports equipment	Falls	No	Yes	No
38. Housing and building codes	Falls	No	Yes	No
39. Rehabilitation	Falls	No	No	No
40. Smoke detectors	Burns	Yes	Yes	Yes
41. Tap water temperature regulation	Burns	No	No	No
42. Child resistant lighters	Burns	No	No	No
43. Fire-safe cigarettes	Burns	No	Yes	No
44. Separating cooking areas from living areas	Burns	No	Yes	No
45. Fire resistant clothing	Burns	No	No	No
46. Safe lamps	Burns	No	Yes	No

Table 2. Selected Interventions for the Prevention of Unintentional Child Injuries

Intervention Strategy	Type of injury addressed	Age group at risk	Child Population at risk for fatality& currently unprotected	Effectiveness Estimates (reduction in risk of death)			
				Point Estimate	Lower Bound	Upper Bound	Source(s)
ROAD TRAFFIC:							
Motorcycle helmets	Motorcyclist	0-18	133,305	36%	20%	48%	Liu B et al. 2003
Stricter traffic codes	All road traffic	0-18	298,419	25%	22%	27%	Aeron-Thomas AS & Hess S. 2005; Poli de Figueiredo et al. 2001
Rumble strips & Speed Bumps	Pedestrian	0-18	88,674	55%	50%	60%	Afukaar FK. 2003
Bicycle helmets	Bicyclists	0-18	61982	55%	50%	60%	Thompson DC et al., 1999; Li G & Baker SP., 1997; Thompson DC et al., 1996; Thomas S et al., 1994
Restraint mechanism: Car/booster seat, seat belt	Car occupants	0-18	71773	53%	45%	60%	Harris GT & Olukoga IA, 2005; Dinh-Zarr T, Sleet D, et al., 2001; Evans L, 1986, WHO 2004, NHTSA 2002
Daytime Running Lights:motorcycles	Motorcyclist	0-18	134723	29%	26%	31%	Radin UR et al., 1996
Speed enforcement detection devices	All road traffic	0-18	298,419	15%	13%	17%	Wilson C et al., 2006
Exclusive MC lanes	Motorcyclists	0-18	134,723	39%	35%	42%	Sohadi RUR et al., 2000
Alcohol control	Car occupants	0-18	71773	20%	18%	22%	WHO 2007; Dellinger AM et al., 2007
POISONING:							
Childproof Kerosene containers	Poisoning	0-4	16,236	48%	43%	53%	Krug et al., 1994
DROWNING:							
Fencing/Barriers	Drowning	0-7	144,473	73%	66%	80%	Thompson DC and RivaraFP, 1998
BURNS:							
Smoke detectors	Burns	0-18	89,931	60%	50%	70%	Ruynan CW et al. 1992; Ahrens M, 2003; Ballesteros MF et al., 2005

Road traffic injuries

The largest number of interventions with effectiveness data were among those targeting fatal road traffic injuries comprising nine of the twelve strategies identified (table 2). These included personal (motorcycle helmets), enforcement (speed limits), and environmental (exclusive motorcycle lanes) interventions. The greatest reductions could result from the strengthening of traffic codes by specifying primary faults and increases in penalties, which if implemented worldwide, could result in the prevention of 80,573 (74,605 – 86,542) child deaths. The use of speed detection devices to enhance enforcement of speed limits also shows great promise and could result in the prevention of 44,763 (38,795 – 50,731) child deaths (24). Another regulatory measure is the establishment of legal blood-alcohol (BAC) limits for drivers (25). Introducing legal BAC limits could potentially save 16,318 (12,277-20,750) children's lives.

Table 3. Estimated number of Children's Lives Saved Annually by Single Interventions by Age Group

Injury Type/Intervention	AGE GROUP				TOTAL		
	0 to 4 Yrs	5 to 9 Yrs	10 to 14 Yrs	15 to 18 Yrs		Range	
	Estimate	Estimate	Estimate	Estimate	Estimate	LB	UB
Road Traffic							
Motorcycle helmets	8,869	6,682	6,903	11,615	34,069	16,833	55,641
Stricter traffic codes	20,753	16,372	15,856	27,593	80,573	74,605	86,542
Rumble strips	10,062	8,346	8,074	12,273	38,756	19,334	58,096
Bicycle helmets	6,062	4,653	4,710	8,720	24,145	10,696	31,638
Child seats / Seat-belts	9,437	5,713	4,865	7,434	27,450	18,728	36,250
Daytime Running Lights (DRL) - Motorcycles	10,196	7,671	7,909	13,293	39,070	31,334	52,677
Speed enforcement detection devices	11,529	9,095	8,809	15,330	44,763	38,795	50,731
Exclusive lanes for motorcycles	3,428	2,579	2,659	4,469	13,135	10,535	17,711
Alcohol Control (Laws and enforcement)	5,217	4,471	2,472	4,157	16,318	12,277	20,750
Poisoning							
Childproof Kerosene containers	7,793	0	0	0	7,793	4,538	12,459
Drowning							
Fencing/Barriers	45,410	11,195	0	0	56,606	50,945	62,266
Burns							
Working Smoke Detectors/Alarms	24,550	9,446	9,008	10,955	53,959	40,469	69,247

LB: Lower bound (90%); UB: upper bound (110%).

While already in use in some parts of the world, increasing the coverage of motorcycle helmets among children from its current estimated level of 17-21% to an ideal coverage level of 90% could result in an additional 34,069 (16,833 – 55,641) children's lives saved. Similarly, 24,145 (10,696 – 31,638) more children's lives could be saved if the bicycle helmet coverage level of 80% set by Sweden could be met by all countries (26). Another intervention already being implemented in North America and Europe with potential for expansion to other parts of the world is the use of restraint mechanisms (27,28). Even though the number of children riding in passenger vehicles is significantly lower in LMICs than in high income countries, 27,450 children's lives could be saved if 90% of all young occupants in LMICs were appropriately restrained in booster seats and/or seatbelts as they are in North America and Europe (7,29-32).

In addition to these interventions, a number of vehicle and road enhancements have also been shown to have promise in preventing road traffic deaths among children (33). In Malaysia, the use of daytime running lights on motorcycles resulted in 29% reduction in motorcycle crashes; if used worldwide, 39,070 (31,334 – 52,677) child pillion riders could be saved each year (34). Only two intervention strategies targeting environmental modifications have been evaluated. The first is the use of speed bumps or rumble strips to slow traffic speed in identified 'black spots' where a large number of crashes occur(33). This was shown to reduce pedestrian deaths by as much as 55%; if this strategy were adopted by all countries, as many as 38,756 (19,334 – 58,096) child pedestrian deaths could be prevented each year. Another environmental intervention is the use of exclusive motorcycle lanes on highways. The first known exclusive motorcycle lane was built in Malaysia and subsequent evaluations documented a 39% reduction in motorcycle crashes on highways (35). Under the assumption that as much as 89% of passenger-miles-traveled is on highways and factoring in the differences in motorcycle usage across regions, this intervention could result in a net gain of 13,135 (10,535 – 17,711) child passengers saved.

Poisoning

While there are more than ten potential strategies identified for the prevention of poisoning such as improved labeling of chemicals and establishment of poison control centers, this review identified only one intervention strategy that had been evaluated in the scientific literature. Numerous descriptive studies identified risk factors such as lack of adult supervision and the storage of toxic substances in containers easily accessible to children (36-38). Only one study conducted in 1994 by Krug et al. showed that the free distribution of childproof containers to households in South Africa for storage of cleaning supplies and cooking fuels could effectively prevent 48% of all kerosene poisonings (39). Although the Krug study was specific to kerosene used for cooking, the basic principle of securing containers of hazardous materials to prevent access by children can be applied to other settings. As this intervention specifically targets young children, the 48% effect is applied only to children 0-4 years in this analysis. Also, as the 1994 study was conducted at a population level, it is assumed in this analysis that the 48% reduction observed is the intervention effectiveness under field conditions and as such, no additional adjustment were made for coverage. Thus this intervention could potentially save over 7,500 child injury deaths globally (table 3).

Drowning

Despite being one of the leading causes of child mortality in many LMICs such as Bangladesh, China, and Vietnam, few interventions for preventing drowning deaths in children have been evaluated (40). In some high income countries, existing strategies include the use of life jackets (or personal floatation devices) and ensuring the presence of lifeguards; there is however, limited data that demonstrates the effectiveness of such strategies (12,41). The use of barriers is the only intervention strategy that has been shown to be effective at preventing drowning among young children (16). Studies in the United States and other high-income countries show that installing a four-sided fence around a pool can reduce the risk of drowning among young children by 73% (16).

In LMIC such as Vietnam or Bangladesh where rural households often maintain a pond as a water source, similar barriers either around the water body or in the home can be constructed to limit access by children. As the use of such barriers is only effective at preventing young children from accessing bodies of water, this analysis limits the application of the intervention effectiveness to children under 8 years of age (42). Installing a fence or other barriers is an environmental modification; once installed, no additional action is required on the part of the parent or child. In North America, Europe, and Australia where most of the child drowning deaths occur in swimming pools, it is reasonable to expect that all pools can be effectively fenced off from children. However, the authors recognize that in many LMIC settings where households are situated in close proximity to large lakes and rivers creating a complete barrier between the household and the body of water may be difficult or infeasible. As such, in this analysis, we conservatively assume that a barrier can be effectively used in only 50% of all bodies of water accessible by children in LMICs. Even with this restriction this potential intervention could save more than 56,606 (50,945-62,266) child lives each year.

Burns

While the review identified several strategies for the prevention of burn related deaths in children such as childproof lighters, fire-safe cigarettes, safe lamps, regulation of hot water temperature in households, and fire resistant clothing, effectiveness data was only available for the use of smoke detectors in households. Studies from the United States have shown that properly working smoke detectors can reduce the risk of a fire related death by 50-70% (43-45). If this strategy were implemented worldwide, 53,959 (40,469-69,247) children could be saved on an annual basis. Although living conditions in LMICs are vastly different than those in the United States; smoke detectors can be manufactured at a low cost and can be installed in almost all settings as they can be battery operated (43-48). This makes them a feasible intervention for even the poorest households where access to electricity is limited.

Overall

Based on the assumptions described above, each of the 12 interventions is estimated to have the potential to save between 8,000 and 80,000 child injury deaths each year (table 3) in all regions of the world (table 4). Exceptions to this occur where either an intervention is specific to some but not other regions (such as use of child protection containers for kerosene in Africa, South and Southeast Asia) or where current coverage levels were used as the reference (child restraints in North America or Europe). The Western Pacific countries and African LMIC gain considerably relative to other regions in terms of child deaths averted.

Table 4. Estimated number of children's lives saved annually by single interventions by region

	WHO REGION						TOTAL		
	AFR	AMR	EMR	EUR	SEAR	WPR		Range	
	Estimate	Estimate	Estimate	Estimate	Estimate	Estimate	Estimate	LB	UB
Road Traffic									
Motorcycle helmets	1,445	1,674	1,390	520	20,918	8,123	**34,069**	**16,833**	**55,641**
Stricter traffic codes	14,765	6,990	7,190	4,705	31,999	14,924	**80,573**	**74,605**	**86,542**
Rumble strips	15,400	3,987	586	1,073	13,819	3,891	**38,756**	**19,334**	**58,096**
Bicycle helmets	1,240	1,587	2,763	970	7,740	9,845	**24,145**	**10,696**	**31,638**
Child seats / Seat-belts	9,472	0	4,860	0	8,035	5,084	**27,450**	**18,728**	**36,250**
Daytime Running Lights (DRL) - Motorcycles	1,586	1,877	1,622	606	24,402	8,976	**39,070**	**31,334**	**52,677**
Speed enforcement detection devices	8,203	3,883	3,995	2,614	17,777	8,291	**44,763**	**38,795**	**50,731**
Exclusive lanes for motorcycles	533	631	545	204	8,204	3,018	**13,135**	**10,535**	**17,711**
Alcohol Control (Laws and enforcement)	7,767	615	1,811	1,054	3,081	1,990	**16,318**	**12,277**	**20,750**
Poisoning									
Childproof Kerosene containers	4,889	59	1,059	0	1,787	0	**7,793**	**4,538**	**12,459**
Drowning									
Fencing/Barriers	11,434	4,586	2,234	3,160	9,395	25,796	**56,606**	**50,945**	**62,266**
Burns									
Working Smoke Detectors/Alarms	14,286	1,884	7,225	1,941	25,574	3,049	**53,959**	**40,469**	**69,247**

LB: lower bound (90%); UB: upper bound (110%); AFR: African Region; AMR: Region of the Americas; EMR: Eastern Mediterranean Region; EUR: European Region; SEAR: South East Asian Region; WPR: Western Pacific Region

DISCUSSION

Current formulations of child health programs generally ignore the impact of child injuries globally and within countries. The authors acknowledge that these estimates were based on data that were derived in some instances from non-randomized studies as well as the limited applicability of studies carried out in different regions with different populations. However, as suggested by this paper, there are potentially huge gains in child mortality from the implementation of existing injury prevention strategies that are known to be effective; each intervention having the potential to save between 8,000 to 80,000 child deaths annually.

This study did not model the benefits of concurrent implementation of interventions (motorcycle helmet legislation and speed control); it is not possible to determine the collective impact of the twelve interventions discussed in this paper. However, assuming that as much as half of the child deaths averted would be the same children if two interventions such as the motorcycle helmet and speed control were implemented, there would still be large positive gains to society. Even with this assumption, as much as a third to half of all current injury related deaths among children worldwide—up to 1,000 lives each day, could be prevented through the implementation of only twelve of the possible 46 interventions identified in this analysis.

Examination of the geographical distribution of the potential benefits of these interventions reveals that countries in the WHO South-East Asian region can gain the most, followed by countries in the Western Pacific region and countries in the African region (table 4). This is not surprising given that the majority of the injury related mortality occurs in these regions. Since the intent of this paper is to project the additional number of children that could be saved if existing intervention strategies were implemented worldwide, for intervention strategies such as the use of booster seats and seatbelts which are already being implemented in North America and Europe, no additional benefits were shown because current benefits were considered a reference for LMICs.

Although graduated licensing for young drivers has been evaluated in some developed countries, it was not among the interventions included in this analysis due to insufficient data on young drivers in LMICs. It is also suspected that fewer older teens in LMICs would have access to motor vehicles and as such, graduated driver licensing program would have less impact in these settings. Similarly, a wide spectrum of childhood injury prevention measures such as the use of personal floatation devices, regulation of baby walkers, home visits, and poison centers were not included in this analysis because they were currently applicable only to a small proportion of the children at risk for injury related mortality. Many of these interventions were developed specifically for children in high-income countries and cannot be easily adapted for children in LMIC settings.

Post-injury interventions which are not specific to children, such as emergency medical care, have also not been addressed in this analysis. These interventions are important for a holistic approach to child injury prevention and are systems that benefit all age groups. These interventions were the subject of preliminary analysis in DCP2 (49,50). The application of such post-event interventions will also increase the gains for preventing deaths and reducing disability for children compared to the estimates presented here.

Many of the estimates included in this review were from studies carried out in controlled environments, while others were conducted in high-income country settings. For some interventions such as the use of motorcycle helmets, the impact of the intervention on a population is dependent upon the level of intervention up-take in the population. While observed coverage data from one country was applied to other settings in this analysis, it is acknowledged that intervention coverage might differ from one region to another as a result of socio-cultural or other factors. In order to improve the precision of the estimates presented in this analysis, it would be necessary to obtain current coverage data from all countries for each of the intervention strategies described; currently not available but an important research agenda for child injury prevention.

This analysis also applies some data generated from developed countries to LMIC settings. For intervention strategies such the use of vehicle restraint mechanisms and pool barriers, the only effectiveness data come from studies carried out in high-income countries. It is possible that the implementation of similar strategies in LMICs might yield different results than those suggested by this analysis. The feasibility and costs of expanding coverage of these twelve interventions to reach all children at risk for injury-related deaths was not considered. Some interventions, such as the use of motorcycle helmets, may be easier to implement in resource-poor settings than those that require significant amounts of resources and time, such as the creation of exclusive motorcycle lanes.

Since this study only considers the impact of these interventions on mortality, the full health benefits of the interventions have not been counted. For example, in addition to preventing deaths among children, interventions such as helmets and seatbelts can reduce the severity of injury suffered by children in non-fatal crashes, thereby reducing the likelihood of permanent disability (29,30,32,51-53). As a result, the years of life lost were not projected in this analysis, and no count for disability or health status was done. Collection of disability and morbidity data in LMIC is clearly needed if gains in non-fatal health outcomes are to be addressed.

Even if only twelve of the 46 interventions to prevent injury-related child deaths were implemented worldwide, it is estimated that a third to half of all injury related deaths among children might be prevented, up to a 1,000 children saved each day. The lack of inclusion of many existing intervention strategies without sufficient evaluation data clearly suggests a greater need for evaluation research in this domain. More importantly, it is an indication that the numbers reported in this analysis are likely an underestimate of the true potential benefit of child injury prevention. Given the promising benefits suggested by this analysis for children, governments should invest greater resources towards the implementation of child injury interventions.

ACKNOWLEDGMENTS

Funding/Support: Support for this study was provided by the World Health Organization. Dr Peden is a staff member of the World Health Organization; she alone is responsible for the views expressed in this publication and they do not necessarily represent the decisions or policies of the World Health Organization.

REFERENCES

[1] World Health Organization. The injury chart book: a graphical overview of the global burden of injuries. Report. Geneva, Switzerland: World Health Organization, 2002.

[2] World Health Organization. Injury: a leading cause of the Global Burden of Disease. Anonymous, editor. Geneva: WHO, 2002.

[3] World Health Organization. Child and adolescent injury prevention: a global call to action. Report. Geneva, Switzerland: World Health Organization, 2005.

[4] World Health Organization. Youth and Road Safety. Report. Geneva, Switzerland: WHO, 2007.

[5] Linnan M, Anh LV, Cuong PV, Rahman F, Rahman A, Shafinaz S, et al. Child Mortality in Asia: Survey results and evidence. Florence: UNICEF Innocenti Research Centre, 2007.

[6] Schwebel DC, Gaines J. Pediatric unintentional injury: behavioral risk factors and implications for prevention. J Dev Behav Pediatr 2007;28(3):245-54.

[7] World Health Organization. World Report on Road Traffic Injury Prevention. Report. Geneva: WHO, 2004.

[8] Brenner RA. Prevention of drowning in infants, children, and adolescents. Pediatrics 2003;112(2):440-5.

[9] Brenner RA, Saluja G, Smith GS. Swimming lessons, swimming ability, and the risk of drowning. Inj Contr Saf Promot 2003;10(4):211-6.

[10] Brenner RA. Childhood drowning is a global concern. BMJ 2002;324(7345):1049-50.

[11] Schwebel DC, Lindsay S, Simpson J. Brief report: A brief intervention to improve lifeguard surveillance at a public swimming pool. J Pediatr Psychol 2007;32(7):862-8.
[12] Norton R, Hyder AA, Bishai D, Peden M. Unintentional injuries. Disease control priorities in developing countries, 2nd ed. New York: Oxford University Press, 2006:737-54.
[13] Miller TR, Levy DT. Cost outcome analysis in injury prevention and control. Med Care 2000;38(6):570-3.
[14] World Health Organization. Global Burden of Disease (GBD). Geneva: WHO, 2010. Accessed 2011 Sep 18. URL: http://www.who.int/healthinfo/global_burden_disease/en/index.html.
[15] Yan-Hong L, Rahim Y, Wei L, Gui-Xiang S, Yan Y, De Ding Z, et al. Pattern of traffic injuries in Shanghai: implications for control. Int J Inj Contr Saf Promot 2006;13(4):217-25.
[16] Nieves JA, Buttacavoli M, Fuller L, Clarke T, Schimpf PC. Childhood drowning: review of the literature and clinical implications. Pediatr Nurs 1996;22(3):206-10.
[17] Mohammadi R, Ekman R, Svanstrom L, Gooya MM. Unintentional home-related injuries in the Islamic Republic of Iran: findings from the first year of a national programme. Public Health 2005;119(10):919-24.
[18] Mock CN, Abantanga F, Cummings P, Koepsell TD. Incidence and outcome of injury in Ghana: a community-based survey. Bull World Health Organ 1999;77:955-64.
[19] Howe LD, Huttly SR, Abramsky T. Risk factors for injuries in young children in four developing countries: the Young Lives Study. Trop Med Int Health 2006;11(10):1557-66.
[20] Hang HM, Bach TT, Byass P. Unintentional injuries over a 1-year period in a rural Vietnamese community: describing an iceberg. Public Health 2005;119(6):466-73.
[21] Ghaffar A, Hyder AA, Masud TI. The burden of road traffic injuries in developing countries: the 1st national injury survey of Pakistan. Public Health 2004;118(3):211-7.
[22] Bar-Joseph N, Rennert G, Tamir A, Ore L, Bar-Joseph G. Ethnic differences in the epidemiological characteristics of severe trauma due to falls from heights among children in northern Israel. Isr Med Assoc J 2007;9(8):603-6.
[23] Goldman S, Aharonson-Daniel L, Peleg K. Childhood burns in Israel: A 7-year epidemiological review. Burns 2006 6;32(4):467-72.
[24] Afukaar FK. Speed control in developing countries: issues, challenges and opportunities in reducing road traffic injuries. Inj Contr Saf Promot 2003;10(1-2):77-81.
[25] Dellinger AM, Sleet DA, Shults RA, Rinehart CF. Interventions to prevent motor vehicle injuries. In: Doll LS, Bonzo SE, Mercy JA, Sleet DA, eds. Handbook of injury and violence prevention. Atlanta, GA: Springer, 2007:55-80.
[26] Nolen S, Ekman R, Lindqvist K. Bicycle helmet use in Sweden during 1990s and in the future. Health Promot Int 2005;20(1):33-40.
[27] Anund A, Falkmer T, Forsman A, Gustafsson S, Matstoms Y, Sorensen G, et al. Child safety in cars - literature review. Linkoping: Swedish National Road Transport Research Institute, 2003.
[28] Zaza S, Sleet DA, Thompson RS, Sosin DM, Bolen JC. Reviews of the evidence regarding interventions to increase the use of child safety seats. Am J Prev Med 2001;21(4 Suppl):31-47.
[29] Dinh-Zarr TB, Sleet DA, Shults RA, Zaza S, Elder RW, Nichols JL, et al. Reviews of evidence regarding interventions to increase the use of safety belts. Am J Prev Med 2001;21(4 Suppl):48-65.
[30] Evans L. The effectiveness of safety belts in preventing fatalities. Accident Anal Prev 1986;18(3):229-41.
[31] Glassbrenner D. The use of child restraints in 2002. Washington, DC: US Department Transportation, National Highway Traffic Safety Administration, 2003.
[32] Harris GT, Olukoga IA. A cost benefit analysis of an enhanced seat belt enforcement program in South Africa. Inj Prev 2005;11(2):102-5.
[33] Elvik R, Vaa T. The handbook of road safety measures. Amsterdam: Elsevier, 2004.
[34] Radin UR, Mackay MG, Hills BL. Modelling of conspicuity-related motorcycle accidents in Seremban and Shah Alam, Malaysia. Accident Anal Prev 1996;28(3):325-32.
[35] Sohadi RUR, Mackay M, Hills B. Multivariate Analysis of Motorcycle Accidents and the Effects of Exclusive Motorcycle Lanes in Malaysia. Traffic Inj Prev 2000;2(1):11.

[36] Munro SA, van Niekerk A, Seedat M. Childhood unintentional injuries: the perceived impact of the environment, lack of supervision and child characteristics. Child Care Health Dev 2006;32(3):269-79.

[37] Polivka BJ, Casavant MJ, Malis E, Baker D. Evaluation of the Be Poison Smart! poison prevention intervention. Clin Toxicol (Philadelphia, PA) 2006;44(2):109-14.

[38] Ramisetty-Mikler S, Mains D, Rene A. Poisoning hospitalizations among Texas adolescents: age and gender differences in intentional and unintentional injury. Texas Med 2005;101(5):64-71.

[39] Krug A, Ellis JB, Hay IT, Mokgabudi NF, Robertson J. The impact of child-resistant containers on the incidence of paraffin (kerosene) ingestion in children. South Afr Med J 1994;84(11):730-4.

[40] Hyder AA, Borse NN, Blum L, Khan R, El Arifeen S, Baqui AH. Childhood drowning in low- and middle-income countries: Urgent need for intervention trials. J Paediatr Child Health 2008;44(4):221-7.

[41] Quan L, Bennett EE, Branch CM. Interventions to prevent drowning. In: Doll LS BS, Mercy JA, Sleet DA, eds. Handbook of injury and violence prevention. Atlanta, GA: Springer, 2007:81-96.

[42] Rahman A, Giashuddin SM, Svanstrom L, Rahman F. Drowning. A major but neglected child health problem in rural Bangladesh: implications for low income countries. Int J Inj Contr Saf Promot 2006;13(2):101-5.

[43] Ahrens M. U.S. experience with smoke alarms and other fire alarms. Anonymous, editor. Quincy, MA: National Fire Protection Association, 2003.

[44] Ballesteros MF, Jackson ML, Martin MW. Working toward the elimination of residential fire deaths: the Centers for Disease Control and Prevention's Smoke Alarm Installation and Fire Safety Education (SAIFE) program. J Burn Care Rehabil 2005;26(5):434-9.

[45] Runyan CW, Bangdiwala SI, Linzer MA, Sacks JJ, Butts J. Risk factors for fatal residential fires. N Engl J Med 1992;327(12):859-63.

[46] DiGuiseppi C, Higgins JP. Systematic review of controlled trials of interventions to promote smoke alarms. Arch Dis Child 2000;82(5):341-8.

[47] Roberts I. Deaths of children in house fires. BMJ 1995;311(7017):1381-2.

[48] Roberts I. Secretary of state for health declines to promote free distribution of smoke alarms. BMJ 1996;313(7060):814.

[49] Kobusingye OC, Hyder AA, Bishai D, Hicks ER, Mock C, Joshipura M. Emergency medical systems in low- and middle-income countries: recommendations for action. Bull World Health Organ 2005;83(8):626-31.

[50] Kobusingye OC, Hyder AA, Bishai D, Joshipura M, Hicks ER, Mock C. Emergency medical services. Disease control priorities in developing countries, 2nd ed. New York: Oxford University Press, 2006:1,261-80.

[51] Bishai DM, Hyder AA. Modeling the cost effectiveness of injury interventions in lower and middle income countries: opportunities and challenges. Cost Effect Resour Alloc 2006;4(1):2.

[52] Thompson MJ, Rivara FP. Bicycle-related injuries. Am Fam Physician 2001;63(10):2007-14.

[53] Cummings P, Wells JD, Rivara FP. Estimating seat belt effectiveness using matched-pair cohort methods. Accident Anal Prev 2003;35(1):143-9.

In: Child and Adolescent Health Issues
Editor: Joav Merrick

ISBN: 978-1-63463-574-5

Chapter 18

TODDLER SAFETY IN THE HOME ENVIRONMENT

Chaya Greenberger*, PhD[1] and Liat Korn, PhD[1,2]
[1]Department of Nursing, Jerusalem College of Technology, Jerusalem, Israel
[2]Department of Health Management, School of Health Science,
Ariel University Center of Samaria, Ariel, Israel

This chapter examines the risk factors for unintentional injury of Israeli toddlers in the home. It focuses on the Jewish Ultra Orthodox ("Haredim"), a culturally distinct social entity, hypothesized to have higher levels of risk than other sectors of the population. A sample of two hundred and twenty two mothers, 94 Haredim, 69 belonging to the religious and traditional and an additional 59 to the secular sectors, consented to fill in a structured questionnaire containing the study variables. Haredi mothers were found to be significantly less knowledgeable regarding safety issues and less aware of the hazards in their home environment than their counterparts. They were also 3.19 times more likely than mothers of other sectors to perceive no danger from falling out of an unguarded window and 5.19 times more likely to not place hot food beyond toddlers' reach. Additional socio-demographic variables, as well as attitude and mothers' locus of control predicted behavior and home hazards. Risk factors emerging from the study echoed previous research. Strategies for reducing risk factors in the Haredi sector of Israeli society are discussed.

INTRODUCTION

Unintentional injury is a prominent cause of morbidity and mortality in young children in Israel as also seen in other countries with the primary venue for pre-schoolers at the home (1-5). Only limited interventional success has been achieved, perhaps for lack of understanding of the interplay of risk factors in different cultures (6,7). Factors that have shown explanatory power of unintentional injury are of low socioeconomic status (8-11), lack knowledge and awareness regarding dangers in the home (12-14), have numerous children

* Correspondence: Chaya Greenberger, PhD, Dean of the Faculty of Life and Health Sciences, Jerusalem College of Technology, Rehov Bet Hadefus 7, IL-95483 Jerusalem, Israel. E-mail: greenber@jct.ac.il.

per family (15-17), cramped living quarters (18), lack of parental supervision (15, 17) and lack of adherence to safety measures (19).

One prospective study (20) examining over 1,700 families and 2,000 children, revealed a significant relationship between levels of general safety precaution and the subsequent hospitalization for unintentional injury, but did not find a relationship between specific precautions and respective injuries. This would defy specific knowledge or the execution of a given safety measure as the only or perhaps even main mechanism of prevention and may be indicative of a more fundamental complex relationship between overall beliefs, attitudes, and safety behaviors (21). It is also remarkable that general perception of susceptibility to injury and its potential severity were found to be correlates of specific maternal safety behavior (22, 23). Russel and Champion (1996) (24) found that maternal health beliefs regarding injury and its prevention, self efficacy (e.g., belief in one's ability to prevent injury) and perception of social expectations regarding home safety explained 26% of the variance of home hazard accessibility with respect to toddlers.

Parental safety locus of control, that is, the degree to which a parent believes he or she is in control of the occurrence of unintentional injury was found to be a correlate of the latter. In a qualitative study based upon the participation of focus groups composed of individuals residing in southern Israel, external safety locus of control, that is, the belief that non-intentional injury is largely a matter of fate, was identified as a contributing factor to the occurrence of accidents involving children (14). Studies examining correlates of occupational injuries among employees also revealed relationships between locus of control and the incidence of unintentional injury (25).

Risk factors in the ultraorthodox Jewish (Haredi) community

The purpose of this study was to explore the interplay of variables related to unintentional injury in the home with respect to children ages 0-4, focusing especially on the Jewish ultraorthodox community. The latter is a culturally distinct entity also known as "Harerdi", comprising approximately 8% of the Israeli population and steadily increasing in proportion, due to its relatively high birthrate (26). Although composed of several subsets, this community has commonly held basic tenets, many of which have relevance to the subject of the study, as will soon become apparent. To a Haredi, G-d's Law as manifested in the sacred scriptures is perceived as reigning supreme; civil laws, even if not negating the scriptures, are looked upon with suspicion, at best (27, 28). Even safety regulations are not strictly heeded. Rosenbloom et al. (29) for example, found that pedestrian Haredi populations violate traffic regulations three times as often as their general Israeli counterparts, although safety precautions are mandated by several Jewish commandments. Government sponsored services are often viewed as a secular intrusion upon their structured religious life. Some do not adhere to routine health screening and immunization. Haredim self-impose insulation from the "enticing outside world"; electronic media, especially television, cinema, and often internet, are taboo (26). Secular education is, moreover, generally frowned upon. These limit channels for transmission of knowledge and values. Haredi men are ideally meant to be engaged in religious study and many do not seek gainful employment. They are nevertheless perceived by their wives as the authority figure and decision maker for the family. Women often work part time, but salaries are typically low. Haredi families, moreover, tend to be large; ten children or more is not unusual. Often responsibility for supervising younger children falls prematurely on "somewhat" older siblings (30,31). Prayer, meticulous fulfillment of the commandments, and faith in G-d are believed to keep one out of harm's way. This perspective, however, may encourage passivity with respect to safety promotion and cultivate the perception of accidents as punishment for sin (32). Perhaps legitimacy to rely on divine providence is perceived as applying to having large families, which is, as will be recalled, also perceived to be a pivotal commandment (33).

Paradoxically, one is obligated to do all that is humanly possible to save and preserve one's own life and safety as well as that of fellow man- even at the price of transgressing other commandments (Tosefta Shabbat 9, 22) (34). Resorting to miracles begins where man's capabilities end. The Haredi community has its own ambulance service, active seven days and week, 24 hours a day, including on the Sabbath.

Study rationale and hypothesis

Based on the above, it was hypothesized that the Haredi community would demonstrate a higher degree of risk than other sectors of the Israeli community. It was further hypothesized that there would be a relationship, for all sectors, between antecedent variables: socio-demographic characteristics; knowledge; beliefs and attitudes, and variables relating to safety behavior and home environment.

OUR STUDY

A descriptive- epidemiological design was utilized, targeting Israeli mothers of toddlers. A convenience sample of 222 mothers of children ages 0-4, Haredi (n=94), religious, traditional (the latter two groups were combined for statistical power; n=69) and secular (n=59) orientation participated. Subjects were recruited from several venues. Participants were recruited at four Jerusalem well-baby clinics affiliated with the "Macabi Health Service" (comparable to Home Maintenance Organizations (HMO) in the United States) on different days of the week and at different times of the day. Additional participants were recruited from a maternity ward at one of the medical center in Jerusalem, in order to include mothers who may not frequent clinics.

Instruments

After receiving approval of the respective ethical review boards of Macabi and Bikur Holim (medical center in Jerusalem), mothers were approached and invited to anonymously fill out a structured self-report questionnaire. The latter is a modification of the questionnaire designed by Beterem (1), the Israeli National Center for Children's Safety and Health; it focuses on safety standards and hazards as delineated appropriate by "Beterem" for Israel. Data were collected from 2008-2010. Research variables reflect the following domains: Socio-demographics, knowledge, locus of control and additional attitudes, behavior, and home environment. They are detailed in the appendix.

Our Findings

Table 1 presents the socio-demographic data of the population sample according to religious orientation. It is apparent that the mean age of Haredi mothers is the lowest, as is their mean income and level of education; the mean number of children in the Haredi family, on the other hand, is highest among the sectors. Differences between the Haredi and secular sectors reached statistical significance (p<0.001).

Table 1. Description of the sample by religious orientation

Sector	N	Mean age (SD)¹	Mean No. of children in the family (SD)²	Mean level of Education (SD)³	Mean of Income (SD)°
Haredi- ultra-orthodox	94	28.5 (5.7)	4.0 (2.6)	3.8 (1.2)	1.6 (1.1)
Traditional/ Religious	69	29.5 (5.9)	2.4(1.8)	4.2 (1.2)	2.8 (1.3)
Secular	59	32.7 (4.4)	2.1 (1.0)	4.8 (1.0)	3.3 (1.1)

One way ANOVA: ¹F (2,217) =10.844, sig<0.001, ²F (2,218) =19.787, sig<0.001, Kruskal-Wallis: ³$\chi^2(2)$=25.751, sig< 0.001, °$\chi^2(2)$=60.847, sig< 0.001. Significant differences were always found between the Haredi group and the secular group. Differences between traditional/religious sector and other groups were not always significant.

Additional research variables

Table 2 displays the percent of affirmative responses for each item in all categories, according to sector. For items queried on a scale of 1-5 (see appendix), responses of 4 and 5 were related to as affirmative responses.

Knowledge

As is clear from table 2, while only 43.5% of Haredi women answered the first knowledge item question correctly, 53.8% and 73.6% of traditional/religious and secular mothers (respectively) did so (p<0.01). Similarly, 90.9% and 83.1% of secular and traditional/religious mothers, respectively, answered the second question correctly, in contrast to only 74.7% of Haredi mothers (p<0.05).

Table 2. Knowledge, locus of control, behaviors and home environment regarding children's safety by sector

Topic	Measures	Haredi	Traditional/ Religious	Secular
Knowledge	A child must be at least nine old to cross the street independently*	74.7	83.1	90.9
	A child must be at least five years old before staying alone in the bath tub for a few minutes.**	43.5	53.8	73.6
Attitudes	"We do not have a falling danger from our windows" (from mothers who did not install any protection)**	46.2	29.6	12.0
	"My home is safe for children"	75.0	87.6	83.5
	"I think Safety should be promote and educated	81.8	87.5	82.7
Internal locus of control	I have the power to prevent my children from being injured.*	77.3	92.3	88.9
	My children's physical health depends on the way I take care of their health.*	59.1	78.5	81.1
	If I take good care on my children, I could protect them from injury.	61.5	66.2	49.1
	I am responsible to my children's well being and safety.***	34.3	46.9	47.2
	I am directly responsible to my children's injuries.***	82.1	95.4	98.1
External locus of control	When children are injured, one should wait and see if it is necessary to call for help.	14.8	12.1	5.9
	Whether children are injured is a matter of fate.	9.2	4.8	1.9
	Whether my children are not injured, it's only a matter of luck.	11.1	9.7	2.0
	I often feel that no matter what I'll do, if my children are about to get injured, they will.	17.7	15.9	13.2
	If my children will get injured is in god hands and there is no point in preventing this from happening in the future.*	13.8	7.8	0.0
	Whether my children will get injured is totally random; there is no point in trying to prevent it.	7.6	1.6	1.9
	Children injuries are very often influence by accidental occurrences.	36.9	43.8	41.5
Behavior	I always cook in the inner flames at home.	31.8	27.4	47.2
	I place hot food out of children's reach	91.5	93.8	96.2
	I am extra careful during preparation of food for the Sabbath	83.3	81.0	79.5
	My toddler is bathed by one of the older siblings	34.9	40.9	45.8
	I transfer cleaning agents out of their original packages	8.6	4.5	3.4
Home environment	accessibility of toddlers to medicine	6.0	19.1	10.8
	accessibility of toddlers to cleaning agents	19.5	33.3	20.1
	accessibility of toddlers to electrical sockets	49.3	59.7	41.8
	accessibility of toddlers to unguarded windows	7.3	24.1	30.4
	Electricity sockets in my home are exposed**	47.3	40.0	30.4

N= 168-207, P<0.05*, P<0.01**, P<0.001***.

Attitudes

No significant differences were found among sectors with respect to attitudes, as reflected by perceptions of their own home safety and the importance of disseminating safety information. With respect to attitude as reflected in the reasons given by mothers for not installing window guards, 46.2% of Haredi mothers, as opposed to only 29.6 % of the traditional/religious mothers and 12.0% of the secular mothers, replied that there was no danger of falling out unguarded windows. These results were significant ($p< 0.01$), as indicated in the table. When only mothers living on upper floors were queried, the trend remained intact (23.1% of Haredi mothers as opposed to 16.7% traditional/religious and 10.5% secular mothers gave the said response) , but lost its significance (the latter results not shown in table).

Attitudes: Locus of control

As apparent in table 2, Haredi mothers expressed significantly less internality than those of other sectors, with one item reaching $p< 0.001$. Responses of 4 and 5 on a Likert scale (strongly agree to strongly disagree) were considered positive responses for each item. Regarding items addressing external locus of control, results reached significance for only one item- if my child gets injured, it is in G-d's hands- with Haredi mothers reporting more externality ($p< 0.05$). With respect to five of the remaining six items, Haredi mothers also reported higher levels of externality, but these did not reach significance. For one item however, injury is an accidental occurrence, they reported less externality.

Behavior

None of the differences among sectors with respect to risk behaviors were significant. It is nevertheless remarkable that more than twice as many Haredi mothers than those of other sectors tended to transfer detergents out of their original packaging.

Environment

The responses for one environmental item, the presence of exposed electrical sockets within toddler's reach, were significantly different. While 40 % of the religious/traditional, and 30.4% of the secular mothers reported said presence, positive responses reached 47.3% among Haredi mothers ($p<0.01$). In terms of the accessibility of various hazards to toddlers, Haredi mothers reported substantially less accessibility than other mothers with respect to medications and unguarded windows, although these findings were not significant.

Table 3. Odds ratio of different variables to predict attitudes and unsafe environment

	Independent variables	Unsafe home environment					Attitudes		
		Accessibility of toddlers to medicine (0=Low, 1=High)	Accessibility of toddlers to cleaning agents (0=Low, 1=High)	Accessibility of toddlers to electrical sockets (0=Low, 1=High)	Accessibility of toddlers to unguarded windows (0=Low, 1=High)	"Electric sockets are exposed in my home" (0=no, 1=yes)	"There is no danger of falling out of our windows" (from mothers who did not install any protection; 0=no, 1=yes)	"My home is a safe environment for my children" (0=Yes, 1=No)	"I think Safety should be promoted " (0=Agree, 1=Do not agree)
Socio-demographic Characteristics	Age (0=26 years and older , 1=Less than 25 years old)	0.78 (0.16, 3.81)	1.64 (0.58, 4.64)	1.99 (0.95, 4.16)	0.89 (0.23, 3.35)	**1.92 (1.01, 3.64)**	2.51 (0.86, 7.30)	0.73 (0.28, 1.92)	0.75 (0.69, 1.82)
	Num. of children (0=2 or more, 1=1)	1.31 (0.32, 5.28)	2.64 (0.98, 7.13)	1.20 (0.56, 2.57)	2.45 (0.80, 7.47)	1.44 (0.78, 2.69)	0.52 (0.18, 1.55)	**2.50 (1.09, 5.72)**	1.52 (0.13, 17.02)
	Education (0=Academic or higher, 1=High school or less)	1.98 (0.53, 7.33)	0.79 (0.24, 2.52)	0.38 (0.15, 0.98)	**3.18 (1.05, 9.56)**	1.35 (0.72, 2.53)	2.57 (0.88, 7.47)	0.73 (0.28, 1.92)	0.74 (0.64, 2.10)
	Religiosity (0=Secular, traditional, religious, 1= Ultra orthodox)	0.60 (0.15, 2.39)	0.52 (0.17, 1.53)	**1.15 (1.58, 2.27)**	0.22 (0.04, 1.02)	1.66 (0.95, 2.89)	**3.19 (1.15, 8.84)**	1.01 (0.45, 2.25)	0.63 (0.56, 0.70)
	Income (0= Average and above, 1= less than average)	0.86 (0.24, 3.09)	1.10 (0.41, 2.92)	1.11 (0.56, 2.21)	0.47 (0.15, 1.47)	**1.82 (1.03, 3.21)**	**4.13 (1.38, 12.34)**	1.14 (0.51, 2.53)	0.49 (0.42, 0.57)
Knowledge	Crossing the street independently (0=9 or older, right answer, 1=less than 9, wrong answer)	1.15 (0.23, 5.67)	1.49 (0.45, 4.91)	1.26 (0.51, 2.94)	0.32 (0.04, 2.59)	1.84 (0.89, 3.81)	1.99 (0.63, 6.25)	2.07 (0.82, 5.19)	0.82 (0.76, 0.88)
	Staying a few minutes alone in the bathtub (0=5 or older, 1=less than 5)	0.72 (0.16, 3.10)	0.65 (0.23, 1.85)	1.79 (0.89, 3.60)	0.51 (0.15, 1.73)	**1.94 (1.09, 3.44)**	**5.03 (1.68, 15.06)**	1.12 (0.49, 2.54)	0.54 (0.47, 0.62)
External locus of control Index	6 items (α=.66; 0=Low, 1=High)	1.54 (0.29, 8.11)	1.76 (0.43, 7.14)	0.82 (0.25, 2.61)	**6.59 (1.63, 26.50)**	0.59 (0.23, 1.50)	2.17 (0.50, 9.26)	1.89 (0.66, 5.40)	0.81 (0.75, 0.87)
Internal locus of control Index	4 items (α=.61; 0=High, 1=Low)	0.90 (0.18, 4.55)	0.98 (0.25, 3.75)	1.80 (0.80, 4.02)	1.88 (0.52, 6.79)	0.93 (0.45, 1.92)	1.07 (0.18, 6.36)	1.34 (0.51, 3.49)	1.62 (0.14, 18.39)
Behavior Index	2 items (α=.61;0=High, 1=Low)	1.94 (0.49, 7.58)	2.56 (0.78, 8.39)	**2.32 (1.05, 5.13)**	0.98 (0.24, 3.96)	1.54 (0.77, 3.05)	0.34 (0.08, 1.36)	1.01 (0.36, 2.78)	2.50 (0.15, 40.81)

*OR= Odds Ratio (CI= Confident Interval).

Table 4. Predicting behavior from socio-demographic characteristics, knowledge and LOC

	Independent variables	Behaviors Toddler bathed by older sibling (0=No, 1=Yes)	Cleaning agents transferred from it's original packaging (0=No, 1=Yes)	Careful during cooking preparation for Shabbat (0=agree, 1=Do not agree)	Put hot food far from children's reach (0=agree, 1=Do not agree)	Always cook in the inner flames (0=agree, 1=Do not agree)
Socio-demographic Characteristics	Age (0=26 years and older , 1=Less than 25 years old)	0.75 (0.69, 0.81)	1.42 (0.42, 4.83)	1.74 (0.67, 0.81)	0.76 (0.70, 0.82)	1.18 (0.58, 2.41)
	Num. of children (0=2 or more, 1=1)	0.72 (0.66, 0.78)	0.78 (0.20, 2.96)	0.77 (0.71, 0.84)	**0.74** **(1.68, 0.81)**	1.04 (0.52, 2.11)
	Education (0=Academic or higher, 1=High school or less)	0.31 (0.03, 2.57)	1.35 (0.39, 4.57)	0.87 (0.08, 8.62)	0.73 (0.67, 0.80)	0.92 (0.46, 1.84)
	Religiosity (0=Secular, traditional, religious, 1= Ultra orthodox)	2.19 (0.60, 8.02)	2.24 (0.70, 7.08)	0.82 (0.36, 1.84)	5.19 (0.53, 50.93)	1.33 (0.71, 2.47)
	Income (0= Average and above, 1= less than average)	0.44 (0.10, 1.83)	**4.84** **(1.03, 22.07)**	1.56 (0.21, 11.37)	1.02 (0.14, 7.42)	1.28 (0.69, 2.38)
Knowledge	Crossing the street by himself (0=9 or older, right answer, 1=less than 9, wrong answer)	2.07 (0.51, 8.45)	0.81 (0.17, 3.84)	5.36 (0.72, 39.84)	0.83 (0.78, 0.89)	1.27 (0.57, 2.82)
	Staying a few minutes alone in the bathtub (0=5 or older, 1=less than 5)	0.78 (0.21, 2.88)	1.22 (0.38, 3.93)	0.42 (0.43, 4.17)	1.27 (0.17, 9.24)	**3.11** **(1.64, 5.86)**
External locus of control Index	6 items (α=.66; 0=Low, 1=High)	2.32 (0.40, 13.38)	**7.07** **(1.48, 33.71)**	0.79 (0.73, 0.86)	0.81 (0.75, 0.87)	0.47 (0.18, 1.20)
Internal locus of control Index	4 items (α=.61; 0=High, 1=Low)	1.96 (0.45, 8.58)	2.15 (0.57, 8.02)	2.92 (0.39, 21.45)	1.56 (0.13, 17.63)	1.04 (0.51, 2.11)

*OR= Odds Ratio (CI= Confident Interval).

Predicting risk

In order to examine the predictive power of the research variables, odds ratios were computed, with results presented in Tables 3 and 4. As detailed in the appendix, items for internality and externality were each combined into an index; these indices (0.61 and 0.66 Cronbach alpha, respectively) were use for ratio computations. Marked in bold are the statistically significant findings (CI>1). Regarding socio-demographic variables as predictors of attitude (table 3), Haredi mothers were 3.19 times significantly more likely than mothers from other sectors to perceive no danger from falling out of an unguarded window in the home. In the same vein, mothers from families with below average income were 4.13 times significantly more likely than mothers from families with above average income, to perceive no danger. Mothers with only one child had 2.5 the odds of perceiving their home as safe, significantly higher than mothers with two or more children. Mothers with only a high school education or younger than 26 were approximately 2.5 times more likely to perceive no danger from falling out of an unguarded window in the home compare to older and more educated mothers. Although these results did not reach statistical significance, probably because of small sample, they should still be considered strong and meaningful. Knowing the appropriate age for staying a few minutes alone in the bathtub was found to be strong and significant predictor (5.03) for perceiving no danger of falling out of the window (where no protective devices were installed). External locus of control was also found to be a strong predictor of this latter attitudinal item (OR= 6.59).

Regarding behavior (table 4), findings were not statistically significant for religiosity. Nevertheless, being Haredi strongly predicted three out of five risk behaviors, one at a ratio of 5.19. Mothers lacking knowledge with respect to the age appropriate for a child to stay nattended in a bathtub were, however, 3.11 times significantly more likely not to limit cooking to inner flames. Locus of control predicted three out of five risk behaviors, with high externality significantly and strongly (7.07) predicting transferring detergents out of their original packaging.

DISCUSSION

Two thousand deaths a year in Israel result from unintentional injury, two hundred among children. This is just the tip of the pyramid of injury which includes, in addition to death, disability, economic losses and psychological distress (35). The aim of this study was to identify and compare risk for unintentional injury of toddlers in the home among three sectors of the Israeli population: secular, religious/traditional and Haredi, focusing primarily on the latter. The risk factors cited in the literature by and large also emerged from this study.

Analysis of Haredi risk factors and impact

In terms of socio-demographics, Haredi mothers tended to be younger and less educated; their families tended to be larger and their incomes significantly lower than other sectors. Haredi mothers also reported less knowledge and awareness. Abu-Asba et al. (2006) (36) reported similar findings regarding awareness. These results are not surprising given the sector's limited exposure to the general media (26, 37). Although in recent years culturally appropriate periodicals, pamphlets and even internet sites have mushroomed within the Haredi community, these have not as yet given adequately addressed safety issues (33).

Locus of control was significantly less internal among Haredi mothers than among their counterparts. This may in part reflect real life limitations on their ability to enhance prevention. Haredi families tend to have large families with closely spaced children, limited economic means and less education (38). Cultural factors may also be involved in promoting externality. Haredi Women are generally taught to be docile rather than proactive (33). The strong belief in divine providence and that G-d's "decisions" are always for the best, probably contributes to low internality (33). The only external item that reached significance, related to injury of children as being in G-d's hands; this is a basic Haredi belief. On the other hand, with respect to the item referring to injury as being accidental, Haredi mothers reported less externality than others. Although seemingly not consistent with other responses, this result is understandable, as accidents defy divine providence.

Sivan et al. (39) found that a disproportionately high fifty percent of Haredi Israelis do not heed the Health Ministry's guidelines regarding lying infants on their side or back, rather than on the abdomen. This behavior was found to be especially prominent among those with more than five children, perhaps due to lack of time to attend to fussy babies or being lulled into complacency (as pervious children placed on the abdomen knew no harm). The reason most often reported, however, was reliance on G-d. Although a clear commandment to actively care for one's health and safety coexists, this aspect of religious observance may consciously or subconsciously take a back seat in mothers' minds, if they feel unable to take control of safety in the home. This possibility is relevant no less to safety in the home for toddlers.

Although no significant differences were found with regard to safety behavior when measured via Chi Square, being Haredi predicted the tendency to report three unsafe behaviors when measured via odds ratio. For one of the three, keeping hot food out of children's reach, Haredi mothers were 5.19 times more likely not to affirm this behavior. In terms of environment, on the other hand, significant differences ($P< 0.01$) emerged via Chi Square among sectors, with more Haredi mothers reporting the presence of uncovered, accessible electrical sockets in the home than counterparts. Nevertheless, being Haredi did not have predictive value when measured via odds ratio. The apparent discrepancy between significant and insignificant findings may be the result of insufficient statistical power related to this study's relatively small sample. Another possibility is that the differences were not very large, as safety issues are breaking through to the Haredi world. Social desirability cannot, however, be totally discounted, as Haredi mothers may feel the need to impress the "establishment" whom they believed stigmatizes them; social desirability and over- reporting exposure can therefore not be totally discounted.

Analysis of additional risk factors and impact

Other risk factors emerged; being young, less educated and having a below average income were risks for low awareness. Regarding maternal behavior, low income level, less knowledge and awareness, as well as externality were significant predictors. These findings are reflected in the literature (14, 24, 40). With respect to environmental safety, although each specific item had different predictors, the overall profile that emerged for predicting an unsafe environment is that of a young, inexperienced (having less than two children) and less educated and knowledgeable mother, externally controlled and less cautious in performing kitchen chores. Predictors from four variable categories- socio-demographics, knowledge, locus of control and behavior differentially emerged for all four items reflecting an unsafe home. Interestingly, less parenting experience (as expressed by number of children) and lower knowledge levels increased the tendency of mothers to acknowledge the home environment as unsafe and report higher levels of accessibility to hazards, perhaps reflecting a true state.

It should be stressed that prediction does not equal causation. In this study, for example, unsafe cooking (as operationalized in the behavioral index), predicted the presence of exposed, accessible sockets. A direct causal relationship between these two variables defies logic. The predictability may be rooted in a common ground held by the two variables. Perhaps individuals who don't perceive danger and generally don't behave safely are less apt generally to put in effort in removing environmental hazards. Paradoxically, low awareness of danger from falling out of unguarded windows did not predict accessibility of unguarded windows to toddlers, although this would have been logically expected if there was direct causation, as both of these variables are from the same domain. Similarly, Kendrick et al. (20) found that environmental hazards predicted injury, but did not find that the hazards paralleled the specific injuries. He too hypothesized a more fundamental underlying principle to explain both presence of hazard and injury. Further research needs to been done to tease out this issue.

CONCLUSION

In conclusion it may be said that both hypotheses of this study were for the most part sustained. With respect to the first, Haredi mothers displayed more risk than counterparts for unintentional home injury of toddlers. They also tended to be less aware and knowledgeable regarding safety and less internally controlled. These variables were in turn found to be risk factors for unsafe behavior and an unsafe environment. Odds ratio for being Haredi also predicted three out of five behaviors. Regarding the second hypothesis, numerous antecedent variables, of a socio-demographic nature as well as those reflecting attitude and locus of control were in fact found to be significant predictors of behavior and environmental hazards, regardless of sector.

Limitations and avenues for further study

This study was limited to identifying risk and did not research its actual impact on injury per se. The authors are not aware of any studies of the latter nature within the Haredi community and these should indeed be pursued. Other limitations were already alluded to: the possibility of social desirability as a source of bias and insufficient statistical power. An additional factor to consider is the possibility that Haredi mothers who are more attuned to safety tended to consent to participation in the study. If this were indeed to be the case, then results are dampened and Haredi risk factors may in fact be more pronounced than herein apparent. On the other hand, the moderate differences between Haredi and other sectors regarding risk may be indicative of a true phenomenon- a Haredi community in flux. There is indeed evidence that the Haredi community is opening up to the outside world this trend has been reported in the literature and although slow in coming, has begun to snowball (41). Health professionals should take advantage of this opportunity by pursuing avenues for promoting safety. In this regard, it is critical to point out that the Haredi community perceives the rabbinic authority as supreme. Some Haredim give the latter more credence than physician, even with respect to health issues (42). Activities approved by Rabbis will thus have substantially greater chance for success. One readily available avenue for dissemination of information and safety is the Haredi institution "Hatzalah" (e.g., saving life). Under this county-wide umbrella organization, highly trained medics handle emergencies seven days a week, twenty four hours a day. Their efficient ambulance service comes speedily to the aid of any caller, regardless of population sector. It is likely that if the Rabbinic authorities would lend their support, courses in first aid and safety could be initiated through "Hatzalah" for women, as is already quite customary for men.

Life is deemed very precious among Haredim and saving lives is fundamental religious obligation. Nurturing children is also of prime importance, it is in fact the rasion d'etre of the Haredi family (33). In this regard, the Haredi community perhaps differs from other groups of low socio-economic status and this should be capitalized upon when planning interventional strategies.

Acknowledgments

This study was funded by Jerusalem College of Technology research center. This research was conducted in compliance with ethical applicable regulations governing the protection of human subjects in research. The authors would first like to thank the Jerusalem College of Technology for funding and supporting this research with scholarships for exceptional under-graduated students. We would like to thank Miss Renana Shwartz and Miss Sara Babian for their hard work and contribution in data collecting and gathering. And finally, to all mothers participating in this study for their precious time spent in filling the questionnaire.

Appendix

Study variables (Translated from the original Hebrew questionnaire):

- *Socio-demographic data*
- Age
- Formal education- on scale of 1-6 (primary, partial secondary, full secondary matriculation, post-secondary, Baccalaureate, Masters and above)
- Family income- on scale of 1-5 (given that 10000 I.S. is average: well above average, somewhat above average, average, somewhat below average, well below average)
- Number of children in the family

- Religious orientation (secular; traditional; religious; Haredi/ultra- orthodox). Groups with a traditional and religious orientation were combined for greater statistical power.

- *Knowledge*:

What is the minimum age appropriate for a child to stay unattended in the bath tub? (5 years)

What is minimum age appropriate for a child to cross a street independently? (9 years)

- *Attitudes:*

General perception of risk:

"My home is a safe environment for my children"

"Safety knowledge should be promoted." (Likert scale response, 1-5)

Specific perception of risk (only those living in homes without window guards were queried):

- I did not install window safety guards because: no need, children grown, windows locked at all times, expensive, ugly, live in a rental, no danger of falling (open choice, more than one possibility)

- *Attitudes- Locus of control:*

Internal locus of control index (α=.61):

1. I have the power to prevent my children from being injured.
2. My children's physical health depends on the way I take care of their health.
3. If I take good care on my children, I can protect them from injury.
4. I am responsible for my children's well being and safety.

An additional item, "I am directly responsible for my child's injury" was analyzed as an individual item, but not included in the index, because of its negative effect on the alpha score. (Likert scale response, 1-5).

External locus of control index (α=.66):

1. When children are injured, one should wait and see if it is necessary to call for help
2. Whether children are injured is a matter of fate.
3. Whether my children are not injured, is only a matter of luck.
4. I often feel that no matter what I do, if my children are to get injured, they will.
5. Whether my children will get injured is in G-d's hands; there is no point in trying to prevent this from happening in the future.
6. Whether my child will get injured is totally random, there is no point in trying to preventing it.

An additional item, "Chlidren's injuries are very often influenced by accidental occurrences"' was analyzed as an individual item, but not included in the index, because of its negative effect on the alpha score. (Likert scale response, 1-5).

- *Behaviors*:

"I always cook on the inner flames of the stove"; "I place hot food high, out of children's reach"; "I am extra careful when preparing food for the Sabbath".

The latter two items were combined into a Behavioral index (α=.61). (Likert scale response, 1-5).

"My toddler is bathed by one of the older siblings".

"I transfer cleaning agents out of their original packaging". (dichotomous response).

- *Environment*:

Accessibility of toddlers to:

Exposed electrical sockets unguarded windows; abrasive cleaning agents; medications (degree of accessibility on a scale of 1-5).

Presence of exposed electrical sockets (dichotomous response).

REFERENCES

[1] Beterem, National Center for Child Safety and Health. Safe Kids Israel annual report 2009. Accessed 2011 May 02. URL: http://www.beterem.org/template/default.aspx?PageId=236&catId=53&maincat=17.

[2] London Department of Health and Social Services and Public Safety, Price water house Coopers 2001. Accident and emergency survey.

[3] Hendrickson S. Reaching an underserved population with a randomly assigned home safety intervention. Inj Prev 2005;11:313-7.

[4] Kerr K. Prevention of injuries at home. Inj Prev 2007;13:141.

[5] Stewart-Brown S. Promoting health in children and young people. JRSH 2005;125:61-2.

[6] Dixey RA. `Fatalism', accident causation and prevention: issues for health promotion from an exploratory study in a Yoruba town, Nigeria. Health Educ Res 1999;14:197-208.

[7] Savitsky B, Aharonson-Daniel L, Giveon A, Group TI, Peleg K. Variability in pediatric injury patterns by age and ethnic groups in Israel. Ethn Health 2007;12:129-39.

[8] Faelker T, Pickett W, Brison RJ. Socioeconomic differences in childhood injury: a population based epidemiologic study in Ontario, Canada. Inj Prev 2000;6:203-8.

[9] Hippisley-Cox J, Groom L, Kendrick D, Coupland C, Webber E, Savelyich B. Cross sectional survey of socioeconomic variations in severity and mechanism of childhood injuries in Trent 1992-7. BMJ 2002;324:1132.

[10] Laursen B, Nielsen JW. Influence of socio-demographic factors on the risk of unintentional childhood home injuries. Eur J Public Health 2008;18:366-70.

[11] Reading R, Langford IH, Haynes R, Lovett A. Accidents to preschool children: Comparing family and neighborhood risk factors. Soc Sci Med 1999;48:321-30.

[12] Krieger J, Higgins DL. Housing and health: time again for public health action. Am J Public Health 2002;92:758-68.

[13] Morrongiello BA, House K. Measuring parent attributes and supervision relevant to child-injury risk: Examining the usefulness of questionnaire measures. Inj Prev 2004;10:114–8.

[14] Raanan RA, Tarairah J, Wasim A, Jabari EJ, Endi-Findling L, Hemmo-Lotem M, Rockoff Y. 2008 In: Palestinian Incidence of home accidents and Israeli communities (Research Report). Accessed 2011 May 02. URL: Research on: No place like home, empowering communities for home safety, http://www2.jdc.org.il/files/olim/olimpublications/ECHOS-Research-Report.pdf.

[15] Bijur PE, Golding J, Kurzon M. Childhood accidents, family size and birth order. Soc Sci Med 1988;26:839-43.

[16] Schwartz S, Eidelman A, Zeidan A, Appelbaum, D. Childhood Accidents: The relationship of family size to incidence, supervision, and rapidity of seeking medical care. Journal of the Israeli Medical Association 2005;7:558-63.

[17] Howes LD, Huttly SR, Abramsky T. Risk factors for injuries in young children in four developing countries: the Young Lives Study. Trop Med Int Health 2006;11:1557-66.

[18] Center for Disease Control and Prevention, National Safe Kids Campaign 2003. Home safety training manual. Accessed 2011 May 02. URL: http://www.hud.gov/offices/lead/library / outreach/ Safekids.pdf.

[19] Tsoumakas K, Dousis E, Mavridi F, Gremou A, Matziou V. Parent's adherence to children's home-accident preventive measures. Int Nurs Rev2009;56:369-74.

[20] Kendrick D, Caroline M, Burton MP. How useful are home safety behaviors for predicting childhood injury? A cohort study. Health Education Research 2005;20:709-718.

[21] dal Santo JA, Goodman RM, Glik D, Jackson K. Childhood unintentional injuries: factors preceding injury risks among preschoolers. J Pediatr Psychol 2004;29:273-83.

[22] Glik CD, Greaves EP, Kronenfeld JJ, Jackson LK. Safety hazards in households with young children. J Pediatrc Psych 1993;18:115-31.

[23] Greaves P, Glik CD, Kronenfeld JJ, Jackson K. Determinants of controllable in home child safety hazards. Health Educ Res 1994;9:307-15.

[24] Russel MR, Champion VL. Health beliefs and social influence in home safety practices of mothers with preschool children. J Nurs Schol 1996;28:59-64.

[25] Jones JW, Wuebker LJ. Safety locus of control and employees' accidents. J Bus Psych 1993;7:449–57.

[26] Israeli Central Bureau of Statistics, 2009. Social Survey: Religiosity in Israel, Characteristics of Different Groups. Accessed 2011 May 02. URL: http://www.cbs.gov.il/reader/newhodaot/hodaa_template.html?hodaa=201019101.

[27] Rosenbloom T, Shahar A, Perlman M. Compliance of ultra-orthodox and secular pedestrians with traffic lights in ultra-orthodox and secular locations. Accid Anal Prev 2008;40:1919-24.

[28] Yigal D, Ratner A. Between commandments and laws: religiosity, political ideology, and legal obedience in Israel. Crime Law Soc Change 2002;38:185-209.

[29] Rosenbloom T, Nemrodov D, Barkan H. For heaven's sake follow the rules: pedestrians' behavior in an ultra-orthodox and a non-orthodox city. Transportation Research Part F: Traffic Psych Behavior 2004;7:395-404.

[30] Rotem T. I have brothers but I don't have time to play. 2006. Accessed 2011 May 02. URL: http://www.haaretz.co.il/hasite/pages/ShArtWin.jhtml?itemNo=704656&contrassID=2 - 22k. (in Hebrew).

[31] Zeltzberg S. The first commandment is to be normal. Different Country 2007;41:30-36. [Hebrew[

[32] Elor T. Knowledge and Ignorance: from the world of Haredi women. Am Oved, Tel Aviv, 1992. [Hebrew]

[33] Shapira T. For your own sake, therefore be most careful: Household accidents among children in the Haredi sector in Israel (Unpublished Masters' thesis). Paul Beaurwold School of Social Work, Hebrew University, Jerusalem 2009. [Hebrew]

[34] Tosefta Shabbat 9 22. The Tosefta is a supplement to the Mishna (The core of the oral scripture collected and edited into its final written form in 200 A.D. by Rabbi Judah the Prince and the sages of his generation) compiled in its written form in 220 A.D. It is divided into six parts, each addressing a major aspect of halacha (i.e., "holidays) with further subdivisions.

[35] Gittelman V, Hemmo-Lotem M, Endi-Findling L. Child injuries in Israel. Petach Tiqva: Beterem, 2006. [Hebrew]

[36] Abu-Asba C, Kradarh-Ibrahim A, Endi-Findling L, Sikron P, Hemmo-Lotem M. Attitudes and perceptions of Arab parents to issues of home safety. Petach Tiqva: Beterem, 2008. [Hebrew]

[37] Horowitz N. The Haredim and the internet. New Approaches 2000;3:30-7. [Hebrew]

[38] Gurevitz N, Cohen-Castro A. The Haredim: geographic spread and demographic, social and economic characteristics. Jerusalem: Central Bureau Statistics, 2004. [Hebrew]

[39] Sivan Y, Reisner S, Amitai Y, Wasser J, Nehama H, Tauman R. Effect of religious observance on infants' sleep position in the Jewish population. J Pediatr Child Health 2004;40:534–9.

[40] Ingram J, Emond A. Parents' perceptions of home injury risk and attitudes to supervision of pre-school children: a qualitative study in economically deprived communities. Prim Health Care Res Dev 2009;10:98-108.

[41] Rosenfeld C. The Haredi society: A wall with openings. Al HaKav 2000;21-2. [Hebrew]

[42] Shaked M. Children and autism; the rabbinical authority against the medical authority. In: Kaplan K, Shtedler N, eds. Leadership and authority in the Hardei society in Israel. Jerusalem: Van Leer Institute, 2009:57-77. [Hebrew]

SECTION FOUR: AUTISM

In: Child and Adolescent Health Issues
Editor: Joav Merrick

ISBN: 978-1-63463-574-5

Chapter 19

SOMALI REFUGEE MOTHERS AND AUTISM

Shanna Miller-Gairy and Saul Mofya, DVM, MSc*
Department of Veterinary Science and Public Health, Fort Valley State University, Fort Valley, Georgia, United States of America

The objective of this chapter was to examine the elements of culture and tradition that affect perceptions and expectations of Somali refugee mothers regarding Autism Spectrum Disorder (ASD). The study consisted of 25 participant; mothers, children and service providers from Refugee Family Assistance Program's Parent As Teachers program through focus groups, participatory observation and face-to-face-interviews. Results of the study indicated that these mothers perceived ASD to be a new concept and a result of a combination of stringent vaccination administration, the environment, and processed food. Some even referred to the evil-eye. Mothers also indicated that their expectations for treatment were low because service providers failed to understand their culture and as a result were unable to communicate with them both literally and figuratively. They do not expected this situation to change until or unless they returned to Somalia, where their child (ren) can have excess to more sun light, organic foods and relaxed vaccination standards. While on the other hand services providers identified failure to understand the etiology of ASD, education, socioeconomic status, family/community support and language as primary barriers to early diagnoses, retention and overall treatment success. Their expectations of the future were hopeful, in spite of recent increase in diagnosis rates, indicating that health promotion and education were effective tools to impact change.

INTRODUCTION

In recent years, research has found that children from non-English speaking families are more likely to receive a late diagnosis than children from English speaking families. With the increased number of diagnoses of autism spectrum disorder (ASD) among American born Somali children it is important to understand what affects this is having on the community

* Correspondence: Assistant Professor Saul Mofya, DVM, MSc, Department of Veterinary Science and Public Health, Fort Valley State University, Fort Valley, Georgia, United States. E-mail: mofyas@fvsu.edu

and what if anything can be done. There are a number of different barriers that immigrants and refugees face upon arrival into a new country, primary among them is access to healthcare (1). Numerous studies have examined the effects of raising children with ASD in many other communities, researchers have concluded that raising children in a new cultural setting presents greater challenges in and of itself but as immigrants with the absence of kinship and familial networks, it is far more difficult (2).

According to the Centers for Disease Control and Prevention – National Center for Birth Defects and Developmental Disabilities, (CDC-NCBDDD) ASD is defined as a group of disorders that affect social, communication and behavioral skills (3). When autism was first diagnosed and named early infantile autism over 70 years ago it was suspected to be specific to a particular community. In fact, when Leo Kanner (1896-1981) first developed his theory regarding autism, "refrigerator mothers" he asserted that it was more likely to be found among educated families who exhibited extremely dysfunctional mother-child relations (4). The term refrigerator mothers referred to the mother's inability to provide a warm and welcoming environment for the children.

Since then, millions of children have been diagnosed and countless studies have been done not only to fully understand the best ways to manage the disorder but that ASD does not target any specific socioeconomic status. A recent study by the CDC-NCBDDD found that this disorder occurs in 1 in about 68 children and seems to be on the rise worldwide (5). While a cure has not yet been found, medical professionals recommend that children diagnosed be treated as early as possible in order to minimize or reduce the clinical symptoms. However, like so many other medical inequalities, minorities diagnosed with autism receive treatment in far fewer numbers than do their peers of other racial groups (6).

This notion is confirmed by countless studies that have found that minority children access medical services less often than their peers even though their rate of diagnosis is just as high (7). In one study conducted in Minnesota the findings have shown that American born Somali children diagnosed with ASD has drastically increased (8). What many of these studies have also found is that both culture and tradition play an important role in late diagnosis and failure to seek follow-up care. It has long since been acknowledged that culture plays an important role in diagnosis and treatment (9).

The purpose of this study was to examine what aspects of culture and tradition shape the perceptions and expectations of Somali mothers with children with autism. In an effort to break the cycle of health disparities among this population addressing compound risk factors, personal characteristics, health risk factors, environmental characteristics and environmental risk factors.

OUR STUDY

This was a three phase ethnographic case study, that consisted of two focus groups, participatory observations during a summer camp and program meetings and finally, face-to-face interviews with all adult participants. Participants were selected from the Parent as Teachers (PAT) program hosted by Refugee Family Assistance Program (RFAP). Mother's (Appendix A and Table 1) profiles were reviewed to ensure that participants lived within the Atlanta metropolitan area, mothers were born in Somali and that their children were born in the United States and had received a diagnosis of ASD from a developmental pediatrician and licensed psychologist. The child also had to be attending school for at least 4 hours daily (5 days a week) with an Individuated Education Plan. If the child was under 5 years of age, he or she must have an Individualized Family Service Plan completed by a Baby's Can't Wait service coordinator within the last six months. The child needed to have a developmental evaluation/psychological evaluation completed by a developmental pediatrician/psychologist within the last 3 years, and to have seen a licensed therapist within the last year. Invitations to attend RFAP's first Inclusive Summer Camp, 15 invitations were extended and only 10 families agreed to participate, five families would not be in town during the summer to participate in the study. The final sample population consisted of 8 mothers, 11 Children (10 males and 1 female). The two additional families decided not to participate in the study for personal reasons. Invitations were also sent out to local service providers within the Atlanta metropolitan area. Of the 15 invitations only 6 service providers agreed to participate in a face-to-face interview.

Table 1. Mother's characteristics

	No. of years in US	Age	Education (Years)	Marital status	Children	Medical Insurance
	10	28	PS (5)	M	3	G
	12	32	PS (5)	W	5	G
	25	45	PS (5)	M	3	G
	08	44	C (14)	D	3	P
	06	34	SS (13)	M	5	G
	14	32	PS (5)	M	4	G
	30	49	C (14)	D	5	G
	18	46	PS (5)	M	4	G
Average	**15.4**	**38.7**	**8.2**		**3.5**	**N/A**

Source: Refugee Family Assistance Program, Parent As Teachers.
Abbreviations: PS = Primary School, SS = Secondary School, C = College, M= Married, W = Widowed, D = Divorced, G = Government, P = Private.

The researcher completed participatory observations for two months under the supervision of the RFAP through their PAT program and summer camp. During the summer camp children were enrolled in biweekly speech, occupational and/or physical therapy (as per their IEP or IFSP), activities at a local community garden, YMCA, as well as library and several other community events and activities. In order to ensure participation from families, two mothers were required to attend the camp at least half days, twice weekly. While attending the camp mothers were given the opportunity to participate in therapy sessions, tutoring, and development of daily lesson plans. Volunteer students from local universities -- completing course work in Social Work, Psychology, Therapy (all areas), Special Education and other behavioral programs help in the summer camp. All volunteers were asked to meet with each mother and provide information from their area of expertise, during briefing sessions.

Through participatory observations the investigator was able to observe the relationship between mother and child (ren) but also observe their (parent and child) relationships with service providers. While conducting these observations the investigator was able to establish a relationship with the families and specialist. The first focus group (Appendix B) was facilitated by the investigator, to further understand group dynamics within the community. While the second was conducted in July and facilitated by the Centers for Disease Control and Prevention's National Center for Birth Defects and Developmental Disabilities Unit was held in order to translate the "Learn the Signs. Act Early' pamphlet. Questions asked during the focus group, were compiled by Health Communication Specialist from the CDC-NCBDDD and RFAP (Appendix C).

The second phase of the study consisted of individual face-to-face interviews (Appendix D) for each mother, either in their homes or while accompanying them to service provider visits. The interview questions were open ended allowing the interviewee to discuss anything they believed to be pertinent to that particular subject matter. And, the final phase of the study was to conduct interviews with medical professionals and other care service providers. The study was approved by Fort Valley State University's Human Studies Committee.

OUR FINDINGS

When the mothers in the focus group were asked what autism is, they all responded that it was a new disease or disorder that they first heard here in the United States. They believe it is an "American or European disease". They are convinced that it is foreign because they never heard about it or saw a child with it while they were in Somali. They said if it was not the case then they would have had a name for it in Somali. When they were asked how they learned about the condition, Over 50% indicated that they had first learned about the "European man's disease" through their child's pediatrician. While the other 40% had heard about the ASD via a private Somali woman's teleconference. And, the final 10 percent, heard about ASD from other sources such relatives and friends.

Perception about etiology: When asked about the origins of ASD, overwhelmingly, mothers stated vaccinations, the environment, and food are the main contributing factors. They believe there are too many vaccinations given to the children. The chemicals or toxins in these vaccines affect the developments of children leading to this condition. They feel the environmental factors such as air, and sunlight may be different from Somali which may also contribute to children having problems. Many of the mothers strongly believed that because their children were born in the US they were more susceptible to diseases. They mentioned that this was most likely because they lacked the exposure to enough sunlight. Therefore, may have experienced vitamin deficiencies of which none of the children had been diagnosed with any vitamin deficiencies. They also mentioned lack of access to certain traditional fresh foods such as goat's milk, fish, meat, fruits and vegetables. In spite of the fact that most of the mothers still cooked traditional foods on a daily basis and that they shopped primarily in Halal stores that catered to their dietary and religious needs. In fact, many participants believed that the increased number of ASD within the Somali community came as a result of their relocation to the US. One of the participants stated, that she would be taking her 5 children back to Somali the following summer to see if her two eldest children, who were diagnosed with ASD when they were 3 years old and 4 years old, will make any improvements.

A few mothers also mentioned traditional spiritual beliefs that are thought to contribute to autism. The frequently used term to describe the cause is 'evil eye', 'jin' and 'murung'. They indicated that while it may not seem believable it is a traditional belief that really could not be explained. It should be mentioned that none of 8 mothers with children with Autism believed that the evil eye, jin or murung had contributed to their child's condition.

Diagnosis: Nine out of the ten children diagnosed with ASD in this study were born in the US while one was born in Canada. However, her mother had indicated that the child had been exposed to a similar vaccine protocol as that recommend by the American Academy of Pediatrics for children here in the US. When asked about ASD in their family or similar symptoms – all participants were aware of children in their family who were born in the US with similar symptoms or an ASD diagnosis. However, this diagnosis is not well received among families within the community because all the participants stated that they had not heard of this disease prior to relocating to the US. All participants indicated that their husbands or male figures in their lives, along with older people in their community (in general), were less inclined to believe that these symptoms were related to ASD. The reason that this disease primarily affected male child, they were even less inclined to believe it. Instead, they believed that these symptoms were associated with either shyness, unruly behavior of children or just traits that they would eventually grow out of. Most importantly, majority of the members within the Somali refugee community believe, that in spite of the increased diagnoses, there is not a need for specialized treatment or treatment at all. While childrearing is the primary responsibility of the mother, she is inclined to respect the wishes of her family and community. The mothers were all able to recall in specific the instance when their child (or children) were changing. They mention that the first started noticing that their children had problems between the ages of 3 and 4 years old. When probed further, one mother stated that her son went in for vaccinations at 18 months, once she got him home she noticed he was lethargic and believed that it was as a result of having had shots that day. He laid down for a nap and when he woke up he still was not as active as usual. She contacted the doctor's office and was told that this may be normal, give it about 48 hours or so. His lethargy, recounts turned into extreme self-isolation. And, like so many others he began the blank stare and then stopped talking.

When asked how their family reacted to this, most mothers said supportive. Then participants were asked about the support they receive from their community, less than 42% indicated that they received some support. In fact, two participants indicated that the stress of raising a child with a disability contributed to the delineation of their marriage. They were however, very clear in pointing out that their child was not the cause of their divorce. According to their culture men are not traditionally expected to be concerned with childrearing, therefore men do not fully understand how much work is involved into taking care of children especially if they have ASD.

Data concerning childrearing/motherhood determined that 100% of the participants believed their primary purpose in life was to take care of their families (children and home). These duties, participants stated, were passed down from generation to generation. As such, all participants were first and foremost concerned with the outcome of their children. Not only was it an indication of their success as a mother but fulfillment of a traditional role within their communities.

When asked what services their child/ren was currently receiving it was noticed that only 4 of the 10 children who participated in the study were actively enrolled in speech, physical and occupational therapy. None of the 10 children had ever attended any social groups or received any specialized services such as feeding therapy or applied behavioral therapy. However, all the mothers were concerned primarily with how their child would survive if they were not around or when he or she was an adult. Most often, the mothers stated that they would probably take their child (ren) back to Somali as they do not believe that the health services here would cure or help their child.

Experience with providers: When asked about their experience with health providers most mothers mentioned that they had difficult accessing healthcare services. The mothers mentioned that language barrier prevented them engaging fully with their child's provider and that the providers were less likely to take the time to consider them or their perspective. One participant said, that a typically therapy session consisted of the therapy coming out and acknowledging her and taking her child to begin therapy. This mother stated that she is rarely given an opportunity to speak with the therapist and give an updated on her child's progress. From this she perceives that the therapist does not find her opinion or ability to give an opinion creditable. Some mothers felt they and their children were treated or handled different because they are regard as foreign and therefore not give the best care. Another problem that one mother pointed out was the limitation in communicating with male care providers as this conflict with their religious and culture norm which requires that communications with men be minimal and be kept to that of immediate family members only. So this prevents them from engaging too closely with members of the opposite sex.

The other problem which deeply troubles most mothers was they felt alienated or have experienced alienation during school meetings, especially Individual Education Plan meetings. Participants stated that school personnel often rarely acknowledged their opinion or concerns in the meetings. They feel during these meeting the school personnel just tell them an endless list of problems or what their child does wrong. They strongly feel the school personnel do not want their children and them being part of the school. This problem has created mistrust by the Somali community about the school system.

Interviews with providers (Appendix E)

The investigator interviewed 8 service professionals in Dekalb County, Georgia whose client base consisted largely of immigrants and refugees throughout the metropolitan area. Providers consisted of therapist (speech/ST, physical/PT and occupational/OT), primary care physicians (PCP), special education teachers as well as the Director of a mental health organization in Somali. Interviews were conducted primarily by phone with the exception of the special education teachers and OT.

Experience of the care providers with Somali family with children with ASD, All the care providers mention that working with these families is challenging. You only deal with the mothers of these children as fathers or males are not involved. One care provider stated that when treating patients with ASD, he rarely, if ever meet any of the fathers. In fact, he stated that of his Somali clients, he has never seen any of the fathers during the office visits. According to one therapist, "you typically see a young mother coming into the office with three children. She would be holding the hand of the ASD child, a baby in a carrier and another small child walking in front of her. This is a common pattern at my office". He further went on to say, this is why he rarely calls the mother into the office during therapy sessions because there is no one to watch the other children. All practitioners believed that this was the primary cultural barrier to accessing treatment and care. Mothers were experiencing a tremendous amount of stress as well as lack of support from families and community. Lacking of support systems that are sympathetic and knowledge about the needs of a mother raising a child or multiple children with special needs in an unfamiliar environment makes it difficult to provide care that needs these families.

The most common terms that were found throughout each of the provider interviews was overall communication. Of the providers, all of them noted that basic communication was an issue. The special education teacher stated that her primary issues was the language barrier. She noted that in parent meetings (IEP etc.) that the child – typically, the one that is being discussed – has to be present to translate. This is always the fault of the school system for lacking interpreters and requiring the parents to have their own and who else would they bring but the child.

The second communication issue was the parent's ability to understand the specifics of the conversation and provide feedback. For example, parents often times failed to engage in the conversation. The SE teacher said, that this not only minimizes the overall success of the meeting but minimizes the success of the student's treatment.

Third most common issue that was noted throughout the interviews was failure to follow through with recommendations or referrals. Most ironically, when asked what they thought caused parents not to comply with recommendations or referrals. Most of the providers were not sure however, the OT suggest that it maybe because they were not comfortable seeking care from anyone else, they did not believe that those additional services were necessary or that they were financially unable to meet additional commitments.

Similarly, the interview with the Director of the Mental Health facility yield some of the same information. It is important to note that the Mental Health facility in Somali primarily treats male patients from the age of 18 years old and up. When asked why he said, that there was not specific reason. It just so happened to be who they treated most frequently.

When asked if he provided recommendations of referrals, he said, yes. However, if one of the facility representatives did not follow-up, it was highly unlikely that patients would comply with recommendations. In his opinion this was because of the expectation of immediate treatment results. He was not able to provide any concrete reason for this but assumed it was most likely because in most rural communities most of life's energy was not focused on being sick. He said, "it is believed that Allah gives you what you can handle and you do not complain."

DISCUSSION

This study sought to determine what elements of culture and tradition affected the perceptions and expectations of Somali refugee mothers with children diagnosed with ASD. The research findings were divided into two parts; those derived from observations and interviews conducted with mothers and those derived from the interviews with the practitioners. The study found that ASD is a new concept within the community; there is lack of understanding of the etiology and origins of ASD, denial of the diagnosis, inability to access resources and misunderstandings between care providers and Mothers. The study also found that these mothers experiences same problems as non-refugee mothers with children with ASD, however being immigrants in unfamiliar environment make it even more difficult to copy and overcome many barriers (10).

It clear from a number of researches that have being conducted that culture and tradition affected all aspects of the participant's lives (11). The main point that was highly evident throughout the focus groups and interviews was the new concept of ASD within their community. Throughout each focus group and interview regardless of the participant's education level, none of them had ever seen these symptoms among children in Somalia. In fact, the one of the mothers who is also a Social Worker said, "I am very familiar with symptoms and signs of ASD and I have gone over it in my mind a million times. Was there anyone in my family with this behavior? Was there anyone in my community with this behavior? My answers has always been, No! We do not even have a word for ASD within our country. We acknowledge mental health issue, 'waali' (11). Another mother said, "This is unlike anything we have ever seen. We will first have to collectively acknowledge that this does exist within our community before we can truly address the issue."

Numerous studies have proven that culture has a tremendous impact on health outcomes (12, 13). Within the Somali community childrearing is the primary responsibility of the mother. As a result this will affect how people within our community view her and the rest of the people in her family. Often times the fear of the stigma outweighs the disease itself and so there is silence. In other instance, "we stick to traditional beliefs that he or she will grow out of it", one of the mother said. Many fathers and elders in the community fail to acknowledge that children have developmental issues because it is not culturally acceptable (10). The lack of familial and community support contributes a great deal to how well mothers can handle and address the diagnosis. Parents whose children have ASD, specifically mothers, are more likely to experience stress and other psychological issues (13). For many families the shock of ASD diagnosis is tough. Not only because there is no cure but its origins are so uncertain (14).

It is important to note, that the western concept of family and community support is far different than that of the Afrocentric concept for families in Africa (15). The Afrocentric concept within the African community origins from pastoralism where the father/male leaves the home for multiple days at a time to gather food (16). While the mother/female stays behind and maintains the home and daily family chores. In instances where the husband has multiple wives and will be traveling to several different homes, the woman plays a very dominant role in her home. As such, from generation to generation, she has been depending less and less on her husband for assistance with daily actives and mainly for financial support (17). Those customs do not change because Somali mothers move to the US or have a disabled child. They simple remaining in their traditional roles. So when asked if she receives support from her husband most mothers replied yes and meant it. The fact is they do not view support by the same standards as those of Western culture. Support from the husband and the community come into question when mothers continually attend provider appointments on their own or when the father is not seen to play an active role in their child's treatment (18).

During the interview with the PT, he noted that in his opinion one of the greatest barriers that these families face is a lack of spousal support. While the PT's observation and concern was legitimate, there is need to consider familial roles that the mother and father play in this community. Failure to consider this familial role results into failed relationship. The implications of a lack of relations or failed relations are enormous on the overall success of a child with ASD.

CONCLUSION

Despite significant advancements in healthcare cultural competency remains a key competent in healthcare disparities among minorities. The barriers to healthcare among Somali children with ASD include limited healthcare (services), education, income, health literacy, language, empowerment of parents and community, and rights by legal status combined with culture, tradition and mistrust. As a result, children with ASD in this community lack access to resources, early intervention and a positive prognosis (8). These barriers are not unlike many of the barriers that minorities from America already face (12).

In order to address these concerns both the community and healthcare providers need to make a consciences effort to understand a number of different cultural and traditional beliefs. One of the most common beliefs are relationships. People of Afrocentric ethnicities' often tend to think in relation oriented terms as opposed to the Eurocentric task oriented thinking pattern (14). The Afrocentric way of thinking focuses on the collective identity rather than the task oriented. As a Somali patients are more likely to consider their family and community when making decisions. Acknowledging that while service providers have received several years of training in their profession, Somali mothers believe that the traditions and training that they received within their patriarchal society are no less important and have been passed down from generation to generation (15). Through this familial education, mothers regardless of ethnicity and religion, have the ability to understand changes that have taken place and continue to take place within their child's growth and development. Always remember that the parent is the primary gatekeeper of their child's health and that in most case they have their child's best interest at heart (16). Communications during visits may be limited because of language barriers and other cultural differences but they can be eased and improved through acknowledgment and inclusion. Culture involves a number of different aspects however, key among them is ways of communication. It includes communication systems, adherence to a certain religious belief, or the manner in which people interact in society (18).

As providers began to understand one's cultural and traditional beliefs he or she is more likely to understand different ways of thinking and conceptualizing. This allows them to take different perspectives into consideration. Opening up the floor for dialogue regarding concerns of not only origin but acceptance of recommendations and nontraditional remedies that may be incorporated into treatment plans. Although none of these elements of thinking can be built without trust between the provider and the patient. Meeting the needs of the patient and their family where they are is an important component in the successful management of ASD.

In conclusion, it is therefore important for care providers to create a relationship with the family and community. Training in multicultural counseling and advocacy competencies are cardinal in order to break these barriers. Furthermore, there is need for social workers, Somali community leaders, and the health professionals to form a partnership in creating a forum to promote public awareness, in communities and schools.

Appendix A
Demographic Questionnaire

1. Mothers country of birth
    a. United States
    b. Somalia
    c. Other
2. Child (ren)'s country of birth
    a. United States
    b. Somalia
    c. Other
3. Mothers Age
    a. 20-30
    b. 31-40
    c. 41-50
4. Child (ren)'s Age
    a. 0-5
    b. 6-10
    c. 11-15
5. Highest level of education completed by mother
    a. Elementary school
    b. Middle school
    c. High School
    d. College degree
6. Child current level of education
    a. Elementary school
    b. Middle School
    c. High school
7. Has child had developmental evaluation or psychological evaluation in the last three years?
    a. Yes
    b. No
8. Received therapy from a license professional in the last year
    a. Yes
    b. No
9. Language spoken at home
    a. Somali
    b. Arabic
    c. English
    d. Other

APPENDIX B
FOCUS GROUP QUESTIONS

1. People have different ideas about autism. What do you think autism is? I'll go around the table so we hear from everyone.

[Instructions: Go around the table in Round Robin style to get a brief description] We are trying to get at perceptions that facilitate/hinder access; cultural differences in beliefs such as whether it is a spiritual, medical, or mental health condition]

[Transition to Early Identification]

2. Now we want to hear more about when you or someone else first started noticing a difference in your child's behavior or development

a) What were the types of behaviors did you/someone else first noticed?

b) Did you go to see someone – who did you go to see?

[Trying to understand if they waited until school; saw a medical professional or alternative healer and how long they waited; remember this is round robin style; we are hearing from everyone]

Probe [as necessary]: Did your child see a professional at school or a doctor/other health care professional?

Probe [as necessary]: How old was the child then? [How long between when noticed something and saw someone] [We want to get at when child is 1st identified/diagnosed]

Probe [as necessary]: Did you see someone else for your child [spiritual healer; alternative medicine etc.]?

2. People often wait to go to see someone after they notice differences in their child; what are some of the reasons parents wait?

[Trying to get at two things: whether it is information (i.e. don't know development milestones) or problems in connections (insurance, etc.) Would like to get at most important things we can do to improve early identification]

Probe: Is there anything else you think makes people wait?

Probe [as necessary]: Do people wait because of shame or embarrassment [Stigma] – because it is difficult to talk about with family or friends?

Probe [as necessary]: Do people wait because they are confused or unsure of what steps to take next? They don't know what services are available?

Probe [as necessary]: How much is health care insurance a problem? Is it not having insurance or being not sure what it will cover

Probe [as necessary]: Do people wait because they do not know the signs of autism? Do they think that it is just normal behavior?

Probe [as necessary]: Do people wait because they don't trust the schools or doctors?

b) What do you think is the MOST important thing that could be done to help families get to see someone or get them services sooner?

Probe [as necessary]: Provide information about available services

Probe [as necessary]: about signs of autism and importance of early intervention

Probe [as necessary]: Help navigating system that is complex

Probe [as necessary]: Culturally sensitive services/outreach/education

Probe [as necessary]: Better insurance

Probe [as necessary]: If insurance a problem, what other resources have helped

Probe [as necessary]: Transportation/childcare

[Transition to Services]

3. We would like to know about your experiences getting services for your child with autism. We will first go around the table and hear from everyone then we will talk more about the types of problems people have had getting services.

[Trying to understand what they have used in past and now, and what problems they have had] [Trying to understand if they are knowledgeable about range of services available]

a. First, where do you mostly receive services and what types of services have you received/are receiving? [Remember this is round robin style, we are hearing from everyone]

[Details about what they rely upon and the types of services they have received [Examples: speech, occupational therapy, physical therapy, Applied Behavioral Analysis (ABA); school or doctor; Autism/Disability Center; Community etc.]

4. Tell us more about a time when it was difficult or you had problems getting services that your child or family needed?

[Trying to understand the most important barriers and solutions – This is a Key Question – make sure you give them time to explain about the problem – make sure you cover the areas in the Probes] [35 minutes]

Probe: Insurance Problems (is in lack of access or copayments or doesn't cover certain services?

Probe: Language Barriers [staff don't speak language; don't understand forms}

Probe: Interpreters: [access, quality, trust of]

Probe: Problems with service providers; problems with doctors/schools

Probe: Lack of information about what services are appropriate

Probe: Lack of community-based resources [lack of resources specific to the community they are in; run by community members]

Probe: Problems with transportation

Probe: Services only being for a short time; not continuous

Probe: Competing Demands: problems with childcare; time with other children

Probe: Waiting lists are too long

a. What services would you most like to receive that you're not getting that you believe will help your child? (i.e. speech, occupational, applied behavioral analysis (ABA), Personal Care Attendant etc.)

Follow-up: What is getting in the way of him/her getting that service? b. What would most help your family get the services you need? [Transition to specific recommendations]

6. If you could talk to someone making decisions/government/Department of Health [choose words most appropriate for your community], what would you most like to tell them that they should do to improve services/reduce barriers for your child and family? [10 minutes]

[Try to get as specific as possible]

[End question]

7. Is there anything else you would like to tell us about yourself and about how autism has affected your family? [5 minutes]

APPENDIX C

CENTER FOR DISEASE CONTROL, NATIONAL CENTER FOR BIRTH DEFECTS AND DEVELOPMENTAL DISABILITIES FOCUS GROUP QUESTIONS

1. What do you think causes autism? (Do you think there may be different reasons why Somali children get autism than other children?)

Maxaad umalaynaysaa inuu autismka keena, maxaad kale oo aad ugumalaynasaa in caruurta

Somalidu autismku ugu badanyahay?

2. When did you first discover that your child had autism? (Symptoms, age at onset, diagnosis from physician).

Goormaad ilmahaaga ku aragtay cudurka autismka oo uu doctorkuu sheegay?

3. How supportive is your husband and family in helping you with your autistic child?

Abaahii makuulacaawiyaa ilmahaaga autismka qaba sida, anuu kula kaxaayo doctorka, ama wixii kale ee uu baahanyahay?

4. How do others in the community treat you and your child? What would you say is the feeling in the community about autistic children?

Sidee umada Somalida ee aad kunooshahay?

5. Where was your autistic child born (i.e., U.S., refugee camp, Somalia, other). Please describe the prenatal care you received with your children. Was there anything different about the prenatal care you received with your autistic child?

Xagee ilmahaagu ku dhashay?Noo sheeg markaad uurka lahayd xanaanada aad heshay?

6. Please explain to me about how infants and children are fed in Somalia? How does that differ from here in the U.S.?

Noo sheeg sida ilmaha ay hooyada Somalida ahi u habta ama wax usiisa / sidii uga dawayntahay to AMERICAN ?

7. Does your autistic child have a pediatrician? How often do you visit the pediatrician?

Ilmahaagu dhakhtar gaar u ah maleeyahay? Side u tagaa dhaktarkiisa?

8. What other services is your autistic child currently receiving? Do you feel that you understand all of the services that your child is receiving?

Ilmaahaagu mahelaa caawimo ? ma is leedahay waad heshaa caawimada ilmahaagu ubaahanyahay?

9. If your child is in school, where do they attend school? For how long? Are you able to communicate with your child's teacher and the staff at the school? Please describe any problems you've had in dealing with your child's school.

Ilmahaagu school madigtaa?Ilaa intii dheganayey ? ma is fahantaan dadka school u dhega ilmahaaga? Hadaad dhibaata qabta ii sheeg?

10. What types of services or resources would be helpful for you and your child? (Interpreters or therapy: occupational health, speech therapy, recreational programs, etc)

Caawimooyinka aad u baahan antahay noo sheeg?sida turjubaan, occupational health, speech therapy, recreational programs, etc)

11. Can you tell us why you may not be able to access some of the services or resources that you listed in the last question?

Maqabsan kartaa keligaa waxaad u baahantahay ?

12. Would you like to add anything, or is there anything that we have not discussed that you feel is important for us to know?

Maxaad u baahantahay noo sheeg aan kugu caawino ama wixii aad isleedahay waanu ka tagnay oo aad ku daraysaa wada tashigeenan?

APPENDIX D
FACE-TO- FACE INTERVIEW QUESTIONS

1. As a Somali women, how would you describe motherhood?
2. How has having children changed your life?
3. What do you know about Autism?
4. Is there a history of Autism in your family?
5. I assume you know other children with autism. What can you tell me about them?
6. What do you think caused your child to have Autism?
7. Do you believe that your community is supportive of individuals with Autism?
8. What services are available to individuals with Autism or related diagnosis?
9. What services would you like to see made available for individuals with Autism?

APPENDIX E
INTERVIEW QUESTIONS FOR PROVIDERS

An explanation of the study will follow an introduction of the investigator. The participant will be asked if he/she mind if the conversation is recorded.

- How long have you been working with families in the refugee community?
- How many of your clients would you say of Somali?
- How often (many) patients would you say you treat with ASD?
- Are there any particular barriers that you notice with your Somali families?
- What is the typical course of care that you recommend?

Alternative (depending on the profession)

- How much do you believe your parents know about ASD?
- What referrals do you provide?
- How often would you say families follow up with referrals?
- What would you say is the reason that families fail to follow up with referrals?
- What concerns do you most often hear from parents?
- What recommendation would you provide for a family new to America with a child with ASD?

Ask if participants have any recommendations for the investigator. Thank them for their time.

REFERENCES

[1] Burgess A. Health challenges for refugees and immigrants. Refugee Rep 2004; 25(2):1-3.
[2] McKeever P, Miller K. Mothering children who have disabilities: A Bourdieusian interpretation of maternal practices. Soc Sci Med 2004; 59:1177-91.
[3] Center for Disease Control. Autism spectrum disorder (ASD). Facts about ASD, 2014. URL: http://www.cdc.gov/ncbddd/autism/facts.html
[4] Thompson T. Autism research and services for young children: History, progress and challenges. J Appl Res Intellect Disabil 2013;26:81-107.
[5] Centers for Disease Control and Prevention (CDC). Prevalence of autism spectrum disorder among children aged 8 years - autism and developmental disabilities monitoring network, 11 sites, United States, 2010. MMWR Surveill Summ 2014;63(2):1-21.
[6] Hewitt A. Minneapolis Somali Autism Spectrum Disorder Prevalence Project, 2013. URL: http://rtc.umn.edu/autism/#project_docs
[7] Chiao J. and Blizinsky K. Population disparities in mental health insights from cultural neuroscience. Am J Public Health 2013;103:S1.
[8] Broder-Fingert S, Shui A, Pulcini CD, Kurowski D, Perrin JM. Racial and ethnic differences in subspecialty services use by children with autism. Pediatrics 2013;132(1):94-100.
[9] Ennis-Cole D, Durodoye B, Harris H. The impact of culture on autism diagnosis and treatment: Considerations for counselors and other professionals, 2013. URL: http://www.courses.unt.edu/Ennis-Cole/articles/File2.pdf
[10] Pathappillil J, Jessy S. Through our eyes: A qualitative study of Indians mothers and their perceptions of autism. Dissertation. Philadelphia, PA: Philadelphia College of Osteopathic Medicine, 2011.
[11] Carroll JK. Murug, waali, and gini: Expressions of distress in refugees from Somalia. J Clin Psychiatry 2004;6(3):119-25.
[12] Pavlish CL, Noor S, Brandt J. Somali immigrant women and the American health care system: Discordant beliefs, divergent expectations, and silent worries. Soc Sci Med 2010;71(2):335-61.
[13] Hernandez LM, Blazer DG, ed. Genes, behavior, and the social environment: Moving beyond nature/nurture debate. Washington, DC: National Acadrmies Press, 2006:25-43.
[14] Walsh J. The psychological person. In: Hutchinson E, ed. Dimensions of human behavior: Person and environments. Thousand Oaks, CA: Sage, 2003:117-48.
[15] Laird LD, Amer MM, Barnett ED, Barnes LL. Muslim patients and health disparities in the UK and US. Arch Dis Child 2007;92(10):922-6.
[16] Case A, Paxson C. Parental behavior and child health. Health Aff 2002; 21(2):164-78.

[17] Kaimba GK, Njehia BK, Guliye AY. Effects of cattle rustling and household characteristics on migration decisions and herd size amongst pastoralists in Baringo District, Kenya. Pastoralism 2011;1:18.

[18] Carroll J, Epstein R, Fiscella K, Volpe E, Diaz K, Omar S. Knowledge and beliefs about health promotion and preventive health care among Somali women in the United States. Health Care Women Int 2007; 28:360–80.

In: Child and Adolescent Health Issues
Editor: Joav Merrick

ISBN: 978-1-63463-574-5

Chapter 20

AUTISM SPECTRUM DISORDER AND SENSORY PROCESSING CHALLENGES IN CHILDREN AND ADOLESCENTS

Esther B Hess*[*], *PhD
Center for th Developing Mind, Los Angeles, California, United States of America

Interventions for children/adolescents with developmental delays such as autism spectrum disorder have often been limited to behavioral approaches that focus on the successful completion of a task rather than in the joyous reciprocal interaction of individuals relating to one and another. DIR/Floortime (Developmental, Individual Difference, Relationship-based) offers an alternative perspective to therapy that takes into account an individual's intrinsic level of interest and then expands on that initial level of motivation to incorporate mutual interest of others, all the while supporting various neurological differences that may be impeding the actual level of development in the first place. The result is a reciprocal interaction that results in an overall improvement in actual brain development processing. This article offers an overview of the theoretical, conceptual, and practical approach to the assessment, diagnosis and treatment of children/adolescents with developmental delays such as autism through the developmental relationship intervention known as DIR/Floortime. Adaptation of play techniques will be examined for use with those impacted, in individual, and family therapy contexts as the primary area of focus.

INTRODUCTION

Play is a complex phenomenon that occurs naturally for most children; they move through the various stages of play development and are able to add complexity, imagination, and creativity to their thought processes and action. However, for many children with autism spectrum disorder (ASD), the various stages of play are difficult to achieve. Challenges in

[*] Correspondence: Esther B Hess, PhD, Center for the Developing Mind, 2990 South Sepulveda Blvd, #308, Los Angeles, CA 90064 United States. E-mail: Drhess@centerforthedevelopingmind.com.

motor planning, expressive and receptive communication, imitation and fine and gross motor movements are just some of the many obstacles that children with ASD encounter during play (1). The Developmental, Individual Difference, Relationship-based model (DIR®) Floortime model is an interdisciplinary framework that enables play clinicians, parents and educators the ability to construct a holistic assessment and intervention program that comprehensively incorporates the child's and family's unique developmental profile that addresses these core deficits (2).

Floortime™ is the heart of the DIR® Floortime™ model and it is the play component of a comprehensive program for infants, children, adolescents and their families with a variety of developmental challenges including autism spectrum disorders. This comprehensive program includes working on all elements of the DIR® Floortime™ model, the functional emotional developmental levels and the underlying, individual, neurological differences in processing capacities, thus creating those learning relationships that will help the child move ahead in their development. These relationships in turn are tailored to the child's individual differences that move them up the developmental ladder, mastering each and every functional emotional developmental capacity that they are capable of (3). The DIR® Floortime™ model involves often not just Floortime™, but different therapies like speech and language therapy, occupational therapy, physical therapy, educational programs, counseling support for parents, and home programs as well as school programs. For the purposes of this article though, I will focus on the Floortime™ component, which is the heart of both the home and the school component. This paper includes a summary of evidence based research that lends support to this developmental/relational based play intervention for children impacted by autism and their families.

THE DIR FLOORTIME MODEL

Floortime™ is a particular technique where the play partner gets down on the floor and works with the child to master each of their developmental capacities. But to represent this model fairly, you will need to think about Floortime™ in two ways (4):

- A specific technique where for 20 or more minutes at a time a parent gets down on the floor to play with their child.
- A general philosophy that characterizes all of the interactions with the child. All of the interactions have to incorporate the features of Floortime™ as well as the particular goals of that interaction including understanding the child's emotional, social and intellectual differences in motor, sensory, and language functioning, and the existing caregiver, child and family functioning and interaction patterns.

At the heart of the definition of Floortime™ are two of what could be called emphases that sometimes work together very easily and other times may appear to be at opposite ends of a continuum:

- Following the child's lead.
- Joining a child in his world and then pulling them into a shared world to help them master each of his functional emotional developmental capacities (2).

It is critical to be aware of both of these polarities, tendencies or dimensions of Floortime™.

FOLLOWING THE CHILD'S LEAD

The most widely known dimension of Floortime™ is following the child's lead- in other words, harnessing the child's natural interests. But what exactly does that mean? By following a child's interests, or their lead, we are taking the first steps in making what I call a great date with a child, in other words a validating emotional experience. What are the elements of a great date? For most of us, it includes being in the company of someone who is attentive, available, fun. And when we are with a person who incorporates all of these emotionally affirming elements, we obviously want the date to go on forever. Conversely, if we are on a bad date, with someone who does not make us feel good about ourselves or our experience, most of us would attempt to escape that encounter as soon as possible. Following a child's lead, taking the germ of their idea and making that the basis of the experience that you are about to share with the child, actually encourages the child to allow you into their emotional life. Through the child's interests; through the child's natural desires, we get a picture of what is enjoyable for the child. Consequently the child stays regulated and engaged longer is able to learn within the experience and ultimately moves forward developmentally (5).

CASE EXAMPLE

A child appears not to be able to leave their home without holding onto a stick. This seems like something inappropriate and something we might want to discourage. But yet something about this object has meaning for this child. So we first have to start off asking ourselves, what is it about this activity that is so meaningful for the child? It is minimizing to simply attribute what we assume to be aberrant behavior to the fact that a child has a developmental delay like autism. Not only is this short sighted, but it does little to help us understand the underlying causes that are potentially fueling the odd behavior. The key to understanding the child is to follow their lead as an entry point into their world, create an emotional connection, a relationship that allows us to pull that child into a shared emotional experience. This might mean that the adult facilitator picks up his own stick and attempts to mimic the gestures of the original item. Then it is up to the adult to expand the initial gesture into something socially appropriate and mutual, say taking the two sticks and gently pretending to fence with them and/or helping the child with developmental delays enter the world of symbolism by pretending that the stick is actually the body of an airplane, the play facilitator guiding by making the appropriate sounds and gestures of a gliding plane.

Here the two philosophies behind DIR® Floortime™ are at work. We are accepting the child and their beloved object knowing that there is something intrinsically valuable in the relationship that that child has with the object and we are also encouraging a child to leave their preferred world of isolation in favor of an experience where his original idea of holding onto a stick has magically emerged into a shared play experience.

JOINING THE CHILD'S WORLD

Following the child's lead is only one half of the equation; one half of this dynamic that we call Floortime™. There is another half; joining the child in their world and pulling them into a shared emotional experience in order to help them master each of their Functional Emotional Developmental Capacities. These are the fundamentals of emotional, social, language and intellectual development. When we talk about Functional Emotional Capacities, we're talking about the fundamentals of relating, communicating and thinking (3).

The larger goal is joining the child in their world. We want to then pull them into our shared world to teach them and help them learn how to focus and attend, how to relate with real warmth, how to be purposeful and take initiative, and have a back-and-forth set of communications with us through non-verbal gestures, and eventually through words. We want to teach them how to problem solve and sequence and get them involved in a continuing interaction with the environment and the people in their environment. We want to teach them to use ideas creatively and then we want to teach them to use ideas logically and then progress up the developmental ladder until they are not only using ideas logically but actually showing high degrees of reflective thinking and high degrees of empathy and high degrees of understanding the world so that they can evaluate their own thoughts and feelings. Not every child is capable of achieving the highest level of reflective thinking, but almost all children are capable of moving up the developmental ladder, mastering their own Functional Emotional Developmental Capacities in regards to optimum social, emotional, and intellectual, linguistic and academic growth (6). Some concerns expressed by play clinicians is whether or not DIR® Floortime™ is applicable to children who have moderate to severe forms of developmental delays. The direct answer is yes, even with children who are severely impacted with developmental delays, with the right kind of support, you can move that child forward and upward.

CASE EXAMPLE

Jane is five years old chronologically, although her current developmental age is about 6 months old. She has no functional language and does not appear to have the interest or the capacity to play with toys. In addition to the diagnosis of severe autism, the child also has a co-morbid diagnosis of moderate to severe mental retardation. She enters the playroom mostly aimless, not able to stay engaged with anything or any person for any length of time. Characteristic of the disorder, the child flaps her arms in a self-stimulatory gesture in a continuous horizontal pattern.

The difficulty that play clinicians often face with severely impacted children is the confusion of how to follow a child's lead when the child appears to not be able to offer any lead to follow. This is the art of Floortime™. You cannot do Floortime™, the play therapy portion of this intervention, unless you understand the child's DIR® (the developmental capacity, the underlying, neurological, processing differences and how to use the child's relationship in the world to woo that child into a shared experience). By knowing a child's DIR®, the interventionist knows how and where to enter the child's world in such a way as to create a validating experience- in other words, the great date. To move a child forward developmentally, to become a more complex thinker, despite overt cognitive delays, we need to make sure they possess the basic capacity to be regulated and stay engaged.

Since Jane is only offering her hand movements as "the lead", this is where the clinician must enter. Playfully, the therapist puts her own hands within the child's self stimulatory hand and arm movements. Notice, that the clinician is not entering the play encounter thinking that she is with a 5 year old child; rather the therapist joins Jane at the little girl's developmental capacity. In other words, in the clinician's mind, she is now playing with a child who is 6 months old and must drop her intervention and her level of expectation to that level, while she uses her relationship to support the child's underlying processing challenges. Consequently, the therapist slows the child's flapping gesture down, creating a regular opening and closing rhythm to what was a moment before, a chaotic gesture. As the interventionist slows and regulates to the beat of the activity, the clinician also uses her voice and her facial gestures to create a high affective encounter. The clinician begins to sing a classic child's song, "Open shut them, open shut them, give a little clap". Suddenly, Jane, who up until this time appeared not to be able to focus and attend, looks with curiosity into the face of her play partner. She appears intrigued and curious. The clinician has just taught this child the first fundamental game of play, pat-a-cake. The developmental age of this child and subsequently her ability to be a more complex thinker, has improved within one play session from 6 month of age to 9 months of age.

PROGRESSING FROM FOLLOWING A CHILD'S LEAD TO MASTERY

How do we use "following the child's lead" to actually mobilize and help the child master these critical developmental milestones? To help children master the first stage of shared attention, when they are, for example, wandering away from our interaction with them, we may play a game that places the play partner in front of the child essentially blocking the child's exit from the interaction. The blocking gesture necessitates the child creating some kind of engagement with their play partner, even if it's a gesture of annoyance. This will form the foundation of the first act of shared attention that they are providing. The play partner is encouraged to continue to up the ante by creating more playful obstructions (like asking for a ticket or a token from the child to assure passage). These types of maneuvers create multiple opportunities for shared attention as well as sustained engagement, because the child is otherwise involved with the therapist. Interestingly, this is also the beginning of purposeful action because the child is trying to move the obstruction (in this case the therapist) out of the way. As they continue to attempt to maneuver the obstacle out of the way, the therapist "plays dumb," forcing the children to solve their way out of the current obstacle. These strategies are called playfully obstructive strategies and they are for the most aimless of children or the most avoidant child.

CASE EXAMPLE

A 5-year-old boy named Ian, impacted with a moderate degree of autism, enters the play room and appears to absent mindedly pick up a piece of chalk, before dropping the drawing material randomly on the floor. Previously, his mother has expressed concern that her son is not showing any age- appropriate interest in drawing, coloring, or cutting, and she fears that the child is progressively falling further and further behind his classmates. The clinician, keeping in mind the parent's concern, decides to take the play activity out of the playroom and into an outdoor play area. She follows Ian's lead by attempting to incorporate the child's fleeting interest in the chalk and then attempting to expand that germ of an idea into a sustained play encounter by doing some chalk drawing on the sidewalk. Once outside, she places Ian in her lap, both to prevent flight and also to help the child become more regulated and engaged by providing proprioceptive input (deep pressure) around which he can organize and reduce the anxiety that is potentially fueling his resistance to the play activity. She hands the child a piece of chalk, while mimicking hand- over -hand gestures in its use. Ian completely rejects the activity and withdraws his hand from any attempt to handle the chalk.

One of the basic principles of Floortime™ is "never take no for an answer." In other words, try not to back away from the resistance that is going to be presented when you try to initially move a child forward developmentally. The first step in this case, is to clarifying the child's actual capacities to see if he has the physical ability to hold a piece of chalk in his hand. Using occupational therapy strategies, the therapist explores whether or not the child has an adequate pincher grasp (the ability to pinch together the thumb and the forefinger) by seeing if the child is capable of handing the clinician's therapy dog a dog biscuit. The thinking is that the child's resistance to drawing can be overcome by his greater love for the clinician's dog. Ian is readily able to feed the dog with the appropriate grasp. This encourages the clinician to further expand the interaction by having the child draw the letters of the dog's name in chalk and then having him use his pincher grasp to again dot the letters of the dog's name with muffin (left over from a previous social skills baking activity) while instructing the dog to "eat up her name" on command. This time around, the request to draw with the chalk is met with absolutely no resistance as Ian delights in the use of this "living puppet" to playfully overcome his resistance to the task and ultimately move him forward developmentally.

The goal of playfully obstructive strategies is to follow the child's lead on the one hand but then create opportunities and challenges that help the child master each of his functional emotional developmental goals on the other. That is the dialectic, the two opposite polarities of Floortime™: joining the child in his rhythms while creating systematic challenges that creates opportunities to master new developmental milestones. It is in those systematic challenges that many of the specific techniques and strategies of Floortime™ come into play.

In conclusion, DIR® Floortime™ requires clinicians, and the parent or caregiver whom they are training to appreciate the polarity between following the child's lead and entering their world. Only then can children be "pulled" into a shared world, by finding their pleasure and joys while continually challenging them to master each of the functional developmental capacities. That means paying attention to the child's underlying neurological differences in the way that they processes sound and sights and movements and modulates sensations. It also means paying attention to the family patterns and to your own reactions as play clinician. This encourages both self awareness and improved techniques as one enters a child's world and tailors interactions to the child's specific nervous system.

EVIDENCE BASE FOR THE DIR® FLOORTIME™ APPROACH

Evidence-base practice integrates the best available scientifically rigorous research, clinical expertise, and the therapist's characteristics to ensure the quality of clinical judgments and delivery of the most cost-effective care (7). A starting point to measure effectiveness of intervention is to determine the factors to be measured. Developmental programs like DIR® Floortime™, in contrast to behavioral approaches that tend to measure specific targeted behaviors, target underlying capacities, or "core deficits" as the focus of intervention, with progress evident in a complex array of changes in interactive behavioral patterns.

Developmental capacities seek to measure changes in an individual's capacity for shared attention, the ability to form warm intimate and have trusting relationships and the ability to initiate using intentioned actions and social engagement that leads to spontaneous communication. Additionally, developmental capacities look at problem- solving strategies by assessing the ability to have co-regulation and consequently being able to adapt to the feelings of others. Developmental capacities also determines individual's ability to be creative as well as the capacity to have logical and analytic thought while developing a sense of self or core values (8).

Developmental models emphasize individual processing differences and the need to tailor intervention to the unique biological profile of children as well as the characteristics of the relationship between parent and child. Because both the factors being measured are complex and because the wide range of individual neurological processes in the population, research on the effectiveness of a developmental framework has progressed by examining the subcomponents of the overall approach. The subcomponents can be summarized by looking at the three major aspects of the DIR® Floortime™ approach:

- D for developmental framework
- I for the underlying, neurological, processing differences of a child
- R for relationship and subsequent affective interactions

D: The developmental framework

A developmental approach considers behavior and learning in the greater context of a developmental or changing process. In 1997, evidence first showed the promise of the DIR® Floortime™ approach when 200 charts of children who were initially diagnosed with autistic spectrum disorder were reviewed. The goal of the review was to reveal patterns in presenting symptoms, underlying processing difficulties, early development and response to intervention in order to generate hypotheses for future studies. The chart review suggested that a number of children with autistic spectrum diagnoses were, with appropriate intervention, capable of empathy, affective reciprocity, creative thinking, and healthy peer relationships (2). The results of the 200 case series led Greenspan and Wieder to publish in 2000 the full description of the DIR® Floortime™ Model (4,9). In 2005, Greenspan and Wieder published a 10-to 15-year follow up study of 16 children diagnosed with ASD that were part of the first 200 case series. The authors described that 10 to 15 years after receiving DIR® Floortime™ as a treatment method, these children had become significantly more empathetic, creative and reflective adolescents with healthy peer relationships and solid academic skills (10).

The DIR® Floortime™ Model has provided a developmental framework that has been studied and found to be accurate in understanding behavior. A common pediatric assessment tool, The Bayley Scale of Infant Development, has adopted the DIR® milestones, specifically configured as the Greenspan Social-Emotional Growth Chart (SEGC) as the measure by which social and emotional development is measured (9Greenspan, 2004). In 2007, Solomon et al., published an evaluation of the Play Project Home Consultation (PPHC), an in-home based version of the DIR® Floortime™ model that trains parents of children with autism spectrum disorder in the DIR® Floortime™ model. The results showed significant increase in the child subscale scored on another pediatric assessment tool the Functional Emotional Assessment Scale (11) after an 8- to 12-month program using DIR® Floortime™ (12).

I: Individual underlying neurological processing differences

In 1979, occupational therapist Jean Ayres, pioneered discoveries about the way in which a child's sensory processing capacities could impact the way in which children learned and integrated themselves into their worlds (13). This revolutionary idea provided a new way to understand the importance of movement and regulatory behaviors in children and began to offer explanations for some of the more worrisome behaviors impacting children with developmental concerns like autism. Over the last 40 years, a large body of research has further illuminated the impact of biologically based differences in regards to both sensorimotor processing and the impact on emotional regulation. In 2001, the National Research Council of the National Academy of Sciences, published a report entitled "Educating Children with Autism" which called for the tailoring of treatment approaches to fit the unique biological profile of the individual child (14). Lillas and Turnball (15), in their published text, described how all behavior is influenced by the sensory systems in the brain. They indicated that an infant's sensory capacities are genetically prepared to respond to human interaction and are shifting in direct relationship to the parent's touch, facial, vocal and movement expressions. Child-parent interactions and sensory activities create nerve cell networks and neural pathways in the development of the child's brain. The exchange of that takes place during child-parent play interactions are seen as an ongoing loop of sensorimotor transformations (15).

R: Relationship and affect

Developmental models have evolved from many years of discovery in the field of infant mental health. Beginning in the 1950s, there was a new understanding of the importance of parent-child interaction (16). Building on these years of research in developmental psychology that underscores the importance of early relationships and family functioning, Dr. Stanley Greenspan and his partner, Dr. Serena Wieder, began their work together studying the interaction of mothers and their babies in the context of infants who were at high risk for attachment problems (17). Subsequently, there have been numerous research studies confirming the importance of parent-child interaction and the value of intervention programs that focus on supporting the parent-child relationship, particularly in the areas of joint attention and emotional attunement (18). In 2006, Gernsbacher published a paper that showed how intervention itself between a parent and child could change the way in which parents interact, in turn increasing reciprocity, and that these changes correlated to positive changes in social engagement and language. And in 2008, Connie Kasari and colleagues at the University of California-Los Angeles (19) used a randomized controlled trial to look at joint attention and symbolic play with 58 children with autism. Results indicated that expressive language gains were greater for treatment groups where a developmental model was utilized as compared with a control group that was based on exclusive behavioral principles.

Discussion

Autism spectrum disorder is now recognized as a dysfunction of integration among various distinct brain functions. Research investigation is currently focused on understanding deficits in neuronal communication as a basis of the wide array of behavioral manifestations of the disorder (8). Developmental intervention has advanced to incorporate the use of affect to enhance integration of sensory-regulatory, communication and motor systems. With that in mind, neuro-imaging research is beginning to provide a deeper understanding as to how emotional experiences are actually impacting developing brain growth. Siegel (20) showed how attuned relationships in infancy change brain structure in ways that later impact social and emotional development, and recently, a research study by Casenhiser, Stieben and Shanker (21) at the York University in Canada, investigated the behavioral and neuro-physiological outcomes of intensive DIR® Floortime™ intervention, using both event-related potential (ERP) and electroencephalography (EEG) measurements. Discussion is also continuing on ways to apply the basic principles of DIR® Floortime™ towards an adult developmentally delayed population (22).

Efforts continue to deepen our understanding of the complexities of autism. The alarming increase in the diagnosis of autism worldwide (23), as well as the lack of specific information about etiology of the disorder demands that play therapists increase their knowledge and understanding of how a child's development is impacted by the individual, underlying, neurological processing differences and the interaction of the relationships that the child has in the world (10). In September 2009, Zero to Three focused an issue on the importance of play, specifically on the role of spontaneous, child-led, social play experiences that support social, emotional, and cognitive growth (24). Although research continues, it is imperative that developmental approaches like DIR® Floortime™ remain a viable option for intervention for children and adolescents with developmental delays and their families.

References

[1] Mastrangelo S. Harnessing the power of play: Opportunities for children with autism spectrum disorders. Teach Excep Child 2009;42(1): 34-44.

[2] Greenspan SI, Wieder S. A functional developmental approach to autism spectrum disorders. JAS 1999;24:147-61.

[3] Greenspan SI. Floor Time™: What it really is, and what it isn't. Accessed 2012 Aug 20. URL http://www.icdl.com/dirFloortime/newsletter/FloortimeWhatitReallyisandisnt.shtml.

[4] Interdisciplinary Council on Developmental and Learning Disorders. Clinical practice guidelines: Redefining the standards of care for infants, children and families with special needs. Bethesda, MD: ICDL, 2000.

[5] Hess E. DIR®/Floor Time™: A developmental/relational approach towards the treatment of autism and sensory processing disorder. Presented at the American Psychological Association Annual Conference, Toronto: CN, 2009.

[6] Greenspan SI. The affect diatheses hypothesis: the role of emotions in the core deficit. In autism and the development of intelligence and social skill. J Dev Learning Dis 2001;5:1-46.

[7] Weisz J, Gray JS. Evidence-based psychotherapy for children and adolescents: Data from the present and a model for the future. ACAMH 2007;27:7-22.

[8] Cullinane, D. Evidence base for the DIR®/Floortime approach. Accessed 2012 Aug 20 URL: http://www.drhessautism.com/img/news/EvidenceBasefortheDIR®Model Cullinane0901

[9] Greenspan SI. The Greenspan Social Emotional Growth Chart: A screening questionnaire infants and young children. San Antonio, TX: Harcourt Assessment, 2004.

[10] Greenspan SI, Wieder S. Can children with autism master the core deficits and become empathic, creative and reflective? A ten to fifteen year follow-up of a subgroup of children with autism spectrum disorders (ASD) who received a comprehensive developmental. individual-difference, relationship-based (DIR®) approach. J Dev Learning Dis 2005;9:39-61.

[11] Greenspan SI, DeGangi G. Research on the FEAS: Test development, reliability, and validity studies. In: Greenspan S, DeGangi G, Wieder S, eds. The functional emotional assessment scale (FEAS) for infancy and early childhood. Clinical and research applications. Bethesda, MD: ICDL, 2001:167-247.

[12] Solomon RS, Necheles J, Ferch C, Bruckman D. Pilot study of a parent training program for young children with autism: The P.L.A.Y. project home consultation program. Autism 2007;11(3):205-24.

[13] Ayres JA. Sensory integration and the child. Los Angeles, CA: Western Psychological Services, 1979.

[14] Lord C, McGee JP, eds. Committee on educational intervention for children with autism. Educating children with autism. Washington, DC: Nat Acad Press, 2001.

[15] Lillas C, Turnball J. Infant/child mental health, early intervention and relationship-based therapists: A neuro-relationship framework for interdisciplinary practice. New York: Norton, 2009.

[16] Bowlby J. Maternal care and mental health. Geneva: WHO, 1951;51.

[17] Greenspan SI, Wieder S. Developmental patterns of outcome in infants and children with disorders in relating and communicating: A chart review of 200 cases of children with autistic spectrum diagnoses. J Dev Learning Dis 1987;1:87-141.

[18] Mahoney G, Perales F. Relationship-focused in early intervention with children with pervasive developmental disorders and other disabilities: a comparative study, J Dev Behav Ped 2004;26:77-85.

[19] Kasari C, Paparella T, Freeman S, Jahromi LB. Language outcome in autism: randomized comparison of joint attention and play interventions, J Consult Clin Psychol 2008;76(1):125-37.

[20] Siegel D. Toward an interpersonal neurobiology of the developing mind: attachment relationships, "mindsight," and neural integration. Infant Ment Health J 2001;22:67-94.

[21] Casenhiser D, Stieben J, Shanker S. Learning through Interaction. Accessed 2013 Mar 10. URL: http://research.news.yorku.ca/2013/03/10/ontarios-lieutenant-governor-visits-yorks.

[22] Samson A. Applying DIR®/Floor Time™ principles to a developmental disabled adult population. Presented at California Association for Disabilities, Los Angeles, 2010.

[23] Kogan MD, Blumberg SJ, Schieve LA, Boyle CA, Perrin JM, Ghandour RM, et al. Prevalence of parent-reported diagnosis of autism spectrum disorder among children in the US. Pediatrics 2009;10:1522-42.

[24] Hirschland D. Addressing social, emotional, and behavioral challenges through play, Zero to Three 2009;30:12-7.

In: Child and Adolescent Health Issues
Editor: Joav Merrick

ISBN: 978-1-63463-574-5

Chapter 21

AUTISM SPECTRUM DISORDERS AND BIPOLAR DISORDER IN YOUTH

Adam S Weissman**, PhD
Child and Family Cognitive Behavioral Psychology,
PLLC and Columbia University, New York,
United States of America

Research suggests a high prevalence of bipolar disorder (BD) in children with autism spectrum disorders (ASD), as well as some striking genetic and neurobiological correlates between the two disorders. However, limited research and knowledge and complex diagnostic issues have rendered a bipolar diagnosis both challenging and controversial in ASD youth. As a result, this comorbid condition often escapes early and accurate detection and safe, timely, and effective treatment, leading to further exacerbation of clinical and neurocognitive functioning, long-term prognosis, and overall quality of life. This paper will briefly review the research on comorbidity and genetic/neurobiological overlap between ASD and BD in youth, as well as clinical and neurocognitive impairment in children diagnosed with both disorders, concluding with a brief discussion of relevant diagnostic challenges and implications for practice.

INTRODUCTION

Research has illustrated a high prevalence of juvenile bipolar disorder (BD; re-conceptualized as temper dysregulation disorder with dysphoria in DSM-V) in children with autism spectrum disorders (ASD) (1), as well as some striking genetic and neurobiological correlates between the two disorders (2-4). Accumulating evidence suggests compromised clinical and neurocognitive functioning in children diagnosed with both disorders (5). However, limited research and knowledge, and complex diagnostic issues, have rendered a bipolar diagnosis both challenging and controversial in ASD youth (3). As a result, this comorbid condition often escapes early and accurate detection and safe, timely, and effective treatment, leading to

* Correspondence: Adam S Weissman, PhD, Child and Family Cognitive Behavioral Psychology, PLLC, 2 Overhill Road, Suite 400, Scarsdale, NY 10583, United States. E-mail: DrAdamWeissman@gmail.com.

further exacerbation of clinical and neurocognitive functioning, long-term prognosis, and overall quality of life (3, 5-8). The present chapter briefly reviews the literature on comorbidity and genetic/neurobiological overlap between ASD and BD in youth, as well as clinical and neurocognitive impairment in children diagnosed with both disorders, concluding with a brief discussion of relevant diagnostic challenges and implications for practice.

Co-occurrence

An emerging literature has documented comorbidity between mood disorders (i.e., bipolar and unipolar depression) and ASD. Komoto and colleagues (9) published a clinical case report describing two autistic children with comorbid mood disorders and a family history of major depressive disorder or bipolar disorder. Gillberg (6) described a 14-year old boy with Asperger disorder, recurrent cycloid psychosis, and an extensive family history of BD. Frazier et al. (3) presented a clinical case study of an Asperger child with comorbid bipolar disorder, who had a marked family history of major depression. Finally, Lainhart and Folstein (7) reviewed all published case reports on comorbid ASD and affective illness (N=17). Thirty-five percent of patients experienced the onset of a mood disorder in childhood with 50% reporting a positive history of affective illness or suicide. Of note, there was a higher proportion of females (47%) in the studies reviewed than in most case series of autistic patients, suggesting a higher prevalence of affective illness in autistic women, paralleling the trend in the general population.

A number of clinical research studies have further illustrated the prevalence of comorbid affective disorders in Asperger and autistic disorders. For example, Wing (10) followed a group of Asperger children (n=18) into adolescence and found that 23% showed signs of affective illness, 11% had attempted suicide, and 17% manifested some form of psychosis. Wozniak et al. (8) reported that out of 727 children evaluated at a pediatric psychopharmacology clinic, 52 met criteria for a pervasive developmental disorder (PDD), 114 met criteria for mania, and 14 met criteria for both. Thus, the comorbid group represented 2% of all referrals, 12% of the mania group, and 27% of the PDD group, suggesting a surprisingly high rate of co-occurrence between the two disorders. Finally, Weissman & Bates (5) reported that out of 76 children diagnosed with either high functioning autistic disorder or Asperger disorder, 21 met at least subthreshold criteria for BD (27.6%).

Genetic and Neurobiological Correlates

In addition to studies of comorbidity, genetics research supports an association between ASD and a family history of bipolar disorder. Herzberg (11) reported that families of individuals diagnosed with autistic disorder had higher rates of BD, schizophrenia, and suicidality than families of non-clinical controls. Delong and Dwyer (12) found that first and second-degree relatives of individuals diagnosed with a pervasive developmental disorder (PDD) had a 4.2% prevalence of BD [39 of 929 relatives], nearly five times greater than the rate reported in the general population. Specifically, the incidence of BD in families with a positive history of Asperger syndrome [19 of 314 relatives; 6.1%] was significantly higher than in families negative for Asperger disorder [20 of 165 relatives; 3.3%], which was assessed via Wing's clinical description (10). One limitation of this study, however, was the overrepresentation of high SES families, which may have biased the results. Delong (2) compared children diagnosed with ASD with and without a family history of BD. 78.4% of the families of ASD youth [29 of 37] reported a history of BD, with a 16.2 % prevalence rate in parents. Of the twenty-nine families positive for BD, the disorder was exclusively on the paternal side in nine families, exclusively on the maternal side in eighteen families, and on both sides in two families. The greater maternal involvement was statistically significant. Of the remaining eight families without a history of BD, other affective syndromes occurred in three fathers and two mothers, raising the total number of families with a parental history of affective illness to 56.8% [21 of 37]. This study also illustrated several striking differences in the behavioral symptom profiles of ASD children with and without a family history of affective illness, implicating a potential genetic component in the interaction between the two clusters of psychiatric disorders. Of note, clinical diagnoses in this study were based on the DSM-III, which does not include diagnostic criteria for Asperger disorder and does not consider atypical symptom presentations of juvenile-onset bipolar disorder.

Finally, a small body of research has targeted common neurobiological substrates of ASD and BD. Both disorders in childhood tend to feature marked aberration of cognitive function, often associated with academic problems, learning disabilities, and mental impairment (2). Although neural abnormalities underlying the expression of both disorders remain crudely defined, the most credible and consistent neuroimaging findings highlight structural and functional abnormalities (i.e., hypofrontality) in the prefrontal cortex and frontostriatal network of both ASD and bipolar youth, independently (13-18). In addition, studies examining emotional processing and affective regulation in both disorders have demonstrated abnormalities in key subcortical structures, including the amygdale and caudate (4,19). For example, neuroimaging studies of bipolar youth using CT (Computed Tomography), MRI (structural magnetic resonance imaging), and fMRI (functional magnetic resonance imaging) techniques have determined that hypoactivity of certain key subcortical structures (i.e., amygdala and caudate) may lead to a loss of modulatory input into the prefrontal cortex, generating unstable hypo and hyperactivated states that could explain the dichotomous expression of bipolar depression and mania (19). Weinberg and colleagues (4) have further implicated the critical involvement of the limbic system and the right hemisphere of the brain in both ASD and bipolar youth

Among the most consistent and unifying findings in children diagnosed with ASD and BD, independently, is the presence of common deficits in executive cognitive functioning, including impulse control, selective/sustained attention, and planning. These deficits have been linked to the underdevelopment or atrophy of the prefrontal cortex, resembling the neurobiological phenomenology of Attention-Deficit/Hyperactivity Disorder (AD/HD; 13-20). Although some of these "executive deficits" (i.e., attentional/inhibitory control) have been found consistently in bipolar children using classic neuropsychological paradigms like the Stroop Color-Word Test (SCWT)(21,22) and the Continuous Performance Test (CPT)(13-16,23-26), these same measures have not detected consistent impairment in ASD youth (18,27). The failure of Stroop and CPT paradigms to detect attentional/inhibitory deficits in ASD children may be attributable to these tests' reasonably simplistic and uniform cognitive demands. Research has indicated that more complex, abstract reasoning tasks do, in fact, reveal impaired executive functioning in ASD youth, as well (18).

CLINICAL AND NEUROCOGNITIVE ASPECTS

In addition to the comorbidity, family history, and neurobiology literature, emerging research has illustrated lower levels of clinical and neuropsychological functioning in children with comorbid ASD and BD when compared with single diagnosis ASD youth. The clinical case reports by Gillberg (6), Frazier and colleagues (3), and Lainhart and Folstein (7) each reported an exacerbation of ASD symptoms and attenuated functioning in the presence of a comorbid mood disorder. For example, in his case study of a fourteen-year-old boy with Asperger syndrome and recurrent episodes of "cycloid/manic-depressive psychosis", Gillberg (6) described "a severe worsening of symptomatology during the first episode after the boy had entered into puberty", and reported that the boy's Autistic Behavior Checklist score was below average relative to other autistic youth. Similarly, in their clinical case report of a thirteen-year-old boy diagnosed with Asperger disorder and BD, Frazier and colleagues (3) illustrated an exacerbation of the child's PDD symptoms (e.g., obsessiveness) during his manic states, suggesting that comorbid BD may, in fact, aggravate the underlying symptoms of ASD. Finally, in Lainhart and Folstein's review (7), the authors suggested that a comorbid mood disorder in an ASD child should be considered in the presence of acute atrophy in cognition, language, or activity. Specifically, they proposed that an episode of depression may precipitate an increase in self-injury and an exacerbation of severe autistic features such as echolalia and hand flapping. Additionally, the review highlights the detriment of behavioral symptoms associated with affective illness with respect to the individual's placement and functioning in the home, school, and workplace. For example, the authors described a boy with autistic disorder who required residential placement for two years and was able to return home only after his mood disorder had been effectively treated.

In addition to qualitative data from clinical case reports, Delong's (2) study also indicated an exacerbation of ASD symptoms and clinical distress in the context of affective illness. The findings underscored several significant differences in the behavioral symptom profiles of ASD children with and without a family history of affective illness. Specifically, ASD children with a family history of mood disorders exhibited more complex obsessive interests, marked cyclic variations in behavior, neurovegetative disturbances, florid agitated, fearful, aggressive, or other extreme affective features, and regression after a period of normal or precocious development (2, 3). Although the children in this sample were not individually diagnosed with a comorbid affective illness, the strong correlation between symptom severity and family history of affective illness is certainly suggestive.

Further, several clinical research studies have demonstrated compromised clinical and/or neurocognitive functioning in ASD children with comorbid bipolar symptomatology. Wozniak and colleagues (8) compared a group of patients diagnosed with comorbid PDD and mania to two single diagnosis groups (i.e., PDD only, mania only) on a number of diagnostic batteries including the Schedule for Affective Disorders and Schizophrenia for School Age Children (K-SADS-IV) and the Child Behavior Checklist (CBCL), two measures of clinical functioning, and the Social Adjustment Inventory for Children and Adolescents (SAICA), a structured assessment of psychosocial functioning. The study revealed marked impairment in the PDD+mania group specifically with regard to attentional, behavioral, and emotional functioning. Children in the comorbid group exhibited higher rates of AD/HD, conduct disorder, oppositional defiant disorder, major depressive disorder, anxiety disorders, and psychosis, relative to PDD children without mania, as well as more impaired scores on the Delinquent Problems, Aggressive Behavior, Withdrawn, Somatization, and Anxious/Depressed CBCL subscales. In assessing psychosocial functioning via the SAICA, the comorbid group once again demonstrated greater impairment than the single diagnosis PDD group on all but three subscales of adaptive functioning (i.e., school academic, school social, social problems, spare-time activities, spare-time problems, peer problems, and home problems). Finally, the comorbid group revealed lower Global Assessment of Functioning (GAF) scores (mean = 38.9) when compared with single-diagnosis PDD children (mean = 44.8) and required hospitalization at a rate of 36%, significantly higher than the PDD group without mania. Even when compared with other comorbid clinical groups (i.e., PDD+anxiety disorders, mania+anxiety disorders, PDD+disruptive disorders, mania+disruptive disorders, PDD+depression), the functioning of the co-occurring PDD+mania group was extremely poor in terms of their SAICA, GAF, and CBCL clinical subscale scores. These impaired scores, indicative of elevated attentional, behavioral, and emotional distress, in conjunction with the high rate of hospitalization reported in this group, suggest that PDD with comorbid mania is a uniquely impairing and financially costly condition, warranting further investigation.

A more recent study by Weissman and Bates (5) compared both clinical functioning via the CBCL and KSADS-IV-R (Schedule for Affective Disorders and Schizophrenia for School Age Children, Present State and Epidemiological Version) and neurocognitive functioning via the Stroop Color-Word Test (SCWT)(21) and the Conners' Continuous Performance Test II (CPT-II)(23), across four groups of children: single-diagnosis bipolar children, single-diagnosis ASD youth, children with comorbid ASD and BD symptomatology, and a nonclinical control group. Relative to the ASD group, the ASD+BD group reported elevated rates of aggression and delinquency via the CBCL, and more symptoms of depression, anxiety, obsessive-compulsive disorder, behavioral disorders, and suicidal ideation, as measured by the KSADS. Although no significant group differences were reported on the CPT, the comorbid group demonstrated poorer performance on the SCWT relative to single-diagnosis ASD youth. This is the only published study, to date, examining both clinical and neuropsychological function in ASD youth with and without concomitant bipolar symptoms. Future research might address how best to improve diagnostic assessment and adapt treatment to meet the unique clinical and neurocognitive needs of this complex and understudied comorbid group.

TREATMENT CONSIDERATIONS

Considered together, the studies summarized above may have important implications for diagnosticians and mental health practitioners involved in the assessment, case conceptualization, and treatment of children with comorbid ASD and BD. The high rate of comorbidity and genetic/neurobiological overlap between these disorders, coupled with increased clinical and neurocognitive impairment and higher rates of hospitalization reported in this group if left untreated (5, 28), suggest the need for timely, accurate detection and targeted treatment of comorbid BD in ASD youth.

Accumulating evidence suggests that planning a safe and effective course of pharmacotherapy may be remarkably complex and require great care and consideration in

ASD youth with co-occurring BD. For example, the misprescription of certain antidepressant medications (e.g., fluoxetine and other SSRI's) to bipolar children may exacerbate manic and aggressive symptoms and induce hypomania in a subset of previously asymptomatic children with a latent propensity for BD (e.g., children with a family history of affective illness)(29-31). In addition, classic neuroleptic medications are known to be depressogenic and thus, may further increase depressive symptomatology in children with comorbid ASD and BD (31). Further, antipsychotic medications may also be counterproductive in treating this population, as they have a tendency to mask mood-related symptoms, further encumbering diagnostic sensitivity.

Notwithstanding this set of challenges, several case reports have demonstrated the effective use of novel antipsychotics such as risperidone in mitigating symptoms of aggression and mania in juvenile bipolar disorder, and aggression and impulsivity in ASD youth (31, 32). These atypical agents are reportedly safer, better tolerated, and associated with fewer movement side effects (e.g., extrapyramidal side effects, tardive dyskinesia, neuroleptic malignant syndrome) than classic neuroleptic drugs. Mood stabilizers, such as lithium and valproate, have also shown promise in treating juvenile bipolar symptoms in children with ASD (2, 9, 29, 33). Further, research suggests that once established on a mood stabilizer, a low dose of SSRI may then be helpful in reducing OCD and depressive symptoms (31).

It is evident from the literature that treatment of ASD youth with concurrent BD is incredibly intricate, often requiring higher doses and a combination of multiple mood stabilizers and atypical antipsychotics to achieve adequate treatment (30, 31). Hence, collaboration among service providers and further investigation of both pharmacological and psychosocial interventions are needed to ensure safe, timely, and effective treatment of children with both disorders.

DIAGNOSTIC CONSIDERATIONS

Of course, appropriate intervention is always contingent on practitioner education, accurate diagnostic assessment, and careful case formulation. In developing an intervention plan for a child with comorbid ASD and BD, several diagnostic challenges may compromise a clinician's ability to accurately discern, and effectively treat, affective illness in the context of ASD (5). First, core features of Asperger and autistic disorders may limit our ability to recognize hallmark symptoms of a concurrent mood disorder. Some of these features include an inability to think abstractly, poor verbal and non-verbal communication skills, and a lack of facial and verbal emotional expression (3, 29, 34, 35). In addition, research suggests that ASD youth may not only have difficulty with expression of feelings and moods but with the comprehension and appreciation of the mental states of self and others, a concept commonly referred to as "Theory of Mind" (36). Furthermore, ASD youth may be extremely sensitive to small changes in their environment, and thus, prone to rapid mood fluctuations that may a) falsely resemble or b) diagnostically overshadow a concurrent mood disorder (7,30). These characteristic limitations in verbal and nonverbal communication, emotional expression, and intra/interpersonal insight, coupled with the complex issues of diagnostic overshadowing and symptom overlap, pose considerable challenges to self-report and direct observational assessment techniques. Symptoms of affective illness may thus, manifest, and subsequently need to be assessed atypically in this population, with a greater emphasis placed on caregiver- and teacher report. The vicarious nature of assessment, coupled with the diagnostic complexities inherent in this population, may suggest the need for a new operational approach in documenting and deciphering signs of affective illness in ASD youth (7).

To complicate things further, these diagnostic considerations may warrant heightened sensitivity with respect to childhood mood disorders, as mood symptoms may present atypically in children and evolve along the developmental trajectory of the disorder (8). Historically considered both rare and controversial, recent work has emerged corroborating the existence of early-onset or prepubertal BD, documenting atypical symptom presentations in this population (37). Specifically, bipolar children often present with a predominantly irritable mood commonly associated with aggression and volatility in lieu of the more prototypical symptoms of adult mania (e.g., euphoria and grandiosity). Additionally, juvenile BD tends to feature rapid cycling and mixed symptoms of mania and depression in a chronic course, in contrast to the more discrete and acute episodic nature of adult BD. Wozniak and colleagues (1995) reported that out of forty-three children under the age of twelve diagnosed with BD (mean age = 4.9 yrs; S.D. = 3.8), 80% were found to present the disorder atypically. A chronic presentation was four times more likely than an episodic course (81% vs. 19%) and 64% presented with irritability, while only 5% manifested a predominantly euphoric mood (28). Another study of twenty-six bipolar children (7-18 years) reported that 81% [22 of 26] featured an atypical rapid cycling course in lieu of more discreet episodes (38).

The atypical presentation of early-onset BD has prompted researchers and mental health practitioners, alike, to question whether juvenile BD is in fact a different developmental expression of the same disorder experienced in adults, or whether it is, perhaps, a different clinical phenomenon altogether. Nonetheless, the diagnosis of juvenile BD has become increasingly common, both in the research arena and in clinical practice. The prevalence of bipolar spectrum disorders (i.e., bipolar I, bipolar II, cyclothymia) in adolescence has been estimated at approximately 1% (37). Although little epidemiological research has been conducted on children with prepubertal BD, the Great Smokey Mountains study of 4,500 youths (9-13 years) reported no cases of threshold mania, but a 0.1% rate of hypomania (39). In addition, a retrospective study of bipolar adults revealed a childhood-onset rate of 0.4%-0.5% (40).

Finally, compounding the atypical presentation and developmental sensitivity of juvenile BD, issues related to differential diagnosis may further complicate accurate classification of BD in ASD youth. The earliest presenting symptoms in prepubertal and early adolescent onset bipolar disorder are commonly hyperactivity or depression (37). As a result, many bipolar children may first be misdiagnosed with either AD/HD or a unipolar depressive disorder, and this clinical overlap may be further clouded in the context of ASD. Considered together, the litany of diagnostic considerations reviewed likely preclude, in many cases, the successful detection of treatable, comorbid bipolar symptoms in ASD youth, compromising clinical and neurocognitive functioning, long-term prognosis, and overall quality of life (3,5- 8).

Conclusion

In summary, there is a high rate of comorbidity and genetic/neurobiological overlap between autism spectrum disorders and bipolar disorder in youth, as well as elevated clinical and neurocognitive impairment in children with both disorders, when compared with single-diagnosis youth (5) as well as other comorbid groups (8). There are also a number of clinical and pragmatic challenges related to timely, accurate diagnosis and safe, effective treatment of children with co-occurring ASD and BD. In light of this, additional studies critically assessing atypical signs and symptoms, differential impairment, long-term prognostic implications, and psychosocial/ psychopharmacological interventions are needed. With continued research, ASD children with comorbid BD may ultimately benefit from a comprehensive multi-modal treatment approach, integrating complex psychopharmacological treatment with behavioral interventions (e.g., individual and/or family-based cognitive-behavioral therapy, applied behavior analysis), affective education, social skills training, speech and language intervention, and vocational training (3). Future study should aim to increase practitioner awareness and improve clinical assessment procedures and targeted treatment of bipolar symptoms in ASD youth, improving the lives of children and families affected by this debilitating dual-diagnosis.

References

[1] Ghaziuddin M. Mental health aspects of autism and Asperger syndrome. London: Jessica Kingsley, 1995.

[2] Delong R. Children with autistic spectrum disorders and a family history of affective disorder. Dev Med Child Neurol 1994;36:674-87.

[3] Frazier JA, Doyle R, Chiu S, Coyle JT. Treating a child with Asperger's disorder and comorbid bipolar disorder. Am J Psychiatry 2002;159:13-21.

[4] Weinberg WA, Harper CR, Brumback RA. Neuroanatomic substrate of developmental specific learning disabilities and select behavioral syndromes. J Child Neurol 1995;10:S78-S80.

[5] Weissman AS, Bates ME. Increased clinical and neurocognitive impairment in children with autism spectrum disorders and comorbid bipolar disorder. Res Autism Spectrum Disord 2010;4:670-80.

[6] Gillberg C. Asperger's syndrome and recurrent psychosis – a case study. J Autism Dev Disord 1985;15:389-97.

[7] Lainhart JE, Folstein S. Affective disorders in people with autism: A review of published cases. J Autism Dev Disord 1994;24:587-601.

[8] Wozniak J, Biederman J, Faraone S, Frazier J, Kim J, Millstein R, et al. Mania in children with pervasive developmental disorder, revisited. J Am Acad Child Adolesc Psychiatry 1997;36:1552-60.

[9] Komoto J, Usui S, Hirata J. Infantile autism and affective disorder. J Autism Dev Disord 1984;14:81-84.

[10] Wing L. Asperger's syndrome: A clinical account. Psychol Med 1981;11:115-29.

[11] Herzberg B. The families of autistic children. In: Coleman M. The autistic syndromes. Amsterdam: Elsevier, 1976.

[12] Delong GR, Dwyer JT. Correlation of family history with specific autistic subgroups: Asperger's syndrome and bipolar affective disease. J Autism Dev Disord 1988;18:593-600.

[13] Altshuler LL, Ventura J, Van Gorp WG, Green MF, Theberge DC, Mintz J. Neurocognitive function in clinically stable men with bipolar I disorder or schizophrenia and normal control subjects. Biol Psychiatry 2004;56:560-69.

[14] Blumberg HP, Martin A, Kaufman J, Leung H, Skudlarski P, Lacadie C, et al. Frontostriatal abnormalities in adolescents with bipolar disorder: Preliminary observations from functional MRI. Am J Psychiatry 2003;160:1345-47.

[15] Borkowska A, Rybakowski, JK. Neuropsychological frontal lobe tests indicate that bipolar depressed patients are more impaired than unipolar. Bipolar Disord 2001;3: 88-94.

[16] Dixon T, Kravariti E, Frith C, Murray M, McGuire PK. Effect of symptoms on executive function in bipolar illness. Psychol Med 2004;34: 811-21.

[17] Reddy LA, Weissman AS, Hale JB, eds. Neuropsychological assessment and intervention for emotional and behavior disordered youth: An integrated step-by-step evidence-based approach. Washington, DC: APA Press, 2010.

[18] Rinehart NJ, Bradshaw JL, Tonge BJ, Brereton AV, Bellgrove MA. A neurobehavioral examination of individuals with high-functioning autism and Asperger's disorder using a fronto-striatal model of dysfunction. Behav Cogn Neurosci Rev 2002;1:164-77.

[19] Strakowski SM, DelBello MP, Adler C, Cecil KM, Sax KW. Neuroimaging in bipolar disorder. Bipolar Disord 2000;2:148-64.

[20] Reddy LA, Weissman AS, Hale JB. Integrated neuropsychological assessment and clinical intervention for youth with Attention-Deficit/Hyperactivity Disorder. In: Reddy LA, Weissman AS, Hale JB. Neuropsychological assessment and intervention for emotional and behavior disordered youth: An integrated step-by-step evidence-based approach. Washington, DC: APA Press, 2010.

[21] Golden JC. Stroop Color and Word Test. Chicago, IL: Stoelting, 1978.

[22] Stroop J. Studies of interference in serial verbal reactions. J Exp Psychol 1935;28:643-62.

[23] Conners CK. Conners' Continuous Performance Test II (CPT-II). Toronto, Canada: Multi-Health Systems, 2004.

[24] Meyer TD, Blechert J. Are there attentional deficits in people putatively at risk for affective disorders? J Affect Disord 2005;84:63-72.

[25] Robertson HA, Kutcher SP, Lagace DC. No evidence of attentional deficits in stabilized bipolar youth relative to unipolar and control comparators. Bipolar Disord 2003;5:330-9.

[26] Swann AC, Pazzaglia P, Nicholls A, Dougherty DM, Moeller FG. Impulsivity and phase of illness in bipolar disorder. J Affect Disord 2003;73:105-11.

[27] Pascualvaca DM, Fantie BD, Papageorgiou M, Mirsky AF. Attentional capacities in children with autism: is there a general deficit in shifting focus? J Autism Dev Disord 1988;28:467-78.

[28] Wozniak J, Biederman J, Kiely K, Ablon JS, Faraone SV, Mundy E, et al. Manic-like symptoms suggestive of childhood-onset bipolar disorder in clinically referred children. J Am Acad Child Adolesc Psychiatry 1995;34:867-76.

[29] Damore J, Stine J, Brody L. Medication-induced hypomania in Asperger's disorder (letter). J Am Acad Child Adolesc Psychiatry 1998;37:248-49.

[30] Duggal HS. Mood stabilizers in Asperger's syndrome (letter). Aust NZ J Psychiatry 2001;35:390-91.

[31] Hellings J. Psychopharmacology of mood disorders in persons with mental retardation and autism. Ment Retard Dev Disabil Res Rev 1999;5:270-8.

[32] Frazier JA, Meyer MC, Biederman J, Wozniak J, Wilens TE, Spencer TJ, et al. Risperidone treatment for juvenile bipolar disorder: A retrospective chart review. J Am Acad Child Adolesc Psychiatry 1999;38:960-5.

[33] Steingard R, Biederman J. Lithium responsive manic-like symptoms in two individuals with autism and mental retardation. J Am Acad Child Adolesc Psychiatry 1987;26:932-35.

[34] American Psychiatric Association. Diagnostic and statistical manual of mental disorders, 4th Ed. Washington, DC: Am Psychiatr Assoc, 1994.

[35] Eisenmajer R, Prior M, Leekam S, Wing L, Gould J, Welham M, et al. Comparison of clinical symptoms in autism and Asperger's disorder. J Am Acad Child Adolesc Psychiatry 1996;35:1523–32.

[36] Brent E, Rios P, Happe F, Charman T. Performance of children with autism spectrum disorder on advanced theory of mind tasks. Autism 2004;8:283-99.

[37] Kaufman J, Blumberg H, Young CM. Neurobiology of early-onset mood disorders. In: Charney DS, Nestler EJ. Neurobiology of mental illness, 2nd Edition. New York: Oxford Univ Press, 2004.

[38] Gellar B, Sun K, Zimerman B, Luby J, Frazier J, Williams M. Complex and rapid cycling in bipolar children and adolescents: A preliminary study. J Affect Disord 1995;18:259-68.

[39] Costello EJ, Angold A, Burns BJ, Stangl DK, Tweed DL, Erkanli, et al. The Great Smoky Mountains study of youth: goals, design, methods, and the prevalence of DSM-III-R disorders. Arch Gen Psychiatry 1996;53:1129-36.

[40] Joyce PR. Age of onset in bipolar affective disorder and misdiagnosis as schizophrenia. Psychol Med 1984;14:145-49.

In: Child and Adolescent Health Issues
Editor: Joav Merrick

ISBN: 978-1-63463-574-5

Chapter 22

PARENTS OF CHILDREN WITH AUTISM: ISSUES SURROUNDING CHILDHOOD VACCINATION

***April M Young**, PhD, MPH*[1], *Abigail Elliston*[2] *and Lisa A Ruble, PhD*[3]**

[1]Department of Epidemiology, University of Kentucky College of Public Health, Lexington, Kentucky, [2]Transylvania University, Lexington, Kentucky and [3]Department of Educational, School, and Counseling Psychology, University of Kentucky College of Education, Lexington, Kentucky, United States of America

Parents of children with autism (PCA) are among those most affected by the controversy surrounding supposed links between vaccines and autism. In this chapter we describe the vaccine attitudes of PCA and their association with satisfaction with their child's healthcare provider. Fifty PCA completed questionnaires on vaccine attitudes, exposure to media discussing links between vaccines and autism ('vaccine-autism media'), and satisfaction with their child's healthcare. These characteristics, as well as autism severity and child cognitive functioning, were examined for their correlation with parents' belief that vaccines caused autism and desire to refuse future vaccination. The majority endorsed vaccines as effective and necessary, yet 56% believed they contributed to autism's cause and 16% would discourage others' vaccination. Nearly 80% discussed concerns with their child's provider and felt they were taken seriously. Attitudes were not associated with parents' demographic characteristics or satisfaction with healthcare, but were associated with trust in health institutions, vaccine safety, exposure to vaccine-autism media, and child's lower cognitive functioning. Conclusions: Although parents reported positive communication with providers, doubts about safety and exposure to vaccine-autism media were common. These findings underscore the importance for targeted campaigns addressing PCA's concerns and to mitigate mistrust.

* Correspondence: April M Young, Department of Epidemiology, University of Kentucky College of Public Health, 111 Washington Avenue, Lexington, KY 40536, United States. E-mail: april.young@uky.edu.

INTRODUCTION

Despite increasing evidence of genetic causes of autism spectrum disorder (ASD) (1-3) and an authoritative review rejecting a causal association between MMR vaccination and ASD (4), fear that childhood vaccines play a key role in the etiology of ASD persists (5). In fact, a review by Brown and colleagues (6) identified a significant association between parents' belief that vaccines cause autism and lower vaccine uptake. The controversy continues to attract media attention and many parents remain skeptical about the safety of childhood vaccines (7,8). The issue is particularly salient for parents of children with autism (PCA) and, with an estimated ASD prevalence of one in 88 (9), vaccine uptake among this group could have a substantive impact on public health.

Online surveys of parents involved with autism organizations in the US and Canada revealed that 40% of parents believed that vaccines were among the most significant contributory factors involved in their child's autism (10). Many factors play a role in producing these beliefs, including the temporal proximity of childhood vaccination and the manifestation of autism, distrust of governmental agencies, perceptions of the risks posed by vaccine-preventable diseases (VPDs), and information from popular media sources (11). Several studies have suggested that the latter, especially web-based sources, may fuel distrust in childhood vaccinations (12-15); yet, given limitations in extant research, developing interventions to address these influences would be challenging (16).

Healthcare providers are on the frontlines in the debate about vaccines and autism, and can have a substantial influence on decisions about childhood vaccination (17-21). Therefore, it remains critical that healthcare providers offer information to caregivers, and to PCA, as early after diagnosis as possible (17). The purpose of this study was to examine attitudes toward childhood vaccination among PCA. The association between various dimensions of healthcare satisfaction, vaccine attitudes, and child autism severity and cognitive ability was explored, as was exposure to media sources portraying a link between vaccines and autism.

OUR STUDY

A convenience sample of PCA were recruited through their participation in randomized controlled trials of a parent-teacher consultation intervention in Kentucky and Indiana (22,23). All children met the diagnostic and statistical manual IV-TR definition of autistic disorder (24) as confirmed by professionally-administered Autism Diagnostic Observation Schedule Modules 1 or 2 (25). Parents (n=79) were mailed two self-administered surveys assessing their attitudes toward childhood vaccines and their satisfaction with their child's medical care. Fifty parents completed the Parent Satisfaction with Care Questionnaire and 49 completed the Vaccine Attitude Questionnaire (described below). Respondents were not significantly different than non-respondents in terms of child's age, parental education level, income, or race. All study procedures were approved by the University's Institutional Review Board.

Demographic information including child age, gender, race, household income, number of siblings, and parent education level was collected (described in table 1). Measures assessing children's severity of autism (Childhood Autism Rating Scale; CARS) and cognitive ability (Differential Abilities Scale; DAS) were administered by the research team (23). The CARS is a valid and reliable, observational scale comprised of 15 items evaluating behaviors such as social relating, resistance to change, communication, and body use (26). The General Conceptual Ability subscore of the DAS, which has strong internal and test-retest reliability (27), was used to assess children's cognitive ability.

Table 1. Bivariate analyses of parents' (n=50) beliefs toward childhood vaccination and experiences with child's healthcare provider

Correlate	Total	Vaccines contributed to cause of child's autism. (n=43)			Would refuse to vaccinate if there were no penalties. (n=47)		
	mean (SD)	Disagree mean (SD)	Agree mean (SD)	p-value	Disagree mean (SD)	Agree mean (SD)	p-value
Demographic and ASD-related characteristics							
White - n(%) (n=47)	34 (68.0)	11 (57.9)	18 (81.8)	0.168	28 (71.8)	6 (85.7)	0.657
Mother attended college - n(%) (n=41)[a]	27 (54.0)	10 (66.7)	13 (65.0)	1.000	21 (61.8)	5 (83.3)	0.399
Income greater than $25,000 - n(%) (n=39)[b]	25 (50.0)	6 (46.2)	15 (75.0)	0.142	20 (62.5)	4 (66.7)	1.000
Child's gender (male) - n (%)	43 (86.0)	17 (89.5)	22 (91.7)	0.806	35 (85.4)	7 (87.5)	0.875
Child's age	5.8 (1.6)	5.4 (1.6)	6.2 (1.6)	0.115	5.8 (1.6)	5.8 (1.7)	0.991
Number of siblings (n=47)	1.2 (1.1)	1.3 (1.3)	1.1 (1.1)	0.625	1.4 (1.1)	0.6 (1.2)	0.094
CARS Score (n=48)	37.7 (8.5)	39.4 (8.4)	37.3 (9.1)	0.455	36.9 (9.0)	41.3 (6.0)	0.194
DAS Score	47.6 (21.2)	50.0 (24.4)	47.3 (20.5)	0.696	51.1 (21.2)	32.8 (13.9)	0.024*
Vaccine Attitudes							
Perception of vaccine safety/efficacy	2.0 (0.5)	2.5 (0.4)	1.8 (0.4)	<0.001†	2.2 (0.5)	1.7 (0.3)	0.002†
Negative consequences of non-vaccination	3.1 (0.5)	3.3 (0.5)	2.9 (0.5)	0.008†	3.2 (0.5)	2.8 (0.7)	0.102
Trust in health institutions	2.3 (0.7)	2.8 (0.6)	2.0 (0.5)	<0.001†	2.4 (0.6)	2.0 (0.7)	0.043*
Vaccine communication with PCP	3.0 (0.7)	3.1 (0.7)	3.0 (0.7)	0.860	3.0 (0.6)	3.0 (0.8)	0.873
Desired autonomy	2.5 (0.7)	2.3 (0.7)	2.8 (0.7)	0.036*	2.4 (0.6)	3.0 (0.6)	0.004†
Sense of responsibility to vaccinate	3.1 (0.6)	3.3 (0.6)	2.9 (0.6)	0.043*	3.2 (0.5)	2.9 (0.7)	0.058
Satisfaction with medical care							
Physician informativeness	2.9 (0.7)	2.9 (0.6)	2.9 (0.8)	0.788	2.9 (0.7)	2.9 (0.7)	0.927
Interpersonal sensitivity	3.2 (0.6)	3.3 (0.6)	3.3 (0.5)	0.864	3.2 (0.5)	3.3 (0.5)	0.875
Partnership building	2.9 (0.6)	3.0 (0.7)	3.1 (0.6)	0.691	3.0 (0.6)	3.0 (0.6)	0.846
Perceived competence	2.7 (0.7)	2.7 (0.7)	2.8 (0.7)	0.584	2.7 (0.7)	2.6 (0.7)	0.730
Accessibility of care	2.9 (0.5)	3.0 (0.5)	3.0 (0.6)	0.720	2.9 (0.5)	2.8 (0.6)	0.343
Affordability of care	2.8 (0.6)	3.1 (0.7)	2.7 (0.6)	0.065	3.0 (0.6)	2.6 (0.7)	0.126
Encountered information provoking fear about vaccine-autism link - n (%)	32 (65.3)	5 (27.8)	22 (91.7)	<0.001†	18 (54.5)	13 (92.9)	0.017*

SD: standard deviation, ASD: Autism Spectrum Disorder, CARS: Childhood Autism Rating Scale, DAS: Differential Ability Scales, PCP: Primary Care Provider.

*p<0.05, †p<0.01.

[a] Response options for parents' education-level included, *"graduate/professional training"*, *"college graduate"*, *"some college"*, *"high school / general equivalence degree"*, *"some high school"*, *"junior high school"*, and *"less than 7 years of education"*. Data were dichotomized at the mean (1 = some college or greater, 0 = no college attendance). Given that 50% of respondents reported that father's education level was "not applicable", mother's educational attainment was used for analysis.

[b] Response options for household income included, *"Less than $10,000"*, *"$10,000 - $24,999"*, *"$25,000 - $49,999"*, *"$50,000 - $100,000"*, and *"Greater than $100,000"*. Data were dichotomized (1= $25,000 or greater, 0 = Less than $25,000) at the mean and to closely correspond with the US Federal Poverty Level for a four person household (US Department of Health and Human Services, 2013).

Participants also completed questionnaires assessing their satisfaction with their child's primary healthcare provider (PCP); Table 2 provides example items and coefficient alphas for subscales. The 24-item Parent Satisfaction with Care Questionnaire contained seven subscales and was based on a modification of two established measures for assessing individuals' satisfaction with medical care (28,29). Five subscales examined parents' perceptions of their child's PCP, including his/her informativeness, interpersonal sensitivity, competence to care for a child with autism, and willingness to engage in partnership building with caregiver. Two additional subscales assessed parents' reported accessibility and affordability of healthcare for their child. Response options were arranged on a 4-point Likert scale ranging from strongly agree to strongly disagree.

Table 2. Description and internal consistency of subscales within the Parent Satisfaction with Care Scale

Scale	Items	Example Item	Coefficient α
Physician's informativeness	5	The doctor thoroughly explains everything to me.	0.87
Physician's interpersonal sensitivity	4	The doctor shows a genuine interest in my child's well-being.	0.81
Physician/caregiver partnership building	4	The doctor asks for my thoughts about autism.	0.80
Physician's Competence	3	The doctor's office has everything needed to provide complete medical care to a child with autism.	0.79
Accessibility of care	4	I can make doctors' appointments at a time that is convenient for my schedule.	0.51
Affordability of care	3	I have to pay for more of my child's medical care than I can afford.	0.71

Parents also completed a 43-item Vaccine Attitude Questionnaire, which was based in part on a study of MMR vaccine attitudes conducted in the United Kingdom (30). The modified questionnaire contained six subscales examining parents' 1) perceived safety and efficacy of childhood vaccines, 2) perceived benefits of childhood vaccination, 3) trust in health institutions such as healthcare providers, the government, and pharmaceutical companies, 4) communication with the child's PCP about vaccination, 5) sense of responsibility to vaccinate their child for his/her welfare and the benefit to society and 6) desire for autonomy in making childhood vaccination decisions. Responses were arranged on a 4-point Likert scale ranging from strongly agree to strongly disagree. Table 3 provides items and coefficient alphas. Likert scale items on both the Parent Satisfaction with Care and Vaccine Attitude Questionnaires were recoded for analysis such that higher values indicated attitudes more positively associated with the subscale construct.

Caregivers were also queried about their exposure to information about links between vaccines and autism. Parents were asked the following three questions: 1) "Have you encountered information on/from [source] about links between vaccines and autism?"; 2) "Was the information useful?"; and 3) "Did the information increase your fears regarding vaccines and autism?" These questions were asked for six different sources (see figure 1). From these data, a binary variable was created in which caregivers with an affirmative response on the third question for any source were assigned a 1 and their counterparts were assigned a 0.

Table 3. Description and internal consistency of subscales within the vaccine attitude questionnaire

Question	n (%)[a]	Coefficient α[b]
Vaccine safety and efficacy		0.85
Childhood vaccines are safe (n=47)	18 (38.3)	
Childhood vaccines are very effective in preventing disease. (n=47)	42 (89.4)	
More research is needed to fully investigate the effects of childhood vaccines. (n=47) [c]	47 (100.0)	
Possible complications of vaccination can be very serious for children. (n=47) [c]	45 (95.7)	
Scientific evidence has shown that vaccines do not cause autism. (n=47)	14 (29.8)	
My child getting autism from vaccines is a major concern for me. (n=49) [c]	35 (71.4)	
Consequences of non-vaccination		0.83
The diseases childhood vaccines prevent are serious. (n=48)	44 (91.7)	
Without vaccines, my child would be at risk for getting the diseases they prevent. (n=48)	42 (87.5)	
People who do not vaccinate their children put others at risk. (n=47)	34 (72.3)	
More kids should be vaccinated so that outbreaks do not occur. (n=48)	32 (66.7)	
Trust in health institutions involved with vaccination		0.80
I trust the opinion of my healthcare provider regarding safety of vaccines. (n=47)	28 (59.6)	
I trust the companies producing my child's vaccines. (n=47)	22 (46.8)	
The government would stop childhood vaccination programs if they were dangerous to children. (n=49)	22 (44.9)	
The government is too defensive about childhood vaccines. (n=48) [c]	35 (47.9)	
Communication about vaccination with healthcare provider		---[a]
I discuss my concerns about vaccination openly with my child's healthcare provider. (n=47)	37 (78.7)	
My concerns about vaccination are taken seriously by my child's healthcare provider. (n=47)	33 (70.2)	
Desired autonomy in vaccination decision		---[a]
Parents should make decisions regarding their child's vaccination rather than healthcare providers or the government. (n=49)	35 (71.4)	
Vaccines should not be required to attend school. (n=49)	11 (22.4)	
Sense of parental/societal responsibility to vaccinate		---[a]
I have a responsibility to vaccinate my children for the protection of all children. (n=49)	41 (83.7)	
As a caregiver, I have a responsibility to vaccinate my child for his/her welfare. (n=49)	45 (91.8)	

[a]Number and percent who indicated that they agreed or strongly agreed with the statement.
[b]Coefficient alpha not computed for scales comprised of fewer than three items.
[c] Items were reverse coded for computation of subscale score and coefficient alpha.

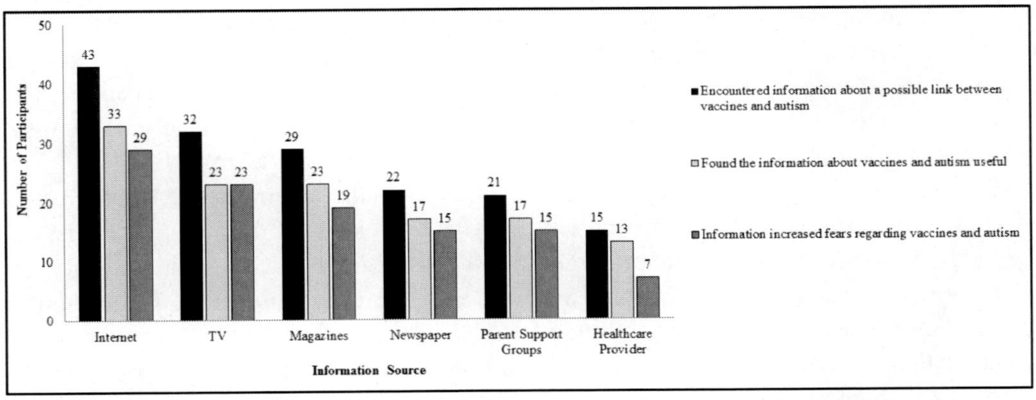

Figure 1. Caregivers' exposure to information regarding a link between vaccines and autism.

Three items on the Vaccine Attitude Questionnaire served as the outcome measures for analysis. Responses to the following three questions were dichotomized (1=strongly agree/agree; 0=strongly disagree/disagree): “Vaccines contributed to the cause of my child’s autism,” “I would recommend to others not to vaccinate their children,” and “If there were no penalties for doing so, I would refuse to vaccinate my children.”

Subscale scores were computed as an average of item ratings. Bivariate associations between the outcome variables and continuous and categorical correlates were assessed through a series of independent samples t-tests and chi-square tests, respectively.

OUR FINDINGS

Demographic characteristics of the sample are described in table 1. The majority of the sample was white (68%), 50% reported a family income of greater than $25,000, and 54% of mothers had attended some college. The majority (86%) of children were male. The average age of children was 5.82 (range: 3 to 9); 22% were under the age of 5 years. Most children (70%) had at least one sibling.

Table 3 describes participants' attitudes toward childhood vaccination. Of note, only 38% believed that childhood vaccines were safe, 30% believed that scientific evidence had shown that vaccines do not cause autism, and 71% reported that they were concerned that their child could get autism from vaccines. However, the majority (89%) did believe that vaccines were effective in preventing disease. Most (92%) believed that VPDs were serious and 88% believed that their children would be at risk for those diseases without vaccination. The majority of parents (72%) also believed that people who do not vaccinate their children put others at risk. Similarly, 84% felt that they had a responsibility to vaccinate their children "for the protection of all children".

Parents' trust in regulatory and health-related institutions involved with vaccination was relatively low. For example, only 60% trusted the opinion of their child's PCP regarding the safety of vaccines, and 47% trusted the pharmaceutical companies producing vaccines. Fewer than half (45%) believed that the government would stop vaccination programs if they were found to be dangerous to children. Despite mistrust, most parents (79%) reported that they did discuss their concerns about vaccination openly with their child's PCP and 70% reported that their concerns were taken seriously. Most parents valued their autonomy in the vaccine decision process, with 71% reporting that vaccination should be a parental decision rather than one mandated by healthcare providers or the government. Moreover, nearly one-fourth (22%) reported that vaccines should not be mandatory for school attendance.

Figure 1 describes parents' exposure to information about the vaccine-autism controversy. The most common source was the internet (reported by 88%), followed by television, magazines, newspaper, parent support groups, and healthcare providers. The majority of parents reported that the information they obtained was useful, ranging from 65% of those receiving information from healthcare providers to 77% for that from parent support groups. Except for those who acquired information from a healthcare provider, the majority of parents reported that the information increased their fears about the association between vaccines and autism. Information obtained from parent support groups provoked fear among proportionally more parents (71%) than did television (70%), internet (67%), magazines (63%), and newspapers (60%). Of note, among those encountering information from healthcare providers, comparatively fewer (37%) reported an increased fear of the links between vaccines and autism.

Over half (56%) of the parents believed that vaccines had contributed to the cause of their child's autism, 30% reported that they would refuse to vaccinate their children if there were no penalties for doing so, and 16% reported that they would recommend others not to vaccinate their children. Most parents (71%) believed that vaccines given later in childhood were less likely to cause autism than those given to children at a younger age and 60% believed that vaccines involving doses that were weeks or months apart were less likely to cause autism than vaccines given all that once.

Bivariate analyses

Table 1 presents results from bivariate analyses. Due to the low number (n=8) of participants who reported that they would recommend others not to vaccinate their children, this variable was not included as an outcome in analyses.

Demographic characteristics and satisfaction with care. None of the demographic variables, including parent education level or child's autism severity, were associated with beliefs of vaccines as a cause of autism or refusal to vaccinate if no penalties existed. Of note, characteristics related to parents' perceptions of their child's PCP and accessibility/affordability of medical care were not significantly associated with parents' belief that vaccines had contributed to their child's autism or to their desire to refuse vaccination.

Belief that vaccines contributed to child's autism. Parents who believed that vaccines had contributed to the cause of their child's autism were significantly more likely to report that they had encountered media that caused them to have fear about the possible links between vaccines and autism ($p<0.001$). These parents had lower average ratings on subscales assessing perceived vaccine safety and efficacy ($p<0.001$), negative consequences of non-vaccination ($p=0.008$), trust in healthcare institutions ($p<0.001$), and sense of responsibility to vaccinate for the welfare of their child and for other children ($p=0.043$). Parents who believed vaccines had contributed to the cause of their child's autism also believed that parents should have more autonomy in childhood vaccination decisions ($p=0.036$). Child autism severity nor child cognitive ability were significantly associated with parents' belief that vaccines had contributed to their child's autism.

Desire to refuse vaccination. Parents who reported that they would refuse to vaccinate their children if there were no penalties for doing so were significantly more likely to report that they had encountered media that caused them to have fear about the possible links between vaccines and autism ($p=0.017$). These parents had a lower average ratings on subscales assessing perceived vaccine safety and efficacy ($p=0.002$), lesser trust in healthcare institutions ($p=0.043$), and believed that parents should have more autonomy in childhood vaccination decisions ($p=0.004$). Parents who reported that they would refuse to vaccinate their children if there were no penalties for doing so had children with significantly lower DAS scores; however, autism severity was not significantly associated.

Discussion

Among this sample of PCA, over half believed that vaccines had contributed to the cause of their child's autism, and over 70% reported that they were concerned that a child could get autism from vaccination. Nearly one-third reported that they would refuse to vaccinate their children if there were no penalties for doing so and nearly one in every six parents reported that they would discourage other parents from vaccinating their children. In this sample, nearly 90% believed that vaccines were effective in preventing disease and over 90% believed that the diseases vaccines prevent are serious. Moreover, nearly 88% of parents reported that, without vaccines, VPDs would pose a risk to their children. These findings are similar to those found in previous research (31). Many studies have reported that low perceived risk of VPDs and doubts about vaccine efficacy contribute to negative attitudes toward childhood vaccination (32-34), though there has been some evidence to the contrary (35).

Perceived safety of childhood vaccines was low, with fewer than 40% reporting that vaccines were safe. Parents who believed that vaccines had contributed to the cause of their child's autism and those who would refuse to vaccinate their children if there were no penalties for doing so reported significantly less confidence in vaccine safety and efficacy than did their counterparts. Distrust of health-related institutions responsible for ensuring safety was common, with fewer than half reporting that they trusted the companies producing vaccines and 45% believing that the government would stop an unsafe vaccination program. Parents who believed that vaccines had contributed to their child's autism and those who would refuse vaccination reported significantly less trust in health institutions. Previous research suggests that institutional trust and perceptions of safety are related. Parental trust in the institutions that develop and regulate vaccines may affect information-seeking behavior and how they receive, process, and react to risk communication from those sources, including material insisting upon vaccine safety (36). As such, vaccine promotion activities involving increased dissemination of information from sources perceived as having questionable credibility is likely to have a limited impact on vaccine attitudes, particularly when the material targets parents' risk: benefit calculus and fails to address underlying mistrust (36).

Of note, the majority of parents believed that alterations in the vaccine schedule would improve the safety of vaccines, specifically delaying vaccines until later in childhood and spacing the doses further apart. Similar attitudes have been identified in previous research (18) and national data suggest that delayed vaccination is not uncommon in the United States (37). These beliefs may be indicative of parents' attempt to educate themselves about vaccination and of their exposure to social discourses, advocated by vaccine-resistant groups and others, suggesting a moral imperative for parents to make empowered, informed, and educated decisions about vaccination to protect their children's health (38). Thus, in a sense, vaccine-resistant groups and public health authorities are promoting the same message: individuals should be informed and empowered to take personal responsibility for their health-related decisions. In this quest, however, individuals are exposed to various information sources and often to 'mixed messages' (38).

While the cross-sectional design precludes ability to draw conclusions about the origins of parents' attitudes, it is notable that 65% reported encountering information from popular media sources, parent support groups, and/or healthcare providers that increased their fear about the links between vaccines and autism. Parents who were exposed to information that provoked fears related to vaccines and autism were significantly more likely to report that vaccines had contributed to the cause of their child's autism and that they would refuse to vaccinate their children in the absence of penalties. Healthcare providers were described as the least frequent source eliciting fear, and the internet was the most common source of exposure to information about the controversy over vaccines and autism. These findings are consistent with those of Woo and colleagues (11) who found that information from magazines/newspapers, healthcare providers, and the internet played important roles in parents' suspicion about links between vaccination and their child's autism.

The implications of these findings for public health practice are complex. Parental mistrust in governmental and pharmaceutical institutions undermines these institutions' ability to discredit and/or counteract information from other sources. Moreover, mistrust may motivate parents to seek information from alternative sources, and circularly, information from alternative sources may contribute to further mistrust. Future longitudinal research is needed to unpack details about the temporality and directionality of these associations. Public health authorities' engagement in an 'information war' with other sources will likely be ineffective if content explicitly or implicitly communicates that vaccine resistance is an 'irrational' and/or ignorant miscalculation of risk without addressing trust, uncertainty, parent's personalized concepts of their children's vulnerability, and the social and political contexts in which scientific evidence is produced and vaccine decisions are made (36,38,39).

With the exception of information received from healthcare providers, information about autism and vaccination encountered from other sources provoked fear in the majority of those parents exposed to it. Interestingly, proportionally more parents who encountered information about autism and vaccines from parent support groups reported that it provoked fear than those who encountered the information from other sources. Previous research has shown that PCA perceive autism organizations to be an equally credible or more credible source of vaccine information than organizations such as the CDC, National Vaccine Information Center, and American Academy of Pediatrics (11). However, dimensions of trust and attitudes regarding credibility and authority are complex. For example, discourses of vaccine-resistant groups frame 'trusting blindly' in traditional scientific authority as symptomatic of disempowerment and entailing a substantive risk (38). Thus, vaccine promotion efforts aiming to improve public trust in traditional health-related institutions may be misguided if 'trust' is in itself seen by consumers as a risk (38). Of note, the present study did not inquire about the specific type of support groups with which parents were involved. Additional research about the types of organizations with which PCA typically affiliate, as well as informal and/or formal discourses about vaccination within these organizations is needed to more fully understand if and how parents' affiliation with these groups affects vaccination behavior. Furthermore, researchers and public health practitioners interested in working with and writing about these groups should be thoughtful in how they frame their language. Specifically, previous research cautions against the tendency to identify these groups with an anti-vaccine 'social movement', as this attribution may inherently grant more social theoretic foundation to their claims by conflating it with broader political transformations focused on individual rights and resistance to authority (40).

Studies have highlighted the important role healthcare providers play in encouraging the uptake of childhood vaccination (17,30). In fact, a literature review revealed that mistrust in healthcare systems and negative experience communicating healthcare providers about vaccination are often associated with lower vaccine uptake (6). In the present study, the vast majority of parents reported that they discussed their concerns about vaccination with their child's healthcare provider and that the provider took their concerns seriously. On average, parents had positive ratings of their healthcare providers' informativeness, sensitivity, competence, and partnership building. Nevertheless, only 60% reported that they trusted their provider's opinion regarding vaccine safety. This percentage is slightly less than that reported in a recent nationally representative survey of parents (41). Although somewhat low, the level of trust in healthcare providers exceeded that reported for other authorities associated with vaccination (pharmaceutical companies, government, etc); thus, the patient-provider relationship may represent an opportunity for effective dialogue about childhood vaccination. Of note, however, none of the measures related to satisfaction with child's PCP or accessibility and affordability of medical care were significantly associated with vaccine attitude outcomes in this study. Given these findings and the logistical constraints faced by healthcare providers (12), immunization campaigns cannot rely solely on healthcare providers to promote vaccination, but must engage other mobilization activities and/or electronic, visual, and print media channels (41) directed at parents and support groups specifically.

Demographic and ASD-related characteristics were generally not associated with vaccine attitudes, with the exception that children of parents who reported they would refuse vaccination had lower cognitive functioning, as assessed by the DAS. Additional research is needed to investigate factors that mediate the association between childhood cognitive functioning and parents' attitudes toward childhood vaccination. For example, mediators may include differences in timing of diagnosis and appearance of symptoms of regression and/or variations in parents' information-seeking behavior according to child's level of cognitive functioning.

Most parents desired autonomy in vaccine decision-making, but the majority reported that they felt a personal obligation to vaccinate for the protection of others and the child. Parents who believed that vaccines contributed to the cause of their child's autism and those who would refuse vaccination desired significantly more decision-making autonomy than their counterparts. The former also felt significantly less responsibility to vaccinate. Interestingly, the concept of societal responsibility to vaccinate often has been ignored in vaccine promotion materials. Although the public health rationale for mitigating vaccine refusal is to maintain coverage levels necessary to achieve herd immunity, many promotional materials focus on presenting the individual-level risks and benefits of vaccination (36). In the present study, 84% of parents believed that they had a responsibility to vaccinate their children for the protection of all children, and parents' sense of societal responsibility to vaccinate was strongly associated with their vaccine attitudes; these findings highlight a pivotal point to target in vaccine promotion. Public health communications and efforts addressing vaccine uptake among PCA should leverage and include information addressing attitudes surrounding the societal implications of individual-level vaccine uptake.

Nevertheless, the tension between individual autonomy and government regulation in immunization has a long and contentious history in the United States and will be difficult to address (42). Nationally, parents are increasingly seeking nonmedical exemptions for vaccination (43), citing religious, ideological, and/or safety concerns (44,45). As discussed above, in the public health arena, vaccine refusal is often assumed to be a matter of miscalculated of risk; however, autonomy in the context of social movements involving 'alternative' concepts of health and responsibility (36), empowered decision-making (38), and tendencies toward a more personalized approach to parenting and vaccine decision-making (39) also play a role. In the coming years, these and other significant health-related issues related to vaccine refusal (46-48) will force the public health community, policy makers, and the public to confront questions surrounding boundaries of personal autonomy and societal responsibility (44).

While this study provides important preliminary insights into the vaccine attitudes of PCA, the study is not without limitations. Though they were based on measures used in previous research in other settings, the questionnaires assessing parent satisfaction with care and vaccine attitudes were self-developed for this formative study and are in need of further evaluation and integration with validated measures developed since the commencement of this study (49). Additionally, although demographic differences between survey respondents and non-respondents were not observed, the response rate (63%) does raise concerns of participation bias. The study was based on a convenience sample of parents participating in a separate autism-related study; given that the vaccine attitudes of participating parents may differ from non-participants, the findings should be generalized with caution. The small sample size also resulted in limited statistical power to detect differences in some pairwise comparisons.

CONCLUSION

PCA are at the center of arguably one of the most heated debates surrounding vaccination in recent history (7,8). The present study highlights the complexity of parents' beliefs about vaccination and underscores the failure of popular narratives dichotomizing attitudes as "pro-vaccine" and "anti-vaccine" to adequately portray nuances. In this study, most parents reported serious concerns about vaccine safety, but the majority viewed vaccines as necessary and effective. Concerns about safety are likely related, in part, to issues of trust, perceived credibility, and exposure to sources of information suggesting a link between vaccines and autism. From a public health perspective, the findings clearly point to a need to reestablish parents' trust in scientific evidence suggesting no link between vaccines and autism and in government-backed immunization programs more generally. This will be an ongoing and tenuous process that should involve transparent and truthful dialogue (50), engage trusted members of the community, and acknowledge the value of parent empowerment and information-seeking.

ACKNOWLEDGMENTS

The authors would like to acknowledge Jennifer Woods for her contribution to the literature search and review, and would like to thank the reviewer for thoughtful suggestions that led to the improvement of this manuscript.

Funding source: No external funding was secured for this study.

Financial disclosure: The authors have no financial relationship relevant to this article to disclose.

Conflict of interest: The authors have no conflicts of interest to disclose.

REFERENCES

[1] Rosenberg RE, Law JK, Yenokyan G, McGready J, Kaufmann WE, Law PA. Characteristics and concordance of autism spectrum disorders among 277 twin pairs. Arch Pediatr Adolesc Med 2009;163(10):907-14.

[2] Hallmayer J, Cleveland S, Torres A, Phillips J, Cohen B, Torigoe T, et al. Genetic heritability and shared environmental factors among twin pairs with autism. Arch Gen Psychiatry 2011;68(11):1095-102.

[3] Ronald A, Happe F, Bolton P, Butcher LM, Price TS, Wheelwright S, et al. Genetic heterogeneity between the three components of the autism spectrum: a twin study. J Am Acad Child Adolesc Psychiatry 2006;45(6):691-9.

[4] National Research Council. Adverse effects of vaccines: Evidence and causality. Washington, DC: National Academies Press, 2012.

[5] Bazzano A, Zeldin A, Schuster E, Barrett C, Lehrer D. Vaccine-related beliefs and practices of parents of children with autism spectrum disorders. Am J Intellect Dev Dsabil 2012;117(3):233-42.

[6] Brown K, Kroll JS, Hudson MJ, Ramsay M, Green J, Long SJ, et al. Factors underlying parental decisions about combination childhood vaccinations including MMR: a systematic review. Vaccine 2010;28(26):4235-48.

[7] Offit PA. Vaccines and autism revisited -- the Hannah Poling case. N Engl J Med 2008;358(20):2089-91.

[8] Smith MJ, Ellenberg SS, Bell LM, Rubin DM. Media coverage of the measles-mumps-rubella vaccine and autism controversy and its relationship to MMR immunization rates in the United States. Pediatrics 2008;121(4):e836-43.

[9] Biao J. Prevalence of autism spectrum disorders. Autism and Developmental Disabilities Monitoring Network, 14 Sites, United States, 2008. MMWR 2012;61(SS03):1-19.

[10] Mercer L, Creighton S, Holden JJA, Lewis MES. Parental perspectives on the causes of an autism spectrum disorder in their children. J Genet Couns 2006;15(1):41-50.

[11] Woo E, Ball R, Bostrom A, Shadomy SV, Ball LK, Evans G, et al. Vaccine risk perception among reporters of autism after vaccination: Vaccine Adverse Event Reporting System 1990–2001. Am J Public Health 2004;94(6):990-5

[12] Pineda D, Myers MG. Finding reliable information about vaccines. Pediatrics 2011;127(Suppl 1):S134-S7.

[13] Kata A. A postmodern Pandora's box: Anti-vaccination misinformation on the Internet. Vaccine 2010;28(7):1709-16.

[14] Zimmerman RK, Wolfe RM, Fox DE, Fox JR, Nowalk MP, Troy JA, et al. Vaccine criticism on the world wide web. J Med Internet Res 2005;7(2):e17.

[15] Nicholson M, Leask J. Lessons from an online debate about measles-mumps-rubella (MMR) immunization. Vaccine 2012;30(25):3806-12.

[16] Brown K, Sevdalis N. Lay vaccination narratives on the web: are they worth worrying about? Med Decis Making 2011;31(5):707-9.

[17] Healy CM, Pickering LK. How to communicate with vaccine-hesitant parents. Pediatrics 2011;127(Suppl 1):S127-S33.

[18] Luthy KE, Beckstrand RL, Callister LC. Parental hesitation in immunizing children in Utah. Public Health Nurs 2010;27(1):25-31.

[19] Vannice KS, Salmon DA, Shui I, Omer SB, Kissner J, Edwards KM, et al. Attitudes and beliefs of parents concerned about vaccines: impact of timing of immunization information. Pediatrics 2011;127(Suppl 1):S120-S6.

[20] Carbone PS, Behl DD, Azor V, Murphy NA. The medical home for children with autism spectrum disorders: Parent and pediatrician perspectives. J Autism Dev Disord 2010;40(3):317-24.

[21] Kennedy A, Lavail K, Nowak G, Basket M, Landry S. Confidence about vaccines in the United States: understanding parents' perceptions. Health Affairs 2011;30(6):1151-9.

[22] Ruble LA, Dalrymple NJ, McGrew JH. The effects of consultation on Individualized Education Program outcomes for young children with autism: The collaborative model for promoting competence and success. J Early Intervent 2010;32(4):286-301.

[23] Ruble LA, McGrew JH, Toland M, Dalrymple NJ, Jung L. A randomized controlled trial of COMPASS web-based and face-to-face teacher coaching. J Consult Clin Psychol 2013;81(3):566-72.

[24] American Psychiatric Association. Diagnostic and statistical manual of mental disorders, 4th ed, text rev ed. Washington, DC: American Psychiatric Association, 2004.

[25] Lord C, Risi S, Lambrecht L, Cook EJ, Leventhal B, DiLavore P, et al. The autism diagnostic observation schedule-generic: a standard measure of social and communication deficits associated with the spectrum of autism. J Autism Dev Disord 2000;30(3):205-23.

[26] Schopler E, Reichler R, DeVellis R, Daly K. Toward objective classification of childhood autism: Childhood Autism Rating Scale (CARS). J Autism Dev Disord 1980;10(1):91-103.

[27] Elliott C. Differential Ability Scales. New York: Harcourt Brace Jovanovitch Psychological Corporation, 1990.

[28] Marshall GN, Hays RD. The patient satisfaction questionnaire short-form (PSQ-18). Santa Monica, CA: Rand, 1994.

[29] Street RL. Physicians' communication and parents' evaluations of pediatric consultations. Med Care 1991;29(11):1146-52.

[30] Casiday R, Cresswell T, Wilson D, Panter-Brick C. A survey of UK parental attitudes to the MMR vaccine and trust in medical authority. Vaccine 2006;24(2):177-84.

[31] Freed GL, Clark SJ, Butchart AT, Singer DC, Davis MM. Parental vaccine safety concerns in 2009. Pediatrics 2010;125(4):654-9.

[32] Salmon DA, Moulton LH, Omer SB, DeHart MP, Stokley S, Halsey NA. Factors associated with refusal of childhood vaccines among parents of school-aged children: a case-control study. Arch Pediatr Adolesc Med 2005;159(5):470-6.

[33] Fredrickson DD, Davis TC, Arnould CL, Kennen EM, Hurniston SG, Cross JT, et al. Childhood immunization refusal: provider and parent perceptions. Fam Med 2004;36(6):431-9.

[34] Allred N, Shaw K, Santibanez T, Rickert D, Santoli J. Parental vaccine safety concerns: results from the National Immunization Survey, 2001-2002. Am J Prev Med 2005;28(2):221-4.

[35] LaVail KH, Kennedy AM. The role of attitudes about vaccine safety, efficacy, and value in explaining parents' reported vaccination behavior. Health Educ Behav 2013;40(5):544-51.

[36] Hobson-West P. Understanding vaccination resistance: moving beyond risk. Health Risk Society 2003;5(3):273-83.

[37] Luman ET, Barker LE, Shaw KM, McCauley MM, Buehler JW, Pickering LK. Timeliness of childhood vaccinations in the United States. JAMA 2005;293(10):1204-11.

[38] Hobson-West P. 'Trusting blindly can be the biggest risk of all': organised resistance to childhood vaccination in the UK. Sociol Health Illness 2007;29(2):198-215.

[39] Poltorak M, Leach M, Fairhead J, Cassell J. 'MMR talk'and vaccination choices: An ethnographic study in Brighton. Soc Sci Med 2005;61(3):709-19.

[40] Blume S. Anti-vaccination movements and their interpretations. Soc Sci Med 2006;62(3):628-42.

[41] Freed GL, Clark SJ, Butchart AT, Singer DC, Davis MM. Sources and perceived credibility of vaccine-safety information for parents. Pediatrics 2011;127(Suppl 1):S107-S12.

[42] Colgrove J. State of immunity: the politics of vacination in twentieth-century America. Berkeley, CA: University of California Press, 2006.

[43] Omer SB, Pan WKY, Halsey NA, Stokley S, Moulton LH, Navar AM, et al. Nonmedical exemptions to school immunization requirements: secular trends and association of state policies with pertussis incidence. JAMA 2006;296(14):1757-63.

[44] Salmon DA, Omer SB. Individual freedoms versus collective responsibility: immunization decision-making in the face of occasionally competing values. Emerg Themes Epidemiol 2006;3:13-3.

[45] Poland GA, Jacobson RM. Understanding those who do not understand: a brief review of the anti-vaccine movement. Vaccine 2001;19(17-19):2440-5.

[46] Salmon DA, Haber M, Gangarosa EJ, Phillips L, Smith NJ, Chen RT. Health consequences of religious and philosophical exemptions from immunization laws: individual and societal risk of measles. JAMA 1999;282(1):47-53.

[47] Omer SB, Enger KS, Moulton LH, Halsey NA, Stokley S, Salmon DA. Geographic clustering of nonmedical exemptions to school immunization requirements and associations with geographic clustering of pertussis. Am J Epidemiol 2008;168(12):1389-96.

[48] Feikin DR, Lezotte DC, Hamman RF, Salmon DA, Chen RT, Hoffman RE. Individual and community risks of measles and pertussis associated with personal exemptions to immunization. JAMA 2000;284(24):3145-50.

[49] Brown K, Shanley R, Cowley NA, van Wijgerden J, Toff P, Falconer M, et al. Attitudinal and demographic predictors of measles, mumps and rubella (MMR) vaccine acceptance: development and validation of an evidence-based measurement instrument. Vaccine 2011;29(8):1700-9.

[50] Poland GA, Spier R. Fear, misinformation, and innumerates: how the Wakefield paper, the press, and advocacy groups damaged the public health. Vaccine 2010;28(12):2361-2.

SECTION FIVE: ACKNOWLEDGMENTS

In: Child and Adolescent Health Issues
Editor: Joav Merrick
ISBN: 978-1-63463-574-5

Chapter 23

ABOUT THE EDITOR

Joav Merrick, MD, MMedSci, DMSc, born and educated in Denmark is professor of pediatrics, child health and human development, Division of Pediatrics, Hadassah Hebrew University Medical Center, Mt Scopus Campus, Jerusalem, Israel and Kentucky Children's Hospital, University of Kentucky, Lexington, Kentucky United States and professor of public health at the Center for Healthy Development, School of Public Health, Georgia State University, Atlanta, United States, the medical director of the Health Services, Division for Intellectual and Developmental Disabilities, Ministry of Social Affairs and Social Services, Jerusalem, the founder and director of the National Institute of Child Health and Human Development in Israel. Numerous publications in the field of pediatrics, child health and human development, rehabilitation, intellectual disability, disability, health, welfare, abuse, advocacy, quality of life and prevention. Received the Peter Sabroe Child Award for outstanding work on behalf of Danish Children in 1985 and the International LEGO-Prize ("The Children's Nobel Prize") for an extraordinary contribution towards improvement in child welfare and well-being in 1987. E-mail: jmerrick@zahav.net.il

In: Child and Adolescent Health Issues
Editor: Joav Merrick

ISBN: 978-1-63463-574-5

Chapter 24

About the National Institute of Child Health and Human Development in Israel

The National Institute of Child Health and Human Development (NICHD) in Israel was established in 1998 as a virtual institute under the auspicies of the Medical Director, Ministry of Social Affairs and Social Services in order to function as the research arm for the Office of the Medical Director. In 1998 the National Council for Child Health and Pediatrics, Ministry of Health and in 1999 the Director General and Deputy Director General of the Ministry of Health endorsed the establishment of the NICHD.

Mission

The mission of a National Institute for Child Health and Human Development in Israel is to provide an academic focal point for the scholarly interdisciplinary study of child life, health, public health, welfare, disability, rehabilitation, intellectual disability and related aspects of human development. This mission includes research, teaching, clinical work, information and public service activities in the field of child health and human development.

Service and Academic Activities

Over the years many activities became focused in the south of Israel due to collaboration with various professionals at the Faculty of Health Sciences (FOHS) at the Ben Gurion University of the Negev (BGU). Since 2000 an affiliation with the Zusman Child Development Center at the Pediatric Division of Soroka University Medical Center has resulted in collaboration around the establishment of the Down Syndrome Clinic at that center. In 2002 a full course on "Disability" was established at the Recanati School for Allied Professions in the Community, FOHS, BGU and in 2005 collaboration was started with the Primary Care Unit of the faculty and disability became part of the master of public health course on "Children and society". In the academic year 2005-2006 a one semester course on "Aging with disability" was started as part of the master of science program in gerontology in our collaboration with the Center for Multidisciplinary Research in Aging. In 2010 collaborations with the Division of Pediatrics, Hadassah Hebrew University Medical Center, Jerusalem, Israel around the National Down Syndrome Center and teaching students and residents about intellectual and developmental disabilities as part of their training at this campus.

RESEARCH ACTIVITIES

The affiliated staff have over the years published work from projects and research activities in this national and international collaboration. In the year 2000 the International Journal of Adolescent Medicine and Health and in 2005 the International Journal on Disability and Human Development of De Gruyter Publishing House (Berlin and New York) were affiliated with the National Institute of Child Health and Human Development. From 2008 also the International Journal of Child Health and Human Development (Nova Science, New York), the International Journal of Child and Adolescent Health (Nova Science) and the Journal of Pain Management (Nova Science) affiliated and from 2009 the International Public Health Journal (Nova Science) and Journal of Alternative Medicine Research (Nova Science). All peer-reviewed international journals.

NATIONAL COLLABORATIONS

Nationally the NICHD works in collaboration with the Faculty of Health Sciences, Ben Gurion University of the Negev; Department of Physical Therapy, Sackler School of Medicine, Tel Aviv University; Autism Center, Assaf HaRofeh Medical Center; National Rett and PKU Centers at Chaim Sheba Medical Center, Tel HaShomer; Department of Physiotherapy, Haifa University; Department of Education, Bar Ilan University, Ramat Gan, Faculty of Social Sciences and Health Sciences; College of Judea and Samaria in Ariel and in 2011 affiliation with Center for Pediatric Chronic Diseases and National Center for Down Syndrome, Department of Pediatrics, Hadassah Hebrew University Medical Center, Mount Scopus Campus, Jerusalem.

INTERNATIONAL COLLABORATIONS

Internationally with the Department of Disability and Human Development, College of Applied Health Sciences, University of Illinois at Chicago; Strong Center for Developmental Disabilities, Golisano Children's Hospital at Strong, University of Rochester School of Medicine and Dentistry, New York; Centre on Intellectual Disabilities, University of Albany, New York; Centre for Chronic Disease Prevention and Control, Health Canada, Ottawa; Chandler Medical Center and Children's Hospital, Kentucky Children's Hospital, Section of Adolescent Medicine, University of Kentucky, Lexington; Chronic Disease Prevention and Control Research Center, Baylor College of Medicine, Houston, Texas; Division of Neuroscience, Department of Psychiatry, Columbia University, New York; Institute for the Study of Disadvantage and Disability, Atlanta; Center for Autism and Related Disorders, Department Psychiatry, Children's Hospital Boston, Boston; Department of Pediatric and

Adolescent Medicine, Western Michigan University Homer Stryker MD School of Medicine, Kalamazoo, Michigan, United States; Department of Paediatrics, Child Health and Adolescent Medicine, Children's Hospital at Westmead, Westmead, Australia; International Centre for the Study of Occupational and Mental Health, Düsseldorf, Germany; Centre for Advanced Studies in Nursing, Department of General Practice and Primary Care, University of Aberdeen, Aberdeen, United Kingdom; Quality of Life Research Center, Copenhagen, Denmark; Nordic School of Public Health, Gottenburg, Sweden, Scandinavian Institute of Quality of Working Life, Oslo, Norway; The Department of Applied Social Sciences (APSS) of The Hong Kong Polytechnic University Hong Kong.

TARGETS

Our focus is on research, international collaborations, clinical work, teaching and policy in health, disability and human development and to establish the NICHD as a permanent institute at one of the residential care centers for persons with intellectual disability in Israel in order to conduct model research and together with the four university schools of public health/medicine in Israel establish a national master and doctoral program in disability and human development at the institute to secure the next generation of professionals working in this often non-prestigious/low-status field of work.

Contact

Joav Merrick, MD, MMedSci, DMSc
Professor of Pediatrics, Child Health and Human Development
Medical Director, Health Services,
Division for Intellectual and Developmental Disabilities,
Ministry of Social Affairs and Social Services, POB 1260, IL-91012 Jerusalem, Israel.
E-mail: jmerrick@zahav.net.il

In: Child and Adolescent Health Issues
Editor: Joav Merrick
ISBN: 978-1-63463-574-5

Chapter 25

ABOUT THE BOOK SERIES "PEDIATRICS, CHILD AND ADOLESCENT HEALTH"

Pediatrics, child and adolescent health is a book series with publications from a multidisciplinary group of researchers, practitioners and clinicians for an international professional forum interested in the broad spectrum of pediatric medicine, child health, adolescent health and human development.

- Merrick J, ed. Child and adolescent health yearbook 2011. New York: Nova Science, 2012.
- Merrick J, ed. Child and adolescent health yearbook 2012. New York: Nova Science, 2012.
- Roach RR, Greydanus DE, Patel DR, Homnick DN, Merrick J, eds. Tropical pediatrics: A public health concern of international proportions. New York: Nova Science, 2012.
- Merrick J, ed. Child health and human development yearbook 2011. New York: Nova Science, 2012.
- Merrick J, ed. Child health and human development yearbook 2012. New York: Nova Science, 2012.
- Shek DTL, Sun RCF, Merrick J, eds. Developmental issues in Chinese adolescents. New York: Nova Science, 2012.
- Shek DTL, Sun RCF, Merrick J, eds. Positive youth development: Theory, research and application. New York: Nova Science, 2012.
- Zachor DA, Merrick J, eds. Understanding autism spectrum disorder: Current research aspects. New York: Nova Science, 2012.
- Ma HK, Shek DTL, Merrick J, eds. Positive youth development: A new school curriculum to tackle adolescent developmental issues. New York: Nova Science, 2012.
- Wood D, Reiss JG, Ferris ME, Edwards LR, Merrick J, eds. Transition from pediatric to adult medical care. New York: Nova Science, 2012.
- Isenberg Y. Guidelines for the healthy integration of the ill child in the educational system: Experience from Israel. New York: Nova Science, 2013.

- Shek DTL, Sun RCF, Merrick J, eds. Chinese adolescent development: Economic disadvantages, parents and intrapersonal development. New York: Nova Science, 2013.
- Shek DTL, Sun RCF, Merrick J, eds. University and college students: Health and development issues for the leaders of tomorrow. New York: Nova Science, 2013.
- Shek DTL, Sun RCF, Merrick J, eds. Adolescence and behavior issues in a Chinese context. New York: Nova Science, 2013.
- Sun J, Buys N, Merrick J, eds. Advances in preterm infant research. New York: Nova Science, 2013.
- Tsitsika A, Janikian M, Greydanus DE, Omar HA, Merrick J, eds. Internet addiction: A public health concern in adolescence. New York: Nova Science, 2013.
- Shek DTL, Lee TY, Merrick J, eds. Promotion of holistic development of young people in Hong Kong. New York: Nova Science, 2013.
- Shek DTL, Ma C, Lu Y, Merrick J, eds. Human developmental research: Experience from research in Hong Kong. New York: Nova Science, 2013.
- Merrick J, ed. Chronic disease and disability in childhood. New York: Nova Science, 2013.
- Rubin IL, Merrick J, eds. Break the cycle of environmental health disparities: Maternal and child health aspects. New York: Nova Science, 2013.
- Rubin IL, Merrick J, eds. Environmental health disparities in children: Asthma, obesity and food. New York: Nova Science, 2013.
- Rubin IL, Merrick J, eds. Environmental health: Home, school and community. New York: Nova Science, 2013.
- Rubin IL, Merrick J, eds. Child health and human development: Social, economic and environmental factors. New York: Nova Science, 2013.
- Merrick J, Kandel I, Omar HA, eds. Children, violence and bullying: International perspectives. New York: Nova Science, 2013.
- Omar HA, Bowling CH, Merrick J, eds. Playing with fire: Children, adolescents and firesetting. New York: Nova Science, 2013.
- Merrick J, Tenenbaum A, Omar HA, eds. School, adolescence and health issues. New York: Nova Science, 2013.
- Merrick J, Tenenbaum A, Omar Ha, eds. Adolescence and sexuality: International perspectives. New York: Nova Science, 2014.
- Diamond G, Arbel E. Adoption: The search for a new parenthood. New York: Nova Science, 2014.
- Taylor MF, Pooley JA, Merrick J, eds. Adolescence: Places and spaces. New York: Nova Science, 2014.
- Greydanus DE, Feinberg AN, Merrick J, eds. Born into this world: Health issues. New York: Nova Science, 2014.
- Greydanus DE, Feinberg AN, Merrick J, eds. Caring for the newborn: A comprehensive guide for the clinician. New York: Nova Science, 2014.
- Rubin IL, Merrick J, eds. Environment and hope: Improving health, reducing AIDS and promoting food security in the world. New York: Nova Science, 2014.

- Greydanus DE, Feinberg AN, Merrick J, eds. Pediatric and adolescent dermatology: Some current issues. New York: Nova Science, 2014.

Contact

Professor Joav Merrick, MD, MMedSci, DMSc
Medical Director, Medical Services
Division for Intellectual and Developmental Disabilities
Ministry of Social Affairs and Social Services
POBox 1260, IL-91012 Jerusalem, Israel
E-mail: jmerrick@zahav.net.il

SECTION SIX: INDEX

#

A

B

C

D

F

G

H

I

J

K

L

M

Q

R

S

T

U

V

W

Y

Z